Modern Management of Acoustic Neuroma

Progress in Neurological Surgery

Vol. 21

Series Editor

L. Dade Lunsford Pittsburgh, Pa.

Modern Management of Acoustic Neuroma

Volume Editors

Jean Régis Marseille
Pierre-Hugues Roche Marseille

70 figures, 14 in color, and 41 tables, 2008

KARGER

Basel · Freiburg · Paris · London · New York · Bangalore · Bangkok · Shanghai · Singapore · Tokyo · Sydney

Progress in Neurological Surgery

Jean Régis

Service de Neurochirurgie Fonctionnelle et Stéréotaxique
Centre Hospitalier Universitaire La Timone Adultes
Assistance Publique – Hôpitaux de Marseille
Marseille, France

Pierre-Hugues Roche

Service de Neurochirurgie
Centre Hospitalier Universitaire Nord
Assistance Publique – Hôpitaux de Marseille
Marseille, France

Library of Congress Cataloging-in-Publication Data

Modern management of acoustic neuroma / volume editors, Jean Régis,
Pierre-Hugues Roche.
p. ; cm. -- (Progress in neurological surgery, ISSN 0079-6492 ; v. 21)
Includes bibliographical references and index.
ISBN 978-3-8055-8370-1 (alk. paper)
1. Acoustic neuroma -- Surgery. I. Régis, Jean. II. Roche, Pierre-Hugues. III.
Series.
[DNLM: 1. Neuroma, Acoustic--surgery. 2. Neurosurgical Procedures. W1 PR673
v.21 2008 / WV 250 M689 2008]
RF260.M64 2008
617.4'8--dc22
2008029727

Bibliographic Indices. This publication is listed in bibliographic services, including Current Contents® and Index Medicus.

www.karger.com
Printed in Switzerland on acid-free and non-aging paper (ISO 9706) by Reinhardt Druck, Basel
ISSN 0079–6492
ISBN 978–3–8055–8370–1

Contents

In Memoriam Prof. Robert Sedan

Prof. Robert Sedan, our mentor, was a creative mind and a humanist heart. He created in 1975 the Timone University Hospital Department of Functional and Stereotactic Neurosurgery. He created a series of new instruments for stereotaxis, including the side-cutting biopsy needle nowadays known under his name and commonly used for the vast majority of the stereotactic brain biopsies worldwide. He taught us the importance of multidisciplinary approach and team work.

His rich personality and legacy remain a permanent source of inspiration for his grateful fellows.

Jean Régis and *Pierre-Hugues Roche*, Marseille

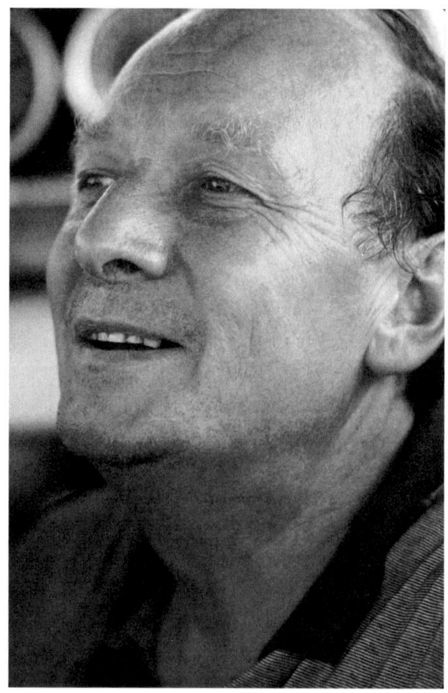

Editors

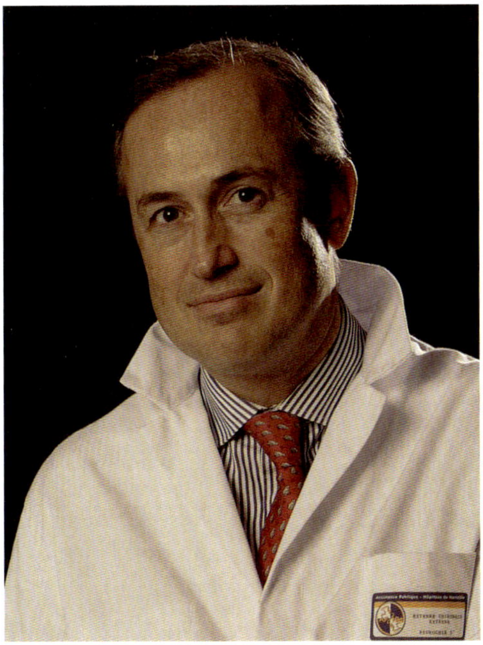

Prof. Jean Régis, MD, PhD
Service de Neurochirurgie Fonctionnelle et Stéréotaxique
Centre Hospitalier Universitaire La Timone Adultes
Assistance Publique–Hôpitaux de Marseille

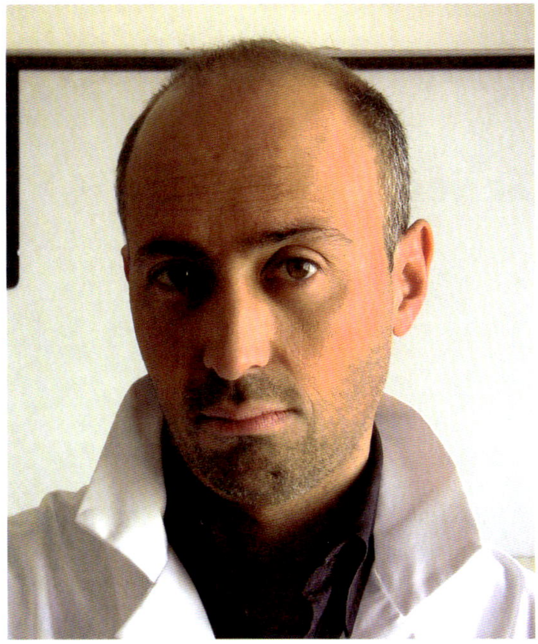

Prof. Pierre-Hugues Roche, MD, PhD
Service de Neurochirurgie
Centre Hospitalier Universitaire Nord
Assistance Publique–Hôpitaux de Marseille

Editorial Assistant

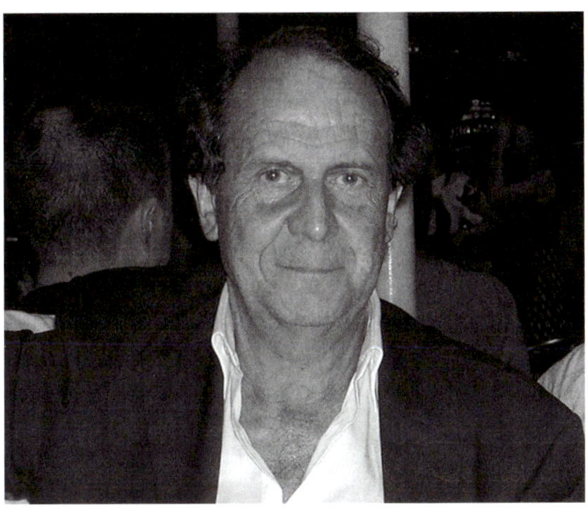

Prof. Jean-Marc Thomassin, MD, PhD
Fédération d'Oto-Rhino-Laryngology
Centre Hospitalier Universitaire La Timone Adultes
Assistance Publique–Hôpitaux de Marseille

Series Editor's Note

Vestibular schwannoma, a more modern update of the original medical term of acoustic neuroma, is a relatively rare and usually benign skull base tumor that has fascinated neurological surgeons for more than 100 years. Surgical pioneers such as Cushing advocated subtotal resection, whereas Dandy recommended complete excision. This set the tone for the sometimes controversial management of this tumor, which has continued to fascinate many generations of neurological surgeons, neuro-otologists, and more recently radiation oncologists. From surgical removal at all cost, evolved a strategy of cranial nerve preservation whenever possible. No tumor provides a greater test of a neurosurgeon's or neuro-otologist's skill than the acoustic neuroma, but the need for improved outcomes proved the driving force in the introduction of stereotactic radiosurgery as a potent management strategy. This volume should help the reader to understand the current spectrum of management strategies, and the enormous strides that have been made on patient's behalves for better outcomes, preservation of cranial nerve function, and even improved quality of life – huge improvement beyond the early years of assessing outcomes by simply noting whether the patient survived or not. There are different operations that are appropriate for different patients. For patients who simply cannot 'live' with a tumor in their head, surgical extirpation should be attempted. For patients who are comfortable with the concept that minimally invasive radiosurgical strategy has a very high chance of achieving tumor dormancy and cranial nerve preservation, surgical removal is not necessary. This volume has taken several years to compile, and represents the current status of management of acoustic neuroma. Over the years, cranial nerve function rates have dramatically improved, and now hearing preservation is a reality.

L. Dade Lunsford, Pittsburgh, Pa.

Foreword

I am honored to be able to provide a foreword to this seminal book by Prof. Régis, who has assembled an excellent list of co-authors.

Acoustic neuroma, despite its relative rarity, continues to fascinate the neurosurgical, otologic, and now radiation oncologic community. Enormous strides have been made in the last two decades relative to enhanced long-term outcomes and reduction in patient morbidity.

History of Radiosurgery in Brief

Lars Leksell, the father of stereotactic radiosurgery, was the Swedish pioneer who was committed to what we now call minimally invasive treatment strategies to deal with difficult problems within the intracranial compartment. While his background was that of a neurophysiologist (who first described the gamma motor system), his training with Olivecrona in the 1930s convinced him that image guidance technology might be able to overcome the occasional operative disasters that he witnessed. His stereotactic fellowship was with the Philadelphia Temple University pioneers, Ernest Spiegel and Henry Wycis. By 1949 when he returned to Stockholm, Leksell had published his first article describing his arc-centered stereotactic guiding device. Two years later in 1951, he coined the term 'stereotactic radiosurgery' after combining his stereotactic guiding device with an orthovoltage dental X-ray unit. He first demonstrated the feasibility of the technique by irradiating the gasserian ganglion of 3 patients with trigeminal neuralgia. During the 1950s and 1960s, Leksell explored various alternative radiation delivery techniques. These ventures included cross-firing cyclotron generated protons in collaboration with Bőrje Larsson at the Gustav Werner Institute in Uppsala, a brief dalliance with the then emerging linear accelerator technology (which he found too unstable for radiosurgery based on the wobble of the gantry) and finally in 1967 the creation of a prototype 179 Cobalt-60 source Gamma Knife. This unit was placed in the Sophia Hospital in Stockholm. It was designed with slit collimators to create discoid-shaped lesions compatible with sectioning of the white matter tracts as required in functional neurosurgery. Its original Swedish name strålkniven or 'the radiation knife', evolved into 'the Gamma Knife'. In 1975, a second prototype unit was developed equipped with circular collimators which created an oblate spheroidal dose profile. It was thereby more suitable for management of intracranial masses.

Leksell delegated various projects to his disciples at the Karolinska Institute where he had become Professor and Chair. The primary acoustic neuroma disciple was Dr. Georg Norén, who pioneered Gamma Knife acoustic neuroma radiosurgery. Georg applied his characteristic Swedish stoicism to withstand the cautious, somewhat skeptical, and always perfectionistic tendencies of Lars Leksell. The first patient was treated in 1969. Imaging was relegated to contrast encephalographic studies performed to outline the borders of the tumor using conventional X-rays. Dose planning was rudimentary, but Norén and Leksell pursued additional experience. It was their collaboration and dedication that now allows us to understand outcomes up to 37 years since the first patient underwent acoustic neuroma radiosurgery. Subsequent installations of additional prototype units in Buenos Aires, Argentina, and Sheffield, UK, ensued. The first efforts in North America were pursued by our group in Pittsburgh in 1987. The first patient treated (of our current 9000) had an acoustic neuroma. At that time, we were in the computed tomography era, and reasonably high resolution imaging was feasible, at least to define the extracanalicular component of the tumor. The new 1987 unit had 201 sources and an even larger collimator helmet (18 mm) was available.

Additional efforts began at other centers across the world, using modifications of linear accelerators, but the initial results from such technologies were not optimal. In part, this was related to a need for greater tumor conformality (the ability to confine the selected treatment to the 3-D volumetric tumor) and in part related to the unknown dosage thought necessary to control tumor growth. These doses were clearly too high, and in the early years were associated with transient facial weakness rates as high as 30–50%. Most centers began a gradual dose de-escalation strategy. At the same time, advances in neuroimaging such as the conversion to magnetic resonance imaging (MRI)-based planning, as well as the great improvements in dose planning facilitated by image integration and rapid computer processing, all contributed to improved outcomes. We recognized that small isocenters not only enhanced conformality, but greatly improved selectivity (the ability to restrict dose to surrounding tissue outside of the target volume). Tremendous improvement in patient outcomes followed earlier recognition of tumors when symptoms were less profound (mild hearing loss, unilateral tinnitus, mild imbalance, episodes of dizziness, etc). Such symptoms fostered early MRI scans as these imaging techniques became widely available. As the size of the tumors diminished at presentation, the need for minimally invasive treatment strategies continued to increase.

The Goals of Radiosurgery

The primary goal of radiosurgery is tumor growth control, a different concept than the traditional surgical goal of tumor removal, as verified by long-term postoperative imaging. After radiosurgery, the tumor looks the same at least initially; long-term control has to be verified with serial follow-up imaging studies. Eventually, we recognized that up to 70% of patients have tumor volumes that gradually regress over the course of 5–7 years. The secondary goal was to enhance neurological outcomes by preservation of first facial nerve function, and subsequently preservation of hearing when appropriate for patients whose hearing status was measurable at the time of the therapeutic option selection. In addition, of course, there are many other outcome measurements for acoustic neuromas such as return to work, reintegration to daily life, and minimization of neuropsychological sequelae of open surgery.

The rapid return to work possible after Gamma Knife radiosurgery and the long-term benefit have facilitated a major transformation in the delivery of patient care for acoustic neuroma patients. Several features have spurred growing interest in radiosurgery: an almost zero risk of facial weakness (a previously dreaded outcome because of its severe effect on personal perception of oneself and integration into the workforce), the opportunity to preserve hearing and the low risk of worsening balance disorders or exacerbating tinnitus. Both surgeons who perform radiosurgery and their patients have to be patient. Compared to microsurgical removal, there is no longer the before and after picture, now you see it, now you don't. Instead, follow-up imaging reveals it is no longer growing, and often shrinks. Early growth of an acoustic neuroma (by a few millimeters) occurs in up to 3–5% of patients before the tumor settles down. In general, 98% of patients after radiosurgery have long-term tumor growth control. Shrinkage tends to develop over the course of time, but it is not necessary in most patients to maintain an adequate outcome. Hearing preservation rates at their preoperative level vary from 50 to 70% of patients. The rare patient may show improvement; however, 30–40% of patients show either hearing deterioration or even deafness over the course of time. Hearing preservation at 2 years after radiosurgery appears to be relatively long-lasting in a significant proportion of patients, although recent evidence suggests that between years 5 and 15, some patients will have further hearing deterioration even in the absence of tumor growth.

Accomplishments of Stereotactic Radiosurgery

Most providers can be confident about long-term tumor growth control outcomes in more than 98% of patients. In addition, we can maintain most neurological function in the vast majority of patients. By emphasizing high conformality and high selectivity, we can efficiently perform the procedure in a 'wheels in to wheels out' approach lasting only a few hours. The efficiency of the procedure has been greatly aided by a long-term commitment to using MRI (as an imaging technique to achieve high 3-D conformality) and to extremely rapid dose planning systems. We must continue to evaluate comparative technologies, including those that have been recently advocated to be able to deliver the beneficial effect using multiple sessions or stages. Ostensibly, such variations in technology and dose delivery are related to goals of enhanced neurological preservation. Unfortunately, from a statistical standpoint, in order to be able to see a 10% improvement in hearing preservation rates at 2 years, a prospective randomized trial with 1,000 patients in each arm might be necessary in order to be able to detect such a differential benefit between one technology and another. Although such a trial is obviously impractical and unlikely to occur, we continue to be assaulted by the claims of various vendors relative to the superiority of their technique. At present, no radiobiological or clinical data show the superiority of staged approaches to that of Gamma Knife radiosurgery.

We also know a great deal now about the radiobiological effect of radiosurgery and the pathological mechanism by which tumor growth control or even involution of the tumor occurs. Radiosurgery results in damage to individual tumor cells, perhaps dose dependent, which leads to the inability of tumor cells to go through mitosis. For slow-growth tumors that act like late-responding tissues, cells do not die until they attempt cell division. This may not occur for months or even years. Secondly, we also know that tumor blood vessel destruction enhances tumor control. This is verified by the striking response to radiosurgery identified on follow-up contrast-enhanced MRI studies. The high-dose areas of the tumor (e.g. 60–70% isodose) appear dark on MRI over several months. This helps to predict eventual shrinkage of the tumor over the course of additional years of observation.

Further Efforts and Issues

One of the major remaining issues has to do with the education of the appropriate providers of radiosurgery. In the United States, most centers work in teams consisting of neurosurgeons, radiation oncologists, and medical physicists. Some centers also rely on the additional input from neuro-otologists with a special interest in the management of acoustic neuromas, as many of them are already the gatekeepers for diagnosis.

How do we continue to educate microsurgeons in the delicate skill of surgical removal, with an increasing percentage of the small tumors relegated to radiosurgery? Unfortunately, this trend means that when tumors are diagnosed in the 30- to 35-mm range, the patient will need microsurgical resection or at least significant tumor debulking.

At centers where neuro-otology provides significant input, should they be the primary providers of this technique? If so, what training and credentialing is required to be able to ensure their appropriate education? If non-neurosurgeons can do acoustic neuromas, can they not do petroclival meningiomas, pituitary tumors, or intracranial metastases? Both various professional societies as well as educational efforts must proceed to analyze this looming credentialing issue. Radiation oncologists need to have neuroanatomic-based radiosurgery as part of their clinical training. Virtually any academic site across the world should now have radiosurgical technologies capable of doing both intracranial, spinal and body radiosurgery.

Who will be the team leaders in these projects? Radiation oncologists bring a skill background in radiobiology education to the table, but do not generally have the same level of neurosurgical neuroanatomy in their background, and are certainly not familiar with the microsurgical options that can be offered as an alternative.

In general, fractionated radiation therapy techniques are rarely alternatives to radiosurgery.

Is the definition of radiosurgery changing? It appears to be evolving from Leksell's original concepts of a single procedure done with image guidance, to a procedure in which image guidance is used and coupled with various radiation techniques to deliver the dose in one or as many as five stages. This is not totally technology dependent, as the concept of stages has been applied not only by linear accelerator centers, but also by the Gamma Knife pioneer, Georg Norén himself, using the most current generation of the robotic Gamma Knife.

Can we really expect to achieve better outcomes by these techniques, and do we have measures actually to compare conformality and selectivity issues between technologies, followed by verifiable patient outcomes to show differences? Patients often become well educated relative to therapeutic options. Since they are the ones that either reap the benefit or pay the price, they are increasingly pro-active in order to obtain as much information as possible. Proper information is widely available. Some information on the internet is even true, but some is not. Patients need to make their own decisions based on adequate informed consent, but it is incumbent upon providers to be able to provide appropriate information over the course of time. In the United States, successful lawsuits have been paid based on incorrect, or frankly false or prejudicial information.

In the past, various largely erroneous pieces of information were told patients: (1) it causes cancer; (2) when it fails, it will be impossible to remove the tumor without major neurologic damage.

How have these issues been resolved? First, we know the theoretical possibility of delayed oncogenesis when radiation is delivered. Using radiosurgical principles, the volume of tissue in a single procedure that receives radiation is very low.

Is one radiation hit more or less risky than two hits? Opinions are divided on this particular issue. It seems, however, that we know of a few 'numerator' cases, perhaps five at the present time, in which new neoplasms within the radiosurgical field have been identified in follow-up of patients who underwent radiosurgery for acoustic neuroma. The 'denominator' is less well known, but assuming that 5 patients with acoustic neuromas fit this criteria (not treated by fractionated radiation), and 25,000 patients have had radiosurgery, the empirical risk is 1/5,000. To put this into perspective, the risk of a major complication or death after surgical removal of an acoustic neuroma at centers of excellence is estimated to be between 1 in 200 to 1 in 500.

What about the outcomes of subsequent microsurgery for a patient who has had prior radiosurgery? This risk is hotly debated. There are those who feel that some tumors are more difficult to remove, and others (usually those with experience), who recognize that tumors in fact are often easier to remove because of the reduction in the number of blood vessels and central necrosis of the tumors. Of course, many patients with minimal growth of their tumor in the first year or two may never need to have anything done. Rarely should those patients be rushed to surgery under the pretense that their tumor is 'growing'. In the early days of radiosurgery, some patients were rushed to early surgery during the time of a maximal radiation reaction in the surrounding tissues (in the era of less conformality and poorer selectivity and higher doses), clearly not an optimal time to try to remove a tumor. With a little bit of patience (a virtue necessary for both acoustic tumor patients and their providers), most such tumors stabilize and subsequently regress, obviating the need for surgery. Less than 2% of patients require surgical intervention.

Can re-treatment be provided? In selected cases, repeat radiosurgery can be performed if a tumor shows defined growth, and the patient is considered to be a poor candidate for microsurgery or is unwilling to consider it. There are little data at the present time as to whether such patients have a greater risk of facial nerve weakness, or the outcomes in terms of vestibular or hearing function. Most patients who have had radiosurgery more than once represent a subgroup that first had microsurgery which failed, and subsequently required radiosurgery for different components of the tumor as it was shown to grow over additional years of observation.

More data from centers with a high volume are warranted. To date, we have very little evidence that various technological procedures are demonstrably superior. Hopefully, answers will come when the data is analyzed by centers with extensive experience, and by those that are not terribly afflicted by preconceived bias.

Many of the questions and comments raised in this introduction will be elucidated in detail by the authors of the chapters of this book. Acoustic neuroma outcomes have been greatly improved by advances first in microsurgical techniques, and now by long-term outcome application of radiosurgery, which is appropriate, verifiable, and extremely clinically relevant treatment strategy. It is no longer an alternative. For most patients of a newly diagnosed acoustic neuroma in the era of high resolution imaging, radiosurgery represents the first-line management for these tumors. Over time, we need to establish whether there is any variation in technologies which further improve results, perhaps assess whether radiation protectors or radiation sensitizers are possible, understand more about the various treatment options for patients with bilateral tumors, and provide appropriate data that allow our patients to select a treatment strategy that is right for them. Our patients take the risks, and they reap the benefits.

L. Dade Lunsford, Pittsburgh, Pa.

Régis J, Roche P-H (eds): Modern Management of Acoustic Neuroma.
Prog Neurol Surg. Basel, Karger, 2008, vol 21, pp 1–5

Introduction

Jean Régis[a] · Pierre-Hugues Roche[c] · Jean-Marc Thomassin[b]

[a]Service de Neurochirurgie Fonctionnelle et Stéréotaxique, et [b]Fédération d'Oto-Rhino-Laryngologie, Hôpital D'Adulte de la Timone, [c]Service de Neurochirurgie, Hôpital Nord, Assistance Publique-Hôpitaux de Marseille, Marseille, France

Vestibular schwannomas (VSs), historically called acoustic neurinomas, are benign neoplasms of Schwann cell origin. They occur predominantly on the vestibular division of the VIIIth nerve at the oligodendroglial/Schwann cell interface, at or within the internal auditory meatus [1]. Due to their benign nature, and the potential surgical morbidity and mortality related to the complex anatomy of the cerebellopontine angle, VSs have always represented a great challenge for neurosurgeons.

The evolution of the surgical management of VSs follows the history of the development of modern neurosurgery (fig. 1). First, during the pioneer era of Harvey Cushing, surgery was undertaken as a life-saving procedure in patients presenting with very large, life-threatening lesions associated with neurological symptoms. Only intracapsular tumor removal was attempted. At that time, the overall mortality in Cushing's series of VSs was 7.7% [2]. Then came the curative era, with Dandy finding that he could achieve complete tumor resection with an acceptably low mortality of around 2.4% [3]. In 1967, the Swedish neurosurgeon Olivecrona proposed to preserve the facial nerve and was able to achieve this in 20% of his 304 patients with a total removal of the tumor in 217. However, the price to pay for the patients was high with the mortality rate rising up to 23% [4].

The microsurgical revolution in the 1960s and 1970s permitted the development of modern neurosurgical strategies with the middle fossa approach by House [5] and the translabyrinthine route by House and Hitselberger [6]. Yasargil [7] refined the microsurgical technique, emphasizing the importance of the brainstem arterial supply (AICA) and the need to optimize the preservation of facial nerve function.

These technical advances have resulted in a 50% reduction in mortality, a rate of complete tumor removal reaching 85% and the successful anatomical preservation of the facial nerve in 80%.

In recent years, owing to the development of new diagnostic instruments (CT, MR, AEP), the average size of VS at diagnosis has decreased drastically. Additionally, the development of multidisciplinary teams and the introduction of intraoperative monitoring (VII, VIII) have led to a dramatic improvement in clinical outcome, with an operative mortality of around 1%, a rate of total tumor removal close to 95%, and in small tumors (Koos I and II) the possibility of preserving normal facial motor function in a significant proportion of cases (House-Brackman 1 or 2). In some expert hands, the preservation of useful hearing (Gardner-Robertson 1 or 2) has been demonstrated to be achievable in selected

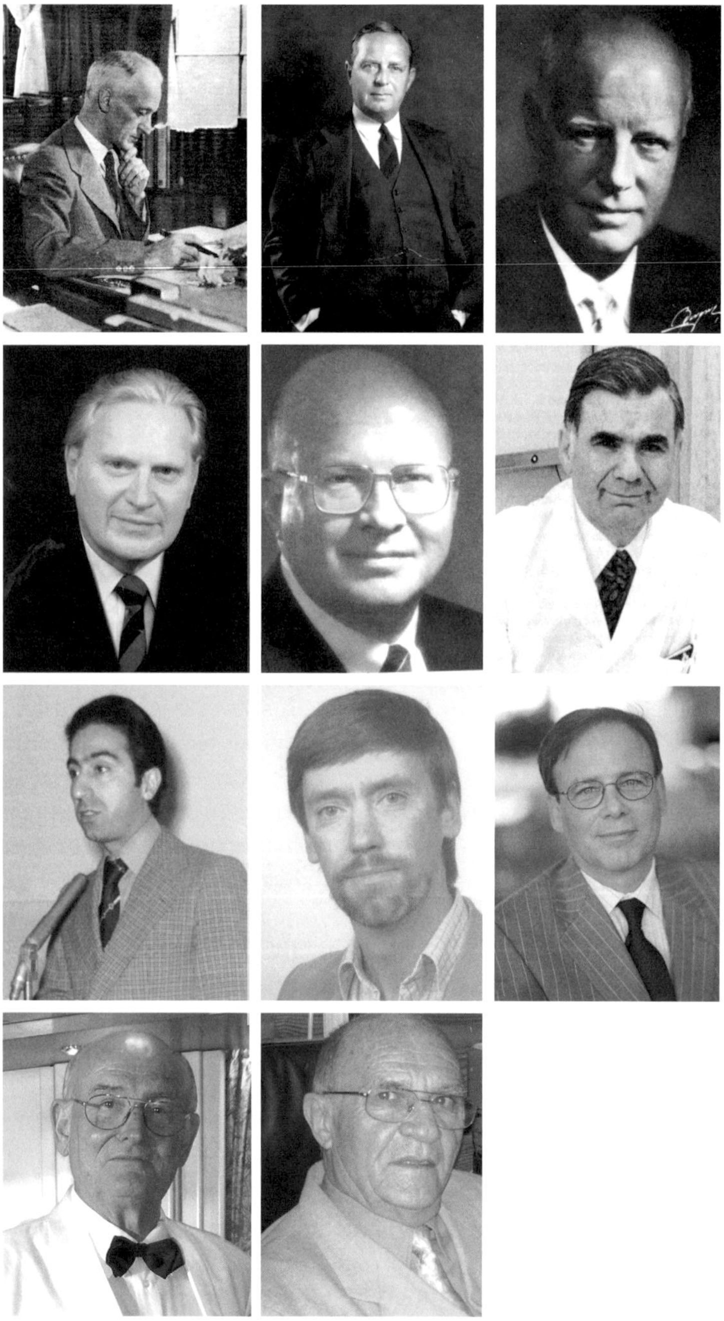

Fig. 1. Some important contributors to the field of neurosurgical management of VSs: Harvey Cushing, Walter Dandy, Herbert Olivecrona, William Koos, Al Rhoton, Gazi Yasargyl, Madji Samii, Georg Noren, Dade Lunsford, and William Pellet and Maurice Cannoni, the founders of the Marseille Otoneurosurgery Team.

small lesions with very good preoperative hearing. In 1997, Samii and Matthies [8] published a series of 962 patients with a tumor control rate of 98% and an impressive functional hearing preservation rate of 39% with an associated mortality of 1.1% and a reasonable complication rate (CSF leak 9%, meningitis 1.2%, hydrocephalus 2.3% and miscellaneous 5%).

Table 1. Prof. Pellet published objective results of microsurgery for VS comparable to the best series in the contemporary literature

Author	Patients	Facial preservation (H-B 1 and 2) %	Functional hearing preservation[1] %	CSF leak %	Lower cranial nerve (IX–XI) deficit %	Mortality %
Hardy, 1989	100	29	ND	13	5	3
Fischer, 1992	102	66	29	3	ND	2.9
Ebersold, 1992	256	64	24	11	2	1
Glasscock, 1993	161	ND	35	13	ND	0
Pellet, 1993	178	66	37.5	7.5	3	1.8
Gormley, 1997	179	77	38	15	2	1
Samii, 1997	1,000	59	40	9.2	5.5	1.1

H-B = House-Brackmann.
[1]For functional hearing preservation results correspond to the subgroup with a conservative approach.

The most recent neurosurgical advance has been radiosurgery, conceived during the 'microsurgical era' of the 1960s and 1970s in the brilliant mind of stereotactic neurosurgeon Lars Leksell [9, 10]. The fantastic image-guided neurosurgical instrument, which Leksell called the Gamma Knife has been able to realize its full potential with the appearance of modern imaging in the late 80s, specifically MRI. In 1992 when Prof. Sedan installed the first French Gamma Knife unit, the local otoneurosurgical team of Prof. Pellet and Cannoni was one of the most experienced in the country, with objective results comparable to those of the best international teams (table 1). This team adopted the translabyrinthine and the middle fossa approaches from the House institute. At this time, not convinced by the radiosurgical data of the literature they considered that a prospective trial was mandatory in order to provide a realistic evaluation of the results of Gamma Knife surgery (GKS). Comparing the functional outcomes evaluated by the patients themselves, this trial demonstrated much better functional preservation in small- to middle-sized VSs treated with GKS instead of microsurgery [11]. These results have been confirmed by all of the subsequent comparative studies [12, 13]. Since this time, more than 2,500 patients presenting with VS have been treated by GKS in Marseille Timone University Hospital. Nowadays, with modern high-resolution imaging, GKS has revolutionized the field of VS management. In experienced hands, 98% of small or middle-sized unilateral VS are controlled by GKS with a less than 1% risk of facial palsy. In patients with subnormal hearing at the time of treatment there is a 75% chance of preserving functional hearing in the long-term [14, 15].

In the 1990s, radiosurgery became the first-line treatment option for small- to middle-sized VS, especially in young patients with few symptoms [14, 15]. However, microsurgery remains the first-line treatment for large VS (Koos IV), and it is still challenging. In the 21st century, the demonstration of the high rate of functional preservation has led us to promote the idea of a combined microradiosurgical approach for large VS, allowing a dramatic reduction in the rate of facial palsy in large VS from 50% to less than 20% [Roche et al., in press].

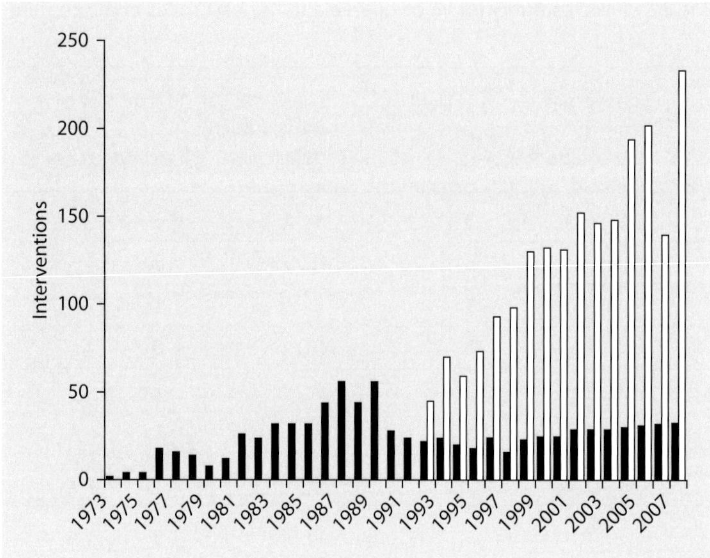

Fig. 2. Global activity of the Timone University Hospital Otoneurosurgery Team (886 microsurgeries and 2,046 GKSs, making up a total of 2,932 interventions). In the 1990s, the demonstration of the better functional outcome with GKS (□) in small- to middle-sized VSs led to a dramatic reduction in the percentage of patients treated microsurgically (■). A second period at the end of the 1990s, certainly due to the wish of the patient to be treated in institutes able to provide them with all the modern solutions available without technical bias, have led to a secondary increase in the microsurgical activity. The creation of a multidisciplinary platform offering all the approaches, including high-precision radiosurgery, explains the continuing exponential expansion of the otoneurosurgical activity in Timone Hospital.

Our experience of more than 3,500 VSs (fig. 2) has led us to consider that, in the modern era, VSs should be managed by experienced multidisciplinary teams able to integrate all the microsurgical and radiosurgical approaches in order to provide the highest level of care and the highest probability of functional preservation and good quality of life. By publishing the results of the whole spectrum of the surgical armamentarium given by leading experts in the field, this book attempts to provide guidelines for the individual and tailored management of VSs. Patients and referring physicians need clarification of the indications for the different techniques. There is also a necessity to improve our knowledge of neurofibromatosis type 2 disease and to offer more satisfactory options to these patients.

References

1 Koos WT, Spetzler RF, Böck FW, Salah S: Microsurgery of cerebellopontine angle tumors; in Koos WT, Spetzler RF, Bock FW (eds): Clinical Microneurosurgery. Sttugart, Georg Thieme Pub, 1976, pp 91–112.
2 Cushing H: Intracranial Tumours. Notes upon a Series of 2,000 Verified Cases with Surgical Mortality Pertaining Thereto. Ilinois, Springfield, Charles C Thomas, 1932.
3 Dandy WE: Results of removal of acoustic tumors by the unilateral approach. A.M.A. Arch Surg 1941;42:1026–1043.
4 Olivecrona H: Acoustic tumors. J Neurosurg 1967;26:6–13.
5 House WF, Gardner G, Hughes RL: Middle cranial fossa approach to acoustic tumor surgery. Arch Otolaryngol 1968;88:631–641.
6 House WF: Translabyrinthine approach; in House WF, Luetje CM (eds): Acoustic Tumors. Baltimore, University Park Press, 1979, pp 43–87.
7 Yasargil MG, Smith RD, Gasser JC: Microsurgical approach to acoustic neurinomas. Adv Tech Stand Neurosurg 1977;4:93–129.

8 Samii M, Matthies C: Management of vestibular schwannomas (acoustic neuromas): hearing function in 1,000 tumor resection. Neurosurgery 1997;40:248–262.
9 Leksell L: The stereotaxic method and radiosurgery of the brain. Acta Chirurgica Scandinavia 1951;102:316–319.
10 Leksell L: A note on the treatment of acoustic tumors. Acta Chirurgica Scandinavia 1969;137:763–765.
11 Regis J, Pellet W, Delsanti C, Dufour H, Roche PH, Thomassin JM, Zanaret M, Peragut JC: Functional outcome after Gamma Knife surgery or microsurgery for vestibular schwannomas. J Neurosurg 2002;97:1091–1100.
12 Pollock B, Lunsford L, Kondziolka D, Flickinger J, Bissonette D, Kelsey S, Jannetta P: Outcome analysis of acoustic neuroma management: a comparison of microsurgery and stereotactic radiosurgery [published erratum appears in Neurosurgery 1995 Feb;36(2):427]. Neurosurgery 1995;36:215–224; discussion 224–219, 1995; erratum Neurosurgery 1995;36:427.
13 Pollock BE, Driscoll CL, Foote RL, Link MJ, Gorman DA, Bauch CD, Mandrekar JN, Krecke KN, Johnson CH: Patient outcomes after vestibular schwannoma management: a prospective comparison of microsurgical resection and stereotactic radiosurgery. Neurosurgery 2006;59:77–85; discussion 77–85, 2006.
14 Lunsford LD, Niranjan A, Flickinger JC, Maitz A, Kondziolka D: Radiosurgery of vestibular schwannomas: summary of experience in 829 cases. J Neurosurg 2005;102(suppl):195–199.
15 Regis J, Delsanti C, Roche PH, Thomassin JM, Pellet W: Functional outcomes of radiosurgical treatment of vestibular schwannomas: 1,000 successive cases and review of the literature. Neurochirurgie 2004;50: 301–311.

Prof. Jean Régis
Service de Neurochirurgie Fonctionnelle et Stéréotaxique
Hôpital d'Adulte de la Timone, 264 bvd Saint Pierre
FR–13385 Marseille Cedex 05 (France)
Tel. +33 4 91 38 65 62, Fax +33 4 91 38 70 56, E-Mail jregis@ap-hm.fr

Régis J, Roche P-H (eds): Modern Management of Acoustic Neuroma.
Prog Neurol Surg. Basel, Karger, 2008, vol 21, pp 6–23

History of Vestibular Schwannoma Surgery

William Pellet

Service de Neurochirurgie, Hôpital Sainte-Marguerite, Marseille, France

Abstract

Attempts of surgical removal of vestibular schwannomas started 150 years ago with major limitations in terms of diagnosis and understanding of the disease but also in respect of surgical technique and instrumentation. Then came Cushing followed by Dandy, two pioneers and legendary neurosurgeons who understood the natural history of the disease and set the landmarks of the current surgery of the cerebellopontine angle. In this century of medicine, results and expectations shifted from a life-threatening affection to the actual standard of cranial nerve preservation and conservation of quality of life. In this overview, it is shown how the standard of the current surgery came from two distinct medical cultures, otologists and neurosurgeons, respectively. Now and in the near future, these competencies will be gathered in multidisciplinary teams who will display the whole panel of the treatment options in order to offer the best individual solutions for the patients.

Although the first case was reported as early as 1777 [1], vestibular schwannoma (VS), at that time called neuroma or neurilemoma or fibroma or even fibrosarcoma, was still an almost unknown tumor at the beginning of the 19th century. Thanks to the anatomoclinical behavior proposed by John Hunter at the end of the 18th century, some very well documented cases [2–9] were reported in the world all along the 19th century, and thus the clinical symptomatology of such tumors gradually became clear. At the end of the 19th century, diagnosis became possible during life and not only at the post-mortem examination.

In 1846, Morton, a dental surgeon working in Boston, proposed narcosis. During the 1860s, Semmelweis and then Pasteur showed the implication of the micro-organisms' involvement in sepsis. Then, in 1875, Lister conceived the antiseptic method with pads impregnated with phenol that were placed into the operative field. As a matter of fact, phenol was aggressive to the patient's as well as the surgeon's tissues. It appeared that the best prevention of operative infections was the preoperative destruction of micro-organisms. The surgical asepsis concept thrust itself with sterilization of instruments, preparation of the skin in the operative field and of the hands of the surgeon, sterile surgical dressing and, from 1890, according to Halsted's advice, use of surgical gloves. During the 1890s, several surgeons attempted to remove VS [10–13] but, as a rule, the operation was fatal. Sir Charles Ballance [14] was the first to successfully remove a cerebellopontine angle tumor on November 19th, 1894. 'A finger had to be insinuated between the pons and the tumor to get it away' specified Sir Ballance in his report, which gives an idea of the adventure. The patient survived but with facial palsy and keratitis which led to eye enucleation. According to

Harvey Cushing [15], this case was a meningioma. Annandale [16] was the first to successfully remove an acoustic neuroma on May 3rd, 1895, in a 25-year-old pregnant woman who had a successful delivery following the operation. Such a success was exceptional, and it seems that Murri's patient [17] operated on by Bendani in 1897 in Bologna was the only other survivor.

Thus, the prehistoric period came to an end. With the beginning of the 20th century, the neurosurgical period of the history of acoustic neurinoma began. These tumors were now defined as a real entity. In 1902, Henneberg and Koch [18] gave a permanent denomination to the clinical presentation of these tumors, the pontocerebellar angle syndrome. Considering that only a limited number of specialists were able to recognize this entity, identification of the disease usually came very late, giving a few chances for survival after a surgery which became technically possible.

The Neurosurgical Period

The neurosurgical period took place during the first 60 years of the 20th century. It was in turn ruled by Harvey Cushing then Walter Dandy. That is why Glasscock [19] then House [20] proposed dividing this period into two eras, each dedicated to each of them. At that time, the main problem was to preserve life.

Harvey Cushing (1869–1939)

After medical studies at the Harvard University, Harvey Cushing graduated in 1895. He then made his surgical training at the Massachusetts Hospital in Boston; then in 1900 he went to the Johns Hopkins Hospital in Baltimore to complete his surgical experience in Halsted's service who taught him rigor and adeptness of the hand. As general surgeon, he became interested in surgery of the brain as early as 1902. At that time, very few surgeons had performed this type of surgery – Sir William Macewen (1848–1924) in Glasgow, Sir Victor Horsley (1857–1916) in London, Fedor Krause (1856–1937) in Berlin and Jaboulay in Lyon.

Cushing operated on his first acoustic neurinoma on January 12th, 1906. His patient was ataxic, bedridden, and blind because of the optical atrophy owing to a severe intracranial hypertension. He was deaf in his right ear and he had suffered a right trigeminal neuralgia. Nobody understood this situation until Cushing thought it was a posterior fossa tumor. The patient was operated on in a sitting position, his head supported by an assistant. He could hardly breathe under the mask. The tumor was 4 cm in diameter and bled significantly. Because of the high amount of blood loss, it was difficult to visualize the operating field and only the inferior part of the tumor could be removed. The patient could not take such an apocalyptical session and died 3 days later of pneumonia. Cushing operated on a second neurinoma 3 months later. The patient was a 25-year-old man who had previously undergone 3 successive occipital craniectomies then a temporal craniectomy which had had no effect on his intracranial pressure. At that time, Cushing already had already learnt from his earlier experiences. The patient was in the prone position and ventilated with a Bennet machine. Widely exposed by his T incision and after large occipital craniectomy, Cushing removed the inferior half part of the tumor. This time, the result was much better. The patient had only transient swallowing troubles, and permanent facial palsy. He was discharged 23 days later and was lost to follow-up. Histology confirmed a neurinoma. Cushing recognized him, 4 years later, in a report of a man who, roughly falling during a seizure, experienced cranial traumatism with a skull fracture and died very soon afterwards. At the autopsy, there was a hemorrhage in the posterior fossa surrounding a tumor. Cushing considered this tumor as a glioma. Subsequently, he thought this case was especially favorable and he would have been able to totally remove the tumor if he had been more experienced. The case of a woman in the same stage operated on 3 months later and who survived for 3 years after a partial removal reinforced his opinion. He carried out his tumor intracapsular hollowing out tactics. Gradually, he refined his technique: the patient in a sitting position to reduce bleeding and to have a cleaner operating field, local anesthesia as Elinhorn and Uhlfelder [21] had disclosed procaine which, when joined with adrenaline, insured a well-anesthetized and hemostatic scalp, ventricular drainage as proposed by Fedor Krause [22], 'cross bow' incision, large bi-occipital craniectomy exposing the two cerebellar hemispheres, total resection of the posterior margin of the occipital foramen and of the posterior arch of the atlas as recommended by Borchart [23] who had perfectly described the herniation of cerebellar tonsilla, careful hemostasis on the scalp with grips on the galea, a method invented by himself and, firstly, cerebral hemostasis with his silver clips and, later, by electrocoagulation which was developed by himself and Bovie. He also invented a lot of instruments such as ventricular probes, ventricular needles or brain movers which made the surgical intervention easier, without speaking about its smoothness, cautiousness and preciseness, his respect of the operative time connection from the incision to the closure with restoration of all the crossed planes or, still, his strict observance of asepsis rules. In 1912, he went to Boston to work in the Department of Surgery of the brand new Peter Bent Brigham Hospital. During the same time, he joined the Harvard Medical School [24] that was to become the 'Mecca' of neurosurgery. There, Harvey Cushing operated on 30 cases. In 1917 [15], he could report a death rate of 15.4% while the death rate reported by other surgeons (Horsley in Dandy [25], Eiselberg [26], Henschen [27], Krause [28] ,Tooth [29]) ranged between 66 and 84%. As, in 1910, Verocay [30] had demonstrated the benign nature of neurinoma, he though his tactics were the best because of the interest in offering some years in an acceptable condition to these patients by a partial removal rather than to hurry their death by an attempt of total resection.

He was faced with another challenge – to more rapidly detect these tumors and, to teach physicians about their symptoms. Krause [31] made the same approach but Cushing, by precise interrogations and examination of his patients, was able to masterfully describe the chronology of the symptoms in his famous monograph [15]; firstly, the auditory and labyrinthine signs, especially the telephone sign, then headaches, then cerebellar incoordination, then palsies of other cranial nerves, then intracranial hypertension signs, especially papilledema and VIth nerve palsy, then phonation and swallowing troubles and finally posterior cerebellar fits. That monograph gave the designation 'acoustic neurinoma' to these tumors born on the vestibular nerve, but whose first sign was hearing loss. His expectations for the future were that diffusion of this knowledge would allow to detect such tumors at the early stage of hearing loss or instability. Diagnosis of course benefited from paraclinical innovations. In 1850, Helmoltz invented the ophthalmoscope thanks to which Von Graefe was able to recognize papilledema. In 1895, Roentgen discovered X-rays, and in 1912 Henschen [32] described the dilatation of the internal auditory canal (IAC) on skull radiography, a determinant sign at that time but difficult enough to disclose on usual X-ray incidence. In 1928, Schuller [33] then Stenvers [34] proposed special incidences that improved the images. In 1875, Graham Bell invented the telephone and in 1878 Hartmann made the first acoumeter in Berlin while Hugues made the first audiometer in the United States. In 1906, Barany developed his caloric method of exploration of the vestibular system. Cushing used all these innovations to better diagnose these types of tumors. Cushing's work was not limited to neurinomas. Management of all intracranial tumors, especially pituitary tumors, benefited from his activity in terms of the treatment of trigeminal pain or the understanding numerous pathophysiological mechanisms such as the action of intracranial hypertension on the systemic arterial pressure (Cushing's reflex) or the importance of craniectomy on intracranial pressure. Indisputably, he was the founder of a new surgical specialty, neurosurgery, and he trained numerous young neurosurgeons among whom Walter Dandy was one. Meanwhile, Panse [35] proposed to reach the neurinoma through the temporal pyramid. He called this approach the translabyrinthine approach, but without magnification, drill or microsurgical instruments, it was rapidly abandoned because of its narrowness and numerous complications owing to bleeding from the lateral sinus injury or to cerebrospinal fluid (CSF) leakages.

Walter Dandy (1886–1945)

He was also Halsted's colleague at the Johns Hopkins Hospital after having begun his medical studies at the Missouri University [36]. He graduated in 1910. He benefited from Cushing's teaching and worked for him in the Hunterian Laboratory of experimental medicine, on vascularization and innervation of the pituitary gland. We know that their strong personalities clashed, and Cushing refused to take Dandy with him when he started his work in Boston. Dandy even lost his position in the Halsted Department but he remained at the Johns Hopkins Hospital thanks to his Director, Dr. Smith, who allowed him to work in the laboratory. With Kenneth Blackfan, he made experimental studies of hydrocephaly and CSF circulation in the dog. As early as 1913, he published a first report [37] that impressed Halsted who reopened his Department to Walter Dandy who became the chief neurosurgeon of the Johns Hopkins Hospital in 1922.

Dandy operated on his two first neurinomas in 1915 [38]. Thanks to Cushing's teaching, these 2 patients came to the operation in good condition with hearing loss, facial numbness and headaches. He used Cushing's hollowing out but both patients died within 12 h. He then operated on 3 additional patients but 2 of them died of meningitis, one within 4 h and the other after 46 h. He operated on a 60-year-old patient in 1917. The woman was well initially, but her condition deteriorated after the 70th day with symptoms of drowsiness, vomiting, dysphonia and dysphagia. In a preliminary report [39], he explained that it could not be a hematoma or meningitis, and he thought that it was due to compression of the brainstem by the remaining piece of tumor. Thus, he operated again on his patient and totally removed the piece of tumor thanks to a skilful maneuver with his forefinger. The patient regained her consciousness within 5 days. Dandy deduced that the remaining piece of tumor could have baneful effects and that it was better to totally remove the tumor if possible. He successfully operated on 2 patients in two stages, hollowing out in a first stage then removing the remnant within a few days. He then thought it was possible to totally remove the tumor in a single stage. Henceforth, he strove to totally hollow out the tumor and then to smoothly dissect its 'capsule', which was achievable on its superior and inferior poles but much more difficult and risky against the brain. Within the 9 following years, he operated on 23 patients and was able to report in 1925 [40] a 30% mortality which was higher than Cushing's rate after partial removal (15.4%) but was better than Cushing's rate after the regrowth (40%) that occurred systematically. Later, Dandy recommended [41] a unilateral narrower approach after a unilateral incision half-way from the mastoid and the external occipital tuberosity. All these initiatives were in contrast to Cushing's certainties. However, Dandy's ideas progressively won. His 1941 report [42] on 41 cases with a 2.4% operative mortality will remain the objective of all neurosurgeons, and for a long time. At that time, this legendary neurosurgeon could already preserve the facial nerve in some cases after drilling in the posterior wall of the IAC.

This man of genius was not only involved in neurinoma surgery. His studies about CSF began in 1913 and led to ventriculography in 1918 [43] then to air encephalography in 1919 [44]. This method gave neurosurgeons adeterminant diagnostic means especially when Sicard and Forestier [45] proposed to replace air by lipiodol. The injection of lipiodol needed less abundant CSF emptying with less morbidity for patients, especially those with intracranial hypertension. With this examination, the neurosurgeon could only visualize the backwards movement of the fourth ventricle. In 1949, Lindgren [46], always based on Dandy's works, conceived fractionated pneumoencephalography. Thus, they were able to display the filling of the pontocerebellar cistern by the tumor. Moniz [47] conceived arteriography as early as 1927, but this test was used only to study the supratentorial arteries until the 1950s and could not be of any help for the diagnosis of neurinoma before that time. Dandy conceived numerous innovative new approaches too, i.e. frontolateral approach to the pituitary gland, trigeminal posterior radicotomy, radicotomy of the IXth nerve, transcallous approach to the third ventricle, and surgery of intracranial aneurysms, etc.

Herbert Olivecrona (1891–1980)

This neurosurgeon from Stockholm was the only neurosurgeon capable of reaching Dandy's results before the advent of microsurgery. In his report published in 1967 [48], he presented a 19.2% mortality rate among a total of 349 removals of 415 operated patients from 1931 to 1960. It is of interest to note that Olivecrona, in that report, thoroughly discussed the respective benefits of total and partial removal. That is the proof that he belonged to Dandy's era when he reported his results after another period had begun, the one of microneurosurgery and otoneurosurgery.

W.J. Atkinson

This author [49] studied lesions of the brain stem that were often found during autopsies of patients after operation for acoustic neurinoma and then considered as traumatic lesions. He described the softening of the lateral part of the pons due to the occlusion of a predominant anteroinferior cerebellar artery (AICA). The AICA shares the vascularization of this region with the posterior-inferior cerebellar artery (PICA). When PICA is of poor caliber, occlusion of the AICA may be responsible for ischemia of the pons. Demonstration of this mechanism indicated the necessity to preserve arteries in the operating field and, to reach this aim, to use magnification during the operation.

The 1950s

These are years of transition to the otoneurosurgical period. Diagnosis was made based on the association of otological and neurological signs, but the latter were moderate, with only facial numbness or cerebellar signs with headaches and papilledema but no longer blindness or cerebellar fits as before. Otologists knew how to easily confirm the unilateral hearing loss or the caloric hypoexcitability on one side. The widening of the IAC was more easily disclosed thanks to the radiological incidences proposed by Chausse [50], but development of linear tomography significantly improved the diagnosis at the end of that decade. Arteriography was not yet used for vertebral artery. Finally, lipiodol ventriculography remained the main examination at that time for making a diagnosis of acoustic neurinomas, but this one had to be large enough to shift the fourth ventricle. That is why diagnosis was very late and the tumor sizes were very large, as in the Olivecrona [48] series where 94% of his tumors were the size and shape of a walnut or a ping pong ball. Ventriculography was performed in a neurosurgical environment, keeping neurinomas in the neurosurgical departments. The operation remained serious and was delayed for the rare cases where the diagnosis was made only based only on otological symptoms. Neurosurgeons preferred to wait for signs of intracranial hypertension before deciding on surgery and risking the lives of their patients. The results reported by

Olivecrona [48] and by McKenzie [51] were the standards to attain.

The Otoneurosurgical Period

The otoneurosurgical period began at the end of the 1950s with the increasing entrusting of VSs to otologists. At that time:

- Diagnosis of VS was made earlier when the patient only complained of hearing loss, dizzines or ear buzz. The patient was no longer a neurosurgical patient but rather an otological one.
- The confirmation of the diagnosis by hearing or vestibular tests was obviously made by an otologist.
- Radiological examinations were less aggressive and not necessarily performed in a neurosurgical environment.
- Otologists have been the first to use microscopy under the impulse of Shambaugh [52] who introduced it in 1940 in the US, while it had been developed by Holmgren in Sweden 10 years earlier.
- Transpetrous approaches to VS were soon to be proposed by otologists.

The 1960s

The main challenge of this period was to preserve the facial nerve. During the first years of this decade, the diagnosis was still made in neurosurgical departments but William House [53] already insisted to his otologist colleagues on the necessity to make instrumental explorations when faced with any unilateral hearing loss or tinnitus, dizziness, vertigo. More effective exploration methods were developed – electronystagmography for vestibule and several audiometric tests (Bekesy, decay test, SISI test) capable of demonstrating a cochlear nerve tiredness that is the proof of a retrocochlear lesion. As a matter of fact, these tests may be negative in 30% of cases when the number of impaired cochlear fibers is not important enough and, not obligatorily, when the tumor is small. Ruben [54] had just proposed transtympanic electrocochleography, and this method would soon allow collecting of auditory evoked responses. Complex helicoidal tomography provided better images of the IAC and the interpretation of these improved especially after Valvassori's [55] publications. Pneumoencephalography, especially when Di Chiro [56] had joined it with helicoidal tomography, could show small tumor occupying the pontocerebellar cistern. When this examination appeared normal although the suspicion of VS was strong, it was possible to try and fill up the IAC with a little bit of lipiodol introduced in the CSF after lumbar or suboccipital puncture. This method proposed by Baker [57] or Scanlon [58], meatocysternography, appeared as the affectedness of examinations that allowed the disclosure of strictly intracanalicular tumors. One had then a new form of neurinoma, a purely otologic form that presented new surgical problems. It is so, as reported by Bradley [59], that Mayfield, at a common otologist-neurosurgeon meeting, would have proposed to distinguish two clinical forms, the small tumors or 'ear tumors' and the other, bigger, or 'brain tumors'. There is nothing better than encouraging the otologists' surgical interest in VS; William House, an otologist, was one of the motivators who showed them the way.

William House

As related by Glasscock [60], William House, an otologist from Los Angeles who did his best to diagnose VS at the earliest, was shocked by the death of a young fireman who just complained of tinnitus and hearing loss and in whom he had discovered a small VS thanks to the dilatation of an IAC and caloric hyporeflexia. He entrusted this patient to a neurosurgeon, but this one preferred to wait for neurological and intracranial hypertension signs before operating on him. These signs appeared 1 year later and the neurosurgeon made the decision to operate on him via a suboccipital approach without optic magnification. This patient died rapidly after the operation.

House who was present at the operation regretted the delay of the operation and the rusticity of the gesture, especially that he himself currently used microscope for his operations. During the following year, he disclosed two other neurinomas and he entrusted the same neurosurgeon with these. Both survived but with important facial and trigeminal disabilities.

At the same time, House was developing the suprapetrous subtemporal approach to the IAC to make vestibular neurectomy after drilling through its roof. He had the idea to combine two approaches, a suprapetrous approach to pull out the facial nerve clear of the tumor in the IAC, then a suboccipital approach to remove the tumor in the posterior fossa. On the 15th of February, 1961, he operated on a first patient with John B. Doyle, neurosurgeon from Los Angeles. The tumor was huge. House drilled out most of the labyrinthine mass. The patient survived with a very incomplete facial palsy, but died 3 years later after having been operated on again by Doyle for a recurrence. Using the same method, this otoneurosurgical team operated on 8 patients during the following year. Half of them benefited from a total removal and one died due to pulmonary embolism.

It was at that time that William House thought of using the translabyrinthine approach of Panse [35]. He made some dissections in the amphitheater and defined the limits of his drilling. Thanks to the microscope, drill and microinstruments, this approach was now feasible with sparing of the external auditory canal, the intrapetrous facial nerve, the jugular bulb and the lateral sinus. John B. Doyle preferred to keep the suboccipital approach and House operated alone on his first patient on the 2nd of June, 1962. It was a middle-sized VS. Its removal was not complete and the patient kept a partial facial palsy. The same day, just before his operation, House operated on another VS through a suprapetrous approach with John B. Doyle [60]. This patient died 7 days later of a hematoma in the posterior fossa. His opinion was made; henceforth, he will use the translabyrinthine approach. He operated on the following tumors with another neurosurgeon, William Hitselberger. Their collaboration will be an example for the ones who decided to treat cerebellopontine angle tumors in otoneurosurgical teams.

In 1964, House reported [61] his 53 first cases. Incomplete removal was achieved in 50% of cases, a rate which decreased to 14% when, 4 years later, he reported his 200 first cases [62]. The mortality rate was then at 7%. In this last series, 1 year after the operation, the facial nerve was normal in 72% of cases, partially paralyzed in 23% of cases and totally paralyzed in 5%. These results were, at that time, already better than those of all the neurosurgeons, and his experience improved all along the following years, 500 cases in 1973 [63], 1,100 in 1979 [64], 1,320 in 1982 [65], 2,157 in 1986 [66].

House's first works raised the interest of neurosurgeons, especially in the US where competition immediately spread out. As a first consequence, neurosurgeons began to use the microscope and, to totally remove the tumor and to try to preserve the facial nerve like House, began to open the posterior wall of the IAC. The suboccipital transmeatal approach was born. According to Bucy [67], Walter Dandy had already made that. As early as 1964, Rougerie and Guyot [68] from Paris began to show their interest in this technique as well as Rand [69] from Los Angeles in 1965, Pool [70] from New York in 1966 or Drake [71] from London, Ont., in 1967. This 'trepanation' of the posterior wall of the IAC was made with a gouge [68, 70–72] or by drilling [69] without anatomical guide marks, the main point being to uncover the distal portion of the intrameatal tumor. Although they were not as good as those of House [62], results reported by neurosurgeons improved with about 50% of preservation of the facial nerve and a mortality rate of about 15%. All these improvements were made thanks to William House's influence, and that is why this period may be named House's period.

The 1970s

The diagnosis was now generally made at an early clinical stage, the otologic stage according to Bebear [73] who distinguished in his thesis of medicine the otologic stage when hearing loss, tinnitus, dizziness or vertigo only exist, the otoneurologic stage when facial numbness, trigeminal pain, phonic or swallowing troubles or cordonal signs appear, and finally the neurosurgical stage when there are signs of intracranial hypertension. Patients were now in a good condition and the operation was not as dangerous as before. It could be decided to operate as soon as the diagnosis was made.

Thanks to Anderson's works [74], the study of the stapedial reflex became usual practice allowing an easy confirmation of cochlear nerve disturbance. In the same way, the study of an auditory brainstem response (ABR) was proposed from 1970 by Jewett [75]; demonstration of a 95% rate of reliability was rapidly done. Likewise, Hounsfield [76] in 1973 developed computerized axial tomography, the CT scanner, which revolutionized radiology of the head with images that seemed a miracle for all who had known those of the 1950s. All these new diagnostic methods allowed earlier diagnosis but one was often surprised by the discrepancy between the important volume of the VS and the discrete clinical symptoms. This anatomoclinical dissociation was now a fact. In the same way, the possibility to make a CT scan to patients enduring a sudden or a fluctuating deafness, a vertigo attack, or dizziness without hearing loss, allowed to disclose not so rare 'atypical' forms of VS.

Some neurosurgeons such as Yasargil from Zurich [77], Malis from New York [78] or Koos from Vienna [79] could now report their important series. They used a suboccipital approach. The tumor was hollowed out, and then generally the posterior wall of the IAC was drilled. Their technique differed only by the method to find the facial nerve. Some searched the facial nerve at the bottom of the IAC then dissected it toward the pons. Others searched it at the pontomedullary junction and dissected it toward the IAC. Others such as Malis [78] preferred to pass through the VS to search the facial nerve on its convexity at the level of the porus, where the nerve is easily dissected because of the presence of an arachnoidal sheet that separates it from the tumor, according to the description of Yazargil [77].

Several otoneurosurgical teams were formed, such as the team from Bordeaux in 1971 [80] or the team from Marseille in 1973 [81], when it appeared to these specialists that the association of their points of view and of their experience may improve the quality of the management of their patients. These otoneurosurgical teams used a translabyrinthine approach or sometimes, as proposed by Morrisson and King [82], a combined translabyrinthine and suboccipital approach as performed by Hitselberger and House [83] at the early stages of their experience when the VS was too large to be exposed with a regular translabyrinthine approach. Maddox [84] proposed to divide the lateral sinus and the tentorium, but this technique was left for giant tumors only.

Several otologists [85], paradoxically, chose to use the suboccipital approach, operating on VS like neurosurgeons and did not take into account the amount of refinements brought by House. Needing to perform like neurosurgeons but willing to remain otologists, they even changed the name of this approach to retrosigmoid transmeatal approach. Surprisingly, neurosurgeons progressively adopted this denomination too, even if the approach they made was globally the one that was performed by Walter Dandy since 1930.

During this decade, discussions were ardent between supporters of the neurosurgical and of the otoneurosurgical attitude, the most passionate even developing deceptive arguments [86, 87] which now appear laughable. More seriously, they argued with statistics, including mortality rate, postoperative hematoma or pontocerebellar infarction rate, CSF leak or meningitis rate and facial nerve preservation rate. However, if House's results at the beginning were better, supporters of the suboccipital approach, with the improvement of their experience, a better knowledge of limits of drilling on the posterior wall of the IAC thanks to the anatomical works of Rhoton [88] and with the use of facial nerve monitoring proposed by Delgado [89], were able to obtain comparable results. Ojeman and Crowel [90], having studied several reports, underlined that the facial nerve may be preserved in 70–80% of cases, all tumor volume mixed. Di Tullio [87], at the same time, reported a mortality rate of 3.7%, normal facial motion in 59% of cases, partial facial palsy in 29%, and total facial palsy in 12%. Bonnal [91] reported normal or near-to-normal facial motion in 81% of cases. Sterkers [92] reported normal facial nerve after the suboccipital approach in 82% of cases. Brackmann [64] who reported House's results in a series of 500 cases operated on between 1968 and 1975, gave a mortality rate of 2.6 and 86.5% of cases had normal or near-to-normal facial nerve. However, it remained important to develop a classification of tumor size to compare these results. The classification proposed by Koos [93] was adopted (table 1).

Table 1. Koos classification

Stage I	Intracanalicular tumor
Stage II	Tumor spreading in the cerebellopontine angle but not reaching the pons
Stage III	Tumor reaching the pons, perhaps deforming it but not shifting it
Stage IV	Tumor deforming the pons and shifting the fourth ventricle

According to this classification, Tarlov [94] reported normal facial nerve in all the cases with Koos stage I or II tumors, normal facial nerve in 57% and partial facial palsy in 43% of cases with Koos stage III tumors and normal facial nerve, partial and total facial palsy in 71, 11 and 18% of cases with Koos stage IV tumors.

Preservation of Hearing

As a matter of fact, preservation of hearing is the main argument when choosing a surgical approach. Such a goal needs to preserve the integrity of the hearing apparatus, the cochlear nerve, the labyrinth and the vascularization of these. Thus, the translabyrinthine approach is to be eliminated. One may then use a suboccipital or a suprapetrous (middle fossa) approach, and it is through that that House [61] was the first to succeed in such an objective as early as 1964. It was his case 46, a woman suffering from dizziness with perception hearing loss (45%) but with a normal IAC and a normal meatocisternography. He wanted to perform a vestibular neurectomy through a suprapetrous approach and found a 3 × 6 mm VS. He removed it totally, and his patient kept a normal facial nerve and recovered 80% hearing perception. In 1968, he reported [95] 4 successes for 5 attempts on intracanalicular tumors and 3 other successes for 14 attempts on lightly spreading VS extending to the pontocerebellar cistern. All his patients had a normal facial motion on awakening. He had a 36.8% rate of preservation of hearing among his 19 attempts, which formed 9.5% of all his operated cases, the preservation of hearing rate among all these cases being 3.5%. In the same year, Hitselberger [96] reported 3 successes among 5 attempts on neurofibromatosis type 2 (NF2) patients and 10 years later, Brackmann [64] reported, among a series of 500 operations, 17 attempts of preservation of hearing and 10 successes. For all the users of the suboccipital approach, preservation of hearing was a decisive argument to choose it. Hullay and Tomis [97] in 1 out of 50 cases and McKissock [98] in 8 cases had reported to have preserved 'some hearing' when operating on patients without the microscope as soon as 1965. One year later, Pertuiset [99] did the same for 2 cases but, curiously, he did not address the problem of hearing preservation in his monograph on VS in 1970 [100]. In 1968,

Rand and Kurze [101] noted that it was possible to preserve nerves when operating on VS using the microscope as an aid. All these observations pointed to the fact that gentle dissection of the cochlear nerve could preserve its function. Some authors had the same success when operating on other lesions – cerebellar cyst [102], meningioma [103] and cholesteatoma [104].

The necessity to master the surgical anatomy of the intrapetrous hearing apparatus appeared to be a prerequisite for an attempt to preserve hearing. In 1977, Gueurking [105] specified all the sizes, distances and positions of the labyrinth according to the external edge of the porus of the IAC, according to the petrous crest and to the posterior aspect of the petrous pyramid. Among all the data provided, there is the fact that the labyrinth overlaps the external third of the IAC, a configuration that obliges the surgeons not to drill up to the fundus of this IAC. When one knows, as we have noted during our operations [106], that 63% of tumors reach the fundus of the IAC and even 17% go up into the fallopian canal, one knows that it is not possible in 80% of cases to totally expose the VS and to easily find the facial nerve downstream the tumor through this approach. The issue of total removal is then settled. Domb and Chole [107] in 1980 confirmed these anatomical data. Smith et al. [108] in 1973 were the first to report a less anecdotal series of preservation of hearing by a suboccipital approach. In 1978, Ojeman et al. [90] underlined that several authors after them (Khirsch, McCarthy, Rhoton, Buchheit) [109] had reported their success too and later Cohen [110] then Sterkers [111] did the same. These results were slightly less good than those obtained by the suprapetrous middle fossa approach, but they demonstrated the possibility to preserve hearing through the suboccipital approach.

The 1980s

In the 1980s, VSs became well known by physicians and especially by otologists who used reliable apparatuses to disclose perception hearing loss and retrocochlear lesions. Scanner images improved and, first of all, magnetic resonance imaging (MRI) was introduced. This method based on Block and Purcell's work made as soon as 1945 and which justified their Nobel prize in 1952 had to wait until the 1980s to become available in clinical practice. Thanks to it, very small VSs may now be identified, as soon as an otological sign appears and even incidentally. The number of these stage I VSs increases among all those disclosed each year. According to epidemiologic studies made by Tos and Thomsen [112], the incidence would be 9.4 per 1 million people per year. However, because of the anatomoclinical dissociation, the rate of these small VSs increases less than the total number. In 1968, House [62] noted a 2.5% rate. In 1991, Dutton et al. [113] reported a 5% rate. In 1998, Koos et al. [114] reported a 3% rate but Harner and Ebersold [115] noted a 13.7% rate. Probably, this rate is between these numbers, perhaps around 10%. The number of Koos stage II and III tumors increases, 46 and 34%, respectively, according to Dutton et al. [113] and 18 and 49% according to Harner and Ebersold [115]. The number of Koos stage IV, is of course decreasing, 64% in the Olivecrona series [48] but 15% in the Dutton series [113] and 20% in the Harner and Ebersold series [115].

Comparisons of facial nerve results were very difficult until now because of the subjectivity of evaluations. In 1983, John House [116], William's nephew, proposed a much more obvious classification which was reported again by Brackmann [117]. This classification is now popularized under the two authors' names. Evans [118] has evaluated and shown its great reliability.

William House, with his transpetrous, translabyrinthine and supra-petrous approaches demonstrated that the facial nerve may be preserved and this preservation had to be attempted in all cases. He also showed that the cochlear nerve might be preserved in some selected cases. His approaches are difficult to achieve without a long and arduous training. That is why neurosurgeons and even some otologists strove to do the same as House by their classical, well-known and much easier, neurosurgical suboccipital approach, and there is no doubt that they succeeded in reaching this aim even if the quality of removal and of results were not exactly the same as House's results. Since preservation of hearing may theoretically always be attempted through the suboccipital approach, it appeared evident to them that their approach was the only approach to be used. Their certainty was reinforced by 3 reports of preservation of hearing after removal of large and extra-large VSs through a suboccipital approach [118–120]. Based on these reports, one could think that preservation of hearing could be attempted in each case of VS, whatever its volume. However, it seems, when attentively studying these cases, that each one had a particular anatomical form with no or little extension of the VS into the IAC. This configuration will be named 'medial' acoustic neurinoma some years later by Tos et al. [121]. In these cases, the facial and cochlear nerves are less injured by the VS and more easily dissected. The attempt to preserve hearing cannot be systematic and should be weighted against several criterions: tumor volume, respective position of the cranial nerves, severity of the hearing loss and the state of hearing on the other side. The quality of the hearing that is to be preserved is indeed an important question. In the case of NF2, this question is not to be posed, but when the ear on the other side is normal this one has all the chances to remain unchanged. It is then useless to try to preserve nonserviceable hearing. From that point of view, one has to note that bi-auricular hearing requires a <25-dB difference between the two ears. Beyond that level, the impaired ear is useless and it may even disturb the normal ear because of the delay of its potentials which, arriving late, disturb integration of the contralateral normal potentials. The level of hearing that is preserved is very important to consider to assess the results

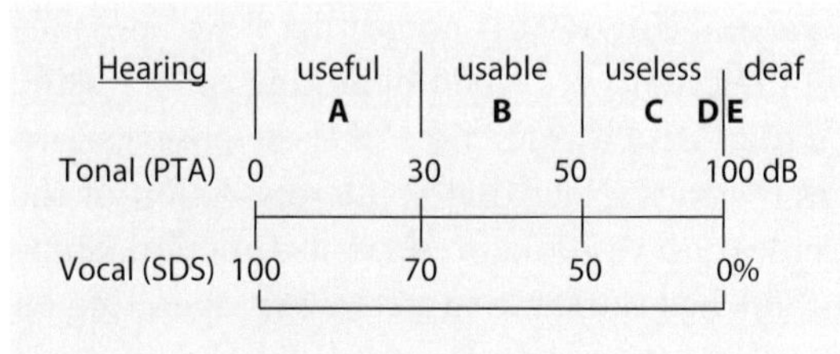

Fig. 1. Gardner-Robertson hearing classification.

and to compare them between different series. In this perspective, one has to know that there usually is an additional postoperative loss of about 10–15 dB. The preoperative hearing level is rarely preserved except in small VSs, medial VSs like in Fischer's case [119] or after sudden deafness, the latter sometimes slowly improving after the operation, as reported by Telian [122]. For all these reasons, it was important to perfectly define a classification of the quality of hearing. Silverstein et al. [123] were the first to propose one (fig. 1) in 1985 but, curiously, it was named 'Gardner and Robertson', probably because of its presentation by these authors in 1987 [124] at a meeting of the American Otological Society in Atlanta where it was adopted.

Just as the dissection of the facial nerve is achieved more safely with the help of perioperative facial nerve monitoring, the dissection of the cochlear nerve may be conducted under perioperative cochlear nerve monitoring and ABR. This method was developed by Levine [125] at the end of the 1970s. It requires the perioperative contribution of neurophysiologists but some teams, such as the one from Lyon [126], have shown its contribution to the improvements of hearing results.

Mainly after the reports of Fisher et al. [119], there was a real eagerness to preserve hearing and, without trying to make an extensive review of the literature, one may easily find numerous reports on attempts to preserve hearing using the suboccipital approach during the two following decades. Of course, those using transpetrous approaches did the same with the suprapetrous approach. One has to insist on the position adopted by Wigand [128, 129] who approached all VS, even the biggest, through a suprapetrous approach with the division of the superior petrosal sinus and tentorium. This approach allowed to well expose the intrameatal part of the tumor and to totally remove it. His results were impressive with 90.5% of total removal, 69.8% of preservation of the continuity of the cochlear nerve, 44.4% of preservation of hearing and 85.7% of normal or near-normal facial motion.

The 1990s Onwards

In respect of diagnosis or surgical treatment, there were no innovating methods. We could signal some refinements such as endoscopy in the cerebellopontine angle [130] but this one gives more beautiful images than real improvements of the operating technique. Dissection of the arachnoid sheaths around the tumor using saline water [131, 132] proved to be valuable. Development of nuclear implants is a very promising method for restoring the huge problem of deafness in NF2 patients. On the other hand, fundamental aspects of this pathology form the subject of unceasing research. Its origin on the vestibular nerve and from Schwann cells is now well demonstrated which justifies its accepted name of vestibular schwannoma. The genetic factors presiding over the development of these schwannomas are gradually being understood. The part of the NF2 gene located on the 22 chromosome and responsible for the control of Schwann cell proliferation is now better known. With the strategies of conservative treatment using sequential MRI control, we know more about the natural history of these tumors. About one third display a very slow growth and appear as stable. In the other two-thirds, the evolution is moderate – less than 2 mm a year in 2 out of 3 cases, but it may be more important, up to 10 mm a year, in the remaining cases. Taking into account the current early diagnosis, the attitude of many specialists has changed. If the patient's hearing is still normal and the VS volume is small, they do not hurry to remove it and favor the conservative attitude with audiometric and MR examinations. In the same way, experience shows us that hearing worsening is very slow (<1 dB/year) in 2 out of 3 cases, but it may be more important (about 7 dB/year) in the remaining case. Taken collectively, these findings indicate that hearing loss is inevitable. If nothing is in a hurry when hearing is already useless or even only usable, one must not wait with the decision to perform removal when hearing is still normal in order to try to save it. When hearing preservation is an important criterion in the evaluation of results, it is essential to adopt a uniform classification of hearing level. If not, it is quite impossible to compare the results of individual publications. That is, for instance, the case for the Samii's very important experience [127] in which the hearing classification is not the Gardner-Robertson one but the Hanover classification only used by this author. In an attempt to solve this problem, a consensus meeting was organized in 2003 in Tokyo [133] to define systems for reporting results in VS. Hearing results were considered and, after a discussion of the weaknesses of the Gardner-Robertson classification (Why the last studied frequency is 3,000 and not 4,000 Hz usually studied by audiometric examinations? Why the upper limit of the functional hearing was stated at 30 dB when one knows the physiological limit of interauricular difference is at 25 dB and even 20 dB when speaking in the crowd?), a new classification was proposed. Tonal valuation must be made on 500, 1,000, 2,000 and 4,000 Hz. Six hearing classes are defined from A (normal hearing) to F (deafness) and are to be considered on a diagram (fig. 2). In this diagram, a hearing result is located on the cross point of the SDS and PTA values. If this one is

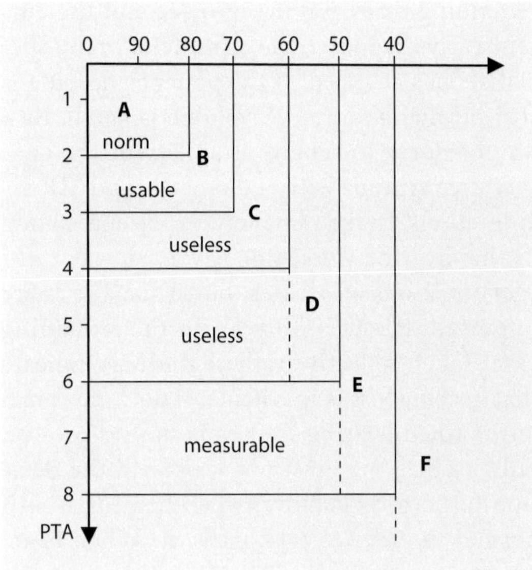

Fig. 2. Classification diagram of hearing according to the Tokyo consensus meeting.

Table 2. Tokyo tumor volume classification

Intracanal tumor		0 (Extracanal)
Extra-canal tumor	Small	1–10 mm
	Middle	11–20 mm
	Moderately big	21–30 mm
	Big	31–40 mm
	Huge	>40 mm
Note if the bottom of the IAC is full:	yes	no

located on the left side of a dotted line because of the better score on SDS than on PTA, it must be put in the upper class.

This Tokyo consensus meeting [133] also defined other classifications in respect of the tumor volume (table 2), the quality of removal (table 3) and a slight modification of the facial motion House-Brackmann grading system (table 4).

Table 3. Tokyo removal quality classification

Removal	Residue
Total	0%
Near total	<2%
Partial	<5%
Subtotal	>5%

At the end of the previous decade, a lot of VSs with very small signs were detected. The technical problems of microsurgery were set down. Even if surgery was generally well tolerated and the facial nerve may be usually well preserved, the operation is the source of permanent side effects and discomfort for the patients. The study we conducted on our patients [134] had underlined that the patients often considered their results were not as good as their surgeon claimed. They suffered from troubles (dizziness, ocular discomfort, varying pains, swallowing difficulties, ...) which were not very serious but sufficiently bothersome to disturb their daily life. Some authors [135–138], in the middle of the previous decade, have justified the rationale of a conservative treatment in patients harboring small tumors. On the other hand, other influential authors [139, 140] had underlined the necessity to always operate on these. Under their authority, the question seemed settled. However, this debate was opened and it led to the search for less aggressive means to treat these patients. That is why we decided to assess the safety and efficacy of radiosurgery as rigorously as possible. Thus, our otoneurosurgical team became an otoradioneurosurgical team in July 1992. We feel that in the era of evidence-based medicine, establishing medical guidelines for individual pathology and emphasizing the necessity to preserve quality of life, our attitude prefigures the attitude of many teams in the future.

Table 4. Facial motion classification (Tokyo; modified House-Brackmann classification)

Grade	Tonus at rest	Mimic				Hemispasm
		global aspect	forehead	eye	mouth	
1. Normal	normal	normal	normal	normal occlusion	normal	absent
2. Light	normal	light asymmetry	light asymmetry	eyelid occlusion: complete without effort	very light asymmetry	absent or very light
3. Moderate A (light)	normal or very light asymmetry	moderate asymmetry	moderate asymmetry	eyelid occlusion: complete with effort confortable eye	clear asymmetry protracted lips occluded	present, moderate
3. Moderate B (heavy)	normal or very light asymmetry	clear asymmetry	clear asymmetry	eyelid occlusion: complete with effort occular discomfort	clear asymmetry protracted lips not occluded	present, clear
4. Real	real asymmetry	real asymmetry	real asymmetry	eyelid occlusion: incomplete	real asymmetry	Present, greater
5. Heavy	greater asymmetry	greater asymmetry	greater asymmetry	eyelid occlusion: roughed	greater asymmetry	absent
6. Total	flaccidity	greater asymmetry	flaccidity	no eyelid occlusion	flaccidity	absent
Note:	crocodile tear: C0 C+		taste troubles: T0 T+		eye: not dry dry	

References

1 Sandifort E: De duro quodam corpusculo nervo auditorio ad haerente. Observatiores anatomico-pathological, Chapitre 9, in *Lugduni Batavorum*, 1777, pp 116–120.

2 Leveque-Lasource A: Observation sur une amaurose et une cophose, avec perte ou diminution de la voix, des mouvements etc, par suite de lesion organique apparente de plusieurs parties du cerveau. J Gen. Med Chir Pharm 1810;37:368–373.

3 Bell C: The nervous system of the human body. appendix of cases; in Longman R (ed): Orme edit. London, 1830, pp 112–114.

4 Boyer M: Tumeur cancereuse de la fosse occipitale comprimant le cervelet, la moelle et la plupart des nerfs qui se distribuent au côté droit de la face. Arch Gen Med 1835;7:91–98.

5 Weiglein C: Einige kran kheitsfalle, beobachtet im siechenhause zu grantz. Med Jahrb Osterr Stantes (wien) 1840;21:569–574.

6 Cruveilhier J: Anatomie Pathologique du corps humain, in. Paris, 1842, pp 1–8.

7 Toynbee J: Neuroma of the auditory nerve. Trans Path Soc Lond 1853;4:259–260.

8 Stevens C: A case of tumor of the auditory nerve occupying the fossa for the cerebellum. Archiv Otol 1879;8:171–176.

9 Oppenhein H: Uber mehrere falle von endo craniellem tumor in welchen es gelang eine genauere localdiagnose zu stellen. Klein Wochenschr 1890;27:38–40.

10 McBurney C, Starr M: A contribution to cerebral surgery: diagnosis, localization and operation for removal of three tumors of the brain: with some comments upon the treatment of brain tumors. Am J Med Sci 1893;361–387.

11 Rosegay H: The Krause operations. J Neurosurg 1992;76:1032–1036.

12 Steiglitz L, Gerster A, Lilienthal H: A study of three cases of tumors of the brain in which operation was per formed- One recovery, two deaths. Am J Med Sci 1896;3:509–531.

13 Ziegenweidt V: Tumor cerebelli. Psychiatr Neurol (Amst) 1899;3: 36–44.

14 Ballance C: Some points in the surgery of the brain and its membranes. London, MacMillan & Co., 1907, p 276.

15 Cushing H: Tumor of the nervus acousticus and the syndrome of the cerebellopontine angle. Philadelphia, WB Saunders Edit., 1917.
16 Ramsden RT: Annandale's case, one hundred years on 'a brillant surgical result, the first recorded; in Sterkers JMCR, Sterkers O (eds): Acoustic Neuroma and Skull Base Surgery. Amsterdam, New York, Kugler Publications, 1996, pp 7–10.
17 Murri A: Upon diagnosis of tumour of the cerebellum. Lancet 1897;1:291–295.
18 Henneber, Koch: Uber 'centrale' neurofibromatose und die gelschwulste des kleinhirnbruckenwinkels (acusticusneurome). Arch F Psychiat 1902;XXXVI:251–304.
19 Glasscock ME: History of the diagnosis and treatment of acoustic neuroma. Arch Otolaryng 1968;88:30–37.
20 House WF, Luetje CM: Acoustic tumors. Volume I: Diagnosis. University Park Press (Baltimore) Edit, Section I: History, 1979, pp 3–32.
21 Elinhorn et Uhlfelder : in Wertheimer P, David M, Sindou M, Redondo A: The birth and development of knowledge in neurosurgery. Neurochirurgie 1979;25:247–263.
22 Krause F: Zur freilegung der hinteren felsenbeinflache und des kleinhirns. Beitr Klein Chir 1903;XXXVII:728–764.
23 Borchart M: Ueber operationen in der hinteren schadelgrube; in: Der operationen der tumoren am kleinhirnbruckenwinkel. Arch Klin Chir 1906;81:386–432.
24 Black PM: Peter Bent Brigham Hospital. J Neurosurg 1991;75:987–988.
25 Dandy W: An operation for the total removal of cerebello-pontine angle (acoustic tumors). Surg Gynecol Obstet 1925;XLI:129–148.
26 Eiselberg A, Ranzi E: Ueber die chirurgische behandlung der hirn-und ruechenmarkstumoren. Verh Dtsch Ges Chir 1913;43:514–521.
27 Henschen F: Zur histolgie und pathogenese der kleinhirnbruckenwinkel tumoren. Arch Psychiatry 1915;56:21–122.
28 Krause F: Discussion of Eiselberg's paper; in: Transactions of the 17th International Congress of Medecine. London, 1913, p 213.
29 Tooth H: The treatment of tumours of the brain and the indications for operation; in: Transactions of the 17th International Congress of Medecine. London, 1913, p 213.
30 Verocay J: Zur Kenntnis der 'neurofibrome'. Beitr Pathol Anat Allg Pathol 1910;XLVIII:1–68.
31 Krause F: Surgery of the brain and spinal cord, based on personal experiences. New York, 1909–1912, Vol 1–3.
32 Henschen F: Die akustikustumoren eine neue gruppe radiographisch darstellbarer hirntumoren. Fortschr A d geb d rontgenstralhen 1912;XVIII:207–216.
33 Schuller A: Acusticus tumoren. Berlin, Springer Verlag, 1928.
34 Stenvers HW: Roentgenologie des felsenbeins und des bitemporalen schdelbildes. Berlin, Springer Verlag, 1928.
35 Panse R: Ein gliom des akustikus. Arch Ohrenh 1904;LVI:251–255.
36 Rizzoli HV, Walter E Dandy: an historical perspective. Clin Neurosurg 1985;32:3–22.
37 Dandy WE, Blackfan KD: An experimental and clinical study of internal hydrocephalus. JAMA 1913;61:2216–2217.
38 House WF, Luetje CM: Acoustic tumors. Volume I: Diagnosis. University Park Press (Baltimore) Edit, Section I: History, 1979, pp 3–32.
39 Dandy WE: An operation for the total extirpation of tumors in the cerebello-pontine angle. A preliminary report. Johns Hopkins Hospital Bull 1922;33:344–345.
40 Dandy W: An operation for the total removal of cerebello-pontine angle (acoustic tumors). Surg Gynecol Obstet 1925;XLI:129–148.
41 Dandy WE: Removal of cerebellopontine (acoustic) tumors through a unilateral approach. Arch Surg 1934;29:337–343.
42 Dandy WE: Results of removal of acoustic tumors by the unilateral approach. AMA Arch Surg 1934;42:1026–1043.
43 Dandy WE: Ventriculography following the injection of air into the cerebral ventricles. Ann Surg 1918;68:5–11.
44 Dandy WE: Roentgenography of the brain after injection of air into the spinal canal. Ann Surg 1919;70:397–403.
45 Sicard JA, Forestier JE: Methode generale d'exploration radiologique par l'huile iodee (lipiodol). Bull Soc Med Hop Paris 1922;46:463–468.
46 Lindgren E: Some aspects on the technique of encephalography. Acta Radiol 1949;31:161–177.
47 Moniz E: L'encephalographie arterielle, son importance dans la localisation des tumeurs cerebrales. Rev Neurol 1927;2:72–90.
48 Olivecrona H: Acoustic tumors. J Neurosurg 1967;26:6–13.
49 Atkinson WJ: Anterior inferior cerebellar artery: its variation, pontine distribution and significance in surgery of cerebello-pontine angle tumors. J Neurol Neurosurg Psychiatry 1949;12:137–151.
50 Chausse C: Premiers resultants d'une methode personnelle de radiodiagnostic des tumeurs de l'auditif. Acta Otolaryng 1948;2:245–251.
51 McKenzie KG, Alexander E Jr: Acoustic neuroma. Clin Neurosurg 1954;2:21–36.
52 Shambaugh GE: Surgery of the ear, ed 2. Philadelphia, W.B. Saunders com., 1967, pp 179–180.
53 House WF: Report of cases. Monograph, transtemporal bone microsurgical removal of acoustic neuromas. Arch Otolaryngol 1964;80:617–667.
54 Ruben RJ, Knickerbocker GG, Sekula J, Nager GT, Bordley JE: Cochlear microphonics in man; a preliminary report. Laryngoscope 1959;69:665–671.
55 Valvassori GE, Pierce RH: The normal internal auditory canal. Am J Roentgenol Radium Ther Nucl Med 1964;92:1232–1241.
56 Di Chiro G: An atlas of pathologic pneumoencephalographic anatomy. USA, Springfield (III), 1967.
57 Baker ML: Myelographic examination of the posterior fossa with positive contrast medium. Radiology 1963;81:791–801.
58 Scanlon RL: Positive contrast medium in diagnosis of acoustic neuroma. Arch Otolaryng 1964;80:698–706.
59 Bradley WH: Appraisal of transtemporal approach in acoustic neuroma surgery. Arch Otolaryngol 1965;82:102–107.

60 Glasscock ME: A history of acoustic tumor surgery: 1961-present; in House WF, Luetje CM: Acoustic Tumors. Volume I : Diagnosis. Baltimore, University Park Press, 1979, pp 33–41.
61 House WF: Report of cases. Monograph, transtemporal bone microsurgical removal of acoustic neuromas. Arch Otolaryngol 1964;80:617–667.
62 House WF: Acoustic neuroma. Case summaries. Arch Otolaryngol 1968;88:586–591.
63 House WF, Graham MD: Surgery of acoustic tumors. Otolaryngol Clin North Am 1973;6:245–266.
64 Brackmann DE: Acoustic neuroma surgery: Otologic Medical Group results; in edit. S (ed): Neurological surgery of the ear. Aesculap Publishing Co., 1979, pp 248–259.
65 House WF, Hitselberger WE: The neuro-otologist's view of the surgical management of acoustic neuromas; in: Clinical Neurosurgery, 1982, pp 214–222.
66 Shelton C, Hitselberger WE, House WF, Brackmann DE: Hearing preservation after acoustic tumor removal: long-term results. Laryngoscope 1990;100:115–119.
67 Bucy PC: Surgical treatment of acoustic tumors. J Neurosurg 1951;8:547–555.
68 Rougerie J, Guyot JF: Essai de conservation du nerf facial dans l'ablation des neurinomes de l'angle ponto-cérébelleux. Neuro-chirurgie Paris 1964;10:13–21.
69 Rand RW, Kurze T: Micro-neurosurgical resection of acoustic tumors by a transmeatal posterior fossa approach. Bull Los Angel Neuro Soc 1965;30:17–20.
70 Pool JL: Suboccipital surgery for acoustic neurinomas: advantages and disadvantages. J Neurosurg 1966;24:483–492.
71 Drake CG: Surgical treatment of acoustic neuroma with preservation or reconstitution of the facial nerve. J Neurosurg 1967;26:459–464.
72 Portmann M: Evolution des moyens diagnostiques du neurinome de l'acoustique. Bordeaux Med 1981;14:231–236.
73 Bebear JP: Apport des techniques récentes dans le diagnostic et le traitement du neurinome de l'acoustique; in: thèse médecine. Bordeaux, 1973.
74 Anderson H, Barr B, Wedenberg E: Intra-aural reflexes in retrocochler lesions. Nobel Symposium 10. Stockholm, Almqvist & Wiksell, 1969.
75 Jewett DL, Romano MN, Williston JS: Human auditory evoked potentials: possible brain stem components detected on the scalp. Science 1970;167:1517–1518.
76 Hounsfield GN: Computerized transverse axial scanning (tomography): Part I. Description of system. 1973. Br J Radiol 1995;68:H166–H172.
77 Yasargil MG, Fox JL: The microsurgical approach to acoustic neurinomas. Surg Neurol 1974;2:393–398.
78 Malis LI: Microsurgical treatment of acoustic neurinomas; in Handa H (ed): Microneurosurgery. Stuttgart, Igaku Shoin Publish edit, 1975, pp 91–112.
79 Koos WT, Spetzler RF, Böck FW, Salah S: Microsurgery of cerebellopontine angle tumors; in Koos WT, Spetzler RF, Bock FW (eds): Clinical Microneurosurgery. Sttugart, Georg Thieme Pub, 1976, pp 91–112.
80 Riemens V, Portmann M, Bebear JP: Les neurinomas de l'acoustiques. A propos d'une série de 40 observations. Neuro-chirurgie Paris 1975;21:527–536.
81 Pellet W, Cannoni M, Pech A: La collaboration oto-neuro-chirurgicale dans l'abord translabyrinthique des neurinomes de l'acoustiques. Neurochirurgie 1979;25:84–90.
82 Morrison AW, King TT: Experiences with a translabyrinthine-transtentorial approach to the cerebellopontine angle. Technical note. J Neurosurg 1973;38:382–390.
83 Hitselberger WE, House WF: A combined approach to the cerebellopontine angle. A suboccipital-petrosal approach. Arch Otolaryngol 1966;84:267–285.
84 Maddox HE 3rd: The lateral approach to acoustic tumors. Laryngoscope 1966;87:1572–1578.
85 Bremond G, Garcin M, Magnan J: Progrès en oto-neurochirurgie : l'abord à minima de l'angle ponto-cérébelleux par la voie rétro-sinusale. Acta Otorhinolaryngol Belg 1976;30:127–144.
86 Rand RW, Kurze T: Micro-neurosurgical resection of acoustic tumors by a transmeatal posterior fossa approach. Bull Los Angel Neuro Soc 1965;30:17–20.
87 DiTullio MV Jr, Malkasian D, Rand RW: A critical comparison of neurosurgical and otolaryngological approaches to acoustic neuromas. J Neurosurg 1978;48:1–12.
88 Rhoton AL Jr: Microsurgery of the internal acoustic meatus. Surg Neurol 1974;2:311–318.
89 Delgado TE, Bucheit WA, Rosenholtz HR, Chrissian S: Intraoperative monitoring of facial muscle evoked responses obtained by intracranial stimulation of the facial nerve: a more accurate technique for facial nerve dissection. Neurosurgery 1979;4:418–421.
90 Ojemann RG, Crowell RC: Acoustic neuromas treated by microsurgical suboccipital operations. Prog Neurol Surg 1978;9:337–373.
91 Bonnal J, Vanderkelen B, Born J: Technique et resultats du traitement neurochirurgical de 42 neurinomes de l'acoustique; in Edit RPV (ed): Livre jubilaire du Pr. Paillas. Marseille, 1979, pp 63–80.
92 Sterkers JM, Corlieu P, Hamann KF, Sterkers O: Chirurgie des tumeurs de l'acoustique par voie rétro-sigmoïde. Technique personnelle. Résultats sur le facial et l'auditiopn (61 cas). Anal Oto Laryng (Paris) 1980;97:519–532.
93 Koos WT, Spetzler RF, Böck FW, Salah S: Microsurgery of cerebellopontine angle tumors; in Koos WT, Spetzler RF, Bock FW (eds): Clinical Microneurosurgery. Sttugart, Georg Thieme Pub, 1976, pp 91–112.
94 Tarlov E: Total one-stage suboccipital microsurgical removal of acoustic neuromas of all sizes: with emphasis on arachnoid planes and on saving the facial nerve. Surg Clin North Am 1980;60:565–591.
95 House WF, Gardner G, Hughes RL: Middle cranial fossa approach to acoustic tumor surgery. Arch Otolaryngol 1968;88:631–641.
96 Hitselberger WE, Hughes RL: Bilateral acoustic tumors and neurofibromatosis. Arch Otolaryngol 1968;88:700–711.
97 Hullay J, Tomits GH: Experiences with total removal of tumors of the acoustic nerve. J Neurosurg 1965;22:127–135.
98 McKissock W: Acoustic tumors. Proc R Soc Med 1965;58:1078–1079.

99 Pertuiset B, Maspetiol R, Semette D, Paychere G: La conservation des fonctions auditive et faciale au cours de l'exérèse totale des neurinomes de l'acoustique par voie sous-occipitale (D'après quatre observations). Presse Médicale 1966;74:2327–2330.
100 Pertuiset B: Les neurinomes de l'acoustiques développés dans l'angle ponto-cérébelleux. Rapport au XXème Congrès de la Société de Neurochirurgie de Langue Française. Neurochirurgie 1970;16(suppl 1):1–147.
101 Rand RW, Kurze T: Preservation of vestibular, cochlear, and facial nerves during microsurgical removal of acoustic tumors. Report of two cases. J Neurosurg 1968;28:158–161.
102 Jerger J, Jerger S, Ainsworth J, Caram P: Recovery of auditory function after surgical removal of cerebellar tumor. J Speech Hear Disord 1966;31:377–382.
103 Christiansen B, Greisen O: Reversible hearing loss in tumors of the cerebello-pontine angle. J Laryngol Otol 1975;89:1161–1164.
104 Schwartz HE, Morgan DE, Calcaterra TC: Recovery of eighth nerve function after cerebellopontine angle surgery. Arch Otolaryngol 1978;104:231–233.
105 Geurking NA: Surgical anatomy of the temporal bone posterior to the internal auditory canal: an operative approach. Laryngoscope 1977;87:975–986.
106 Domb GH, Chole RA: Anatomical studies of the posterior petrous apex with regard to hearing preservation in acoustic neuroma removal. Laryngoscope 1980;90:1769–1776.
107 Pellet W, Cannoni M, Pech A: Otoneuro-chirurgie. Berlin, Heidelberg, Springer Verlag, 1989, p 155.
108 Smith MF, Miller RN, Cox DJ: Suboccipital microsurgical removal of acoustic neurinomas of all sizes. Ann Otol Rhinol Laryngol 1973;82:407–414.
109 Buchheit WA, Gastaldo JA: The posterior fassa approach to acoustic tumors : preservation of hearing; in edit. Sa N (ed): Neurological surgery of the ear. Aesculap Publishing Co., 1977, pp 263–266.
110 Cohen NL: Acoustic neuroma surgery with emphasis on preservation of hearing. Laryngoscope 1979;89:886–896.
111 Sterkers JM, Fentonk JE, Smail M: Intracanalicular acoustic neuromas; in Sterkers JMCR, Sterkers O. Edit (ed): Acoustic neuroma and skull base surgery, Proceedings of the 2nd international conference on acoustic neuroma surgery and 2nd European skull base Society congress, Paris, 22–26 Avril 1995. Amsterdam, New york, Kugler Pub., 1996, pp 207–209.
112 Tos M, Thomsen J, Charabi S: Epidemiology of acoustic neuromas: has the incidence increased during the last years?; in edit. Te T (ed): Acoustic neuroma. Proceeding of the first international conference on acoustic neuroma. Amsterdam, New York, Kugler pub., 1991, pp 3–6.
113 Dutton JE, Ramsden RT, Lye RH, Morris K, Keith AO, Page R, Vafadis J: Acoustic neuroma (schwannoma) surgery 1978–1990. J Laryngol Otol 1991;105:165–173.
114 Koos WT, Day JD, Matula C, Levy DI: Neurotopographic considerations in the microsurgical treatment of small acoustic neurinomas. J Neurosurg 1998;88:506–512.
115 Harner SG, Ebersold MJ: Management of acoustic neuromas, 1978–1983. J Neurosurg 1985;63:175–179.
116 House JW: Facial nerve grading systems. Laryngoscope 1983;93:1056–1069.
117 House JW, Brackmann DE: Facial nerve grading system. Otolaryngol Head Neck Surg 1985;93:146–147.
118 Sugita K, Kobayashi S, Mutsuga N, Suzuki Y, Mizutani T, Shibuya M, Kageyama N, Tanahashi T: Microsurgery for acoustic neurinoma–lateral position and preservation of facial and cochlear nerves. Neurol Med Chir (Tokyo) 1979;19:637–641.
119 Fischer G, Costantini JL, Mercier P: Improvement of hearing after microsurgical removal of acoustic neurinoma. Neurosurgery 1980;7:154–159.
120 Wanxing C: Preservation of facial and acoustic nerves in the total removal of large and small acoustic tumors. Report of two cases. J Neurosurg 1981;54:268–272.
121 Tos M, Drozdziewicz D, Thomsen J: Medial acoustic neuromas. A new clinical entity. Arch Otolaryngol Head Neck Surg 1992;118:127–133.
122 Telian SA, Kemink JL, Kileny P: Hearing recovery following suboccipital excision of acoustic neuroma. Arch Otolaryngol Head Neck Surg 1988;114:85–87.
123 Silverstein H, McDaniel A, Norrell H, Wazen J: Conservative management of acoustic neuroma in the elderly patient. Laryngoscope 1985;95:766–770.
124 Gardner G, Robertson JH: Hearing preservation in unilateral acoustic neuroma surgery. Ann Otol Rhinol Laryngol 1988;97:55–66.
125 Levine RA, Ojemann RG, Montgomery WW: Evoked potential detection of hearing loss during acoustic neuroma surgery. Neurology 1978;28:339–342.
126 Fischer C: Brainstem auditory evoked potential (BAEP) monitoring in posterior fossa surgery; in Desmedt JEe (ed): Neuromonitoring in surgery. Elsevier Science Pub., 1989, pp 191–207.
127 Samii M, Matthies C: Management of 1,000 vestibular schwannomas (acoustic neuromas): hearing function in 1,000 tumor resections. Neurosurgery 1997;40/2:456–461.
128 Wigand ME, Hait CT, Berg M, Wolf SR: Indications and technique for and avantages of the enlarged middle fossa approach; in Sterkers JMCR, Sterkers O. Edit (ed): Acoustic neuroma and skull base surgery, Proceedings of the 2nd international conference on acoustic neuroma surgery and 2nd European skull base Society congress, Paris, 22–26 Avril 1995. Amsterdam, New york, Kugler Pub., 1996, pp 231–234.
129 Wigand ME, Rettinger G, Haid T, Berg M: Removal of acoustic neuromas of the cerebellopontile angle with transtemporal approach by the middle cranial fossa. Hno 1985;33:11–16.
130 Magnan J, Chays A, Caces F, Lepetre C, Cohen JM, Belus JF, Bruzzo M: Apport de l'endoscopie de l'angle pontocérébelleux par voie rétrosigmoïde. Ann Otol Laryng (Paris) 1993;110:259–265.
131 Sterkers JM: Saline serum injection into the arachnoid sheet to improve dissection of the facial nerve?; in: Proceedings of the VIIIth international symposium on the facial nerve. April 13–18 1997. Kugler Pub, 1998, p 431.

132 Tran Ba Huy P, Lot G, Herman P: La dissection'aquatique' du nerf facial dans la chirurgie du neurinome de l'acoustique. A propos de 212 cas. Ann Otolaryngol Chir Cervicofac 1998;115:42–44.
133 Kanzaki J, Tos M, Sanna M, Moffat DA: New and modified reporting systems from the consensus meeting on systems for reporting results in vestibular schwannome. Otology-Neurology 2003;24:642–649.
134 Pellet W, Emram B, Cannoni M, Pech A, Zanaret M, Thomassin M: Les resultats fonctionnels de la chirurgie des neurinomes de l'acoustique unilateraux. Neurochirurgie 1993;39:24–41.
135 Clark WC, Moretz WH Jr, Acker JD, Gardner LG, Eggers F, Robertson JH: Nonsurgical management of small and intracanalicular acoustic tumors. Neurosurgery 1985;16:801–803.
136 Gardner LG, Moretz WH, Robertson JH, Clark WC, Shea JJ: Nonsurgical management of small and intracanalicular acoustic tumors. Otolaryngol Head Neck Surg 1986;94:328–333.
137 Nedzelski JM, Canter RJ, Kassel EE, Rowed DW, Tator CH: Is no treatment good treatment in the management of acoustic neuromas in the elderly? Laryngoscope 1986;96:825–829.
138 Silverstein H, McDaniel A, Norrell H, Wazen J: Conservative management of acoustic neuroma in the elderly patient. Laryngoscope 1985;95:766–770.
139 House JW, Nissen RL, Hitselberger WE: Acoustic tumor management in senior citizens. Laryngoscope 1987;97:129–130.
140 Samii M, Tatagiba M, Matthies C: Acoustic neurinoma in the elderly: factors predictive of postoperative outcome. Neurosurgery 1992;31:615–620.

Prof. William Pellet, MD
Service de Neurochirurgie de l'Hopital Nord
Assistance Publique-Hôpitaux de Marseille, Chemin des Bourrelly
FR-13915 Marseille Cedex 20 (France)
Tel. +33 491968620, Fax +33 491968915, E-Mail wpellet@mail.ap-hm.fr

Régis J, Roche P-H (eds): Modern Management of Acoustic Neuroma.
Prog Neurol Surg. Basel, Karger, 2008, vol 21, pp 24–31

Genesis and Biology of Vestibular Schwannomas

Pierre-Hugues Roche[a] · Corinne Bouvier[c] · Olivier Chinot[b] · Dominique Figarella-Branger[c]

[a]Service de Neurochirurgie, Hôpital Sainte-Marguerite, et [b]Unité de Neuro-Oncologie, Hôpital de la Timone, Assistance Publique-Hôpitaux de Marseille, [c]Laboratoire de Neuropathologie et Biopathologie du Système Nerveux, Faculté de Médecine la Timone, Marseille, France

Abstract

This review chapter is a synthesis of the recent literature about pathogenesis of schwannomas with emphasis on vestibular schwannomas (VSs). The cornerstone of cellular transformation and proliferation of Schwann cells toward schwannomas has been attributed to the nonexpression of normal schwannomin/merlin (S/M) by these cells. The understanding of this mechanism has been gained from molecular genetic studies of neurofibromatosis type 2 (NF2) patients, in whom mutations of a tumor suppressor gene (NF2 gene) was clearly identified. S/M is the normal NF2 gene product. Lack of normal S/M protein in the schwannoma cell is due to gene mutation in 50% of sporadic VSs. In the other cases, epigenetic factors or activation of protease cascade contribute to ineffective S/M. The exact interactions of S/M with extracellular matrix, membranous glycoprotein and cytoskeleton are not fully understood. However, it is recognized that these interactions activate several pathways that might regulate cell-cycle process, apoptosis and intercellular interaction. Apart from the involvement of the S/M pathway, the authors review the potential role of other genetic abnormalities and growing factors that are supposed to be involved in the pathogenesis of VS. Understanding the pathways of action and regulation of S/M may provide the basics for identifying potential therapeutic targets, which is of paramount importance for a better management of NF2 patients.

The term acoustic neuroma has been inappropriately used for decades to name the most frequent tumor of the internal auditory canal (IAC) and cerebellopontine angle. Operative observations under the microscope, data obtained from autopsy and progress in the field of histopathology have permitted to shift this terminology toward a more accurate name, vestibular schwannoma (VS), which is now widely adopted by the scientific community. As a rule, the tumor is histologically benign.

In the majority of cases, the tumor develops from the inferior vestibular nerve but in many cases, both nerves are involved and undistinguishable. It has been suggested that the site of birth of the tumor was the junction zone between central and peripheral myelination [1]. This zone is called the fibrous cone or Obersteiner-Redlich zone. The distance between this zone and the brain stem is more than 1 cm, while it is around 1 mm for the other cranial nerves. In the analysis from Bridger and Farkashidy [2], this zone was at the level of the porus in 56% of cases and inside the IAC in 44%. Several studies have considered that the tumor origin was more peripheral than the junction zone. An electronic microscopic study could show the interpenetration of the

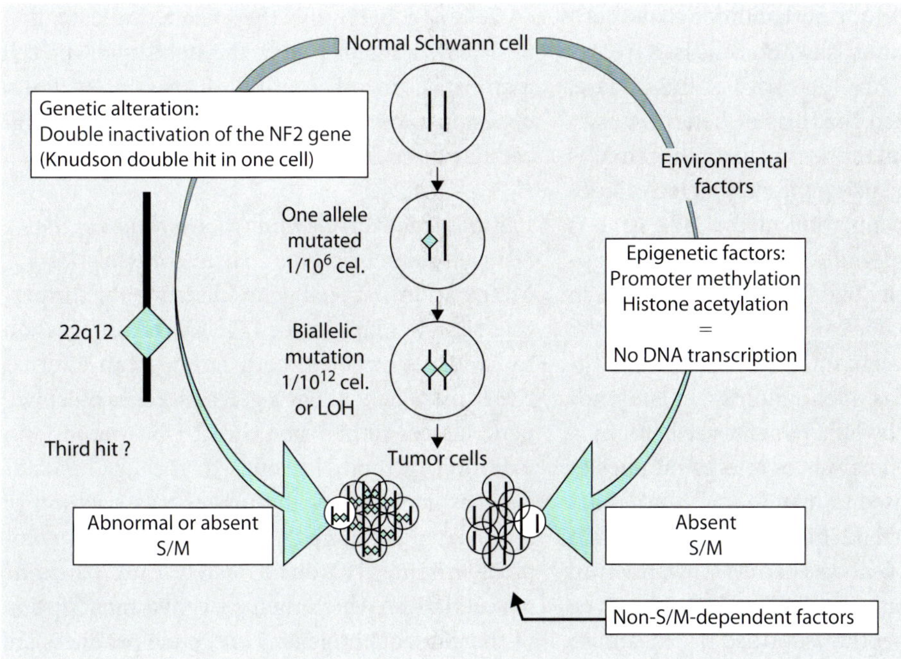

Fig. 1. Pathogenesis of unilateral VSs: the NF2 gene. On the left side, the widely accepted 'Knudson double-hit model' explains the proliferation of abnormal Schwann cells toward schwannomas, while an alternative 'epigenetic' mechanism of schwannoma formation is shown on the right side.

tumor cells and cells from the ganglion of Scarpa at the fundus of the IAC [3]. Based on the histological examination of 112 petrous bones, Pirsig showed that 28 out of them harbored abnormal cellular proliferation (Verocay like) at the close contact with the Scarpa ganglion [4]. More rarely, the schwannoma may take origin from the inside of the vestibule [5] or from the internal auditory meatus (named medial VS), as described by Tos et al. [6].

Mechanisms of Genesis and Growth

Genetic and Epigenetic Factors: The Key Role of the Neurofibromatosis Type 2 Gene Product

The understanding of the mechanism of birth and growth of unilateral VS has been boosted by the comprehension of genetic studies that were conducted in the field of neurofibromatosis type 2 (NF2).

Mutation of the Neurofibromatosis Type 2 Gene, a Tumor Suppressor Gene

From the early stage, it has been postulated that loss of genetic material was at the origin of this disease [7, 8] and the role of the NF2 gene as a tumor suppressor gene was also demonstrated early. In order to induce the proliferation of tumor cells, an alteration of both alleles of the TSG must happen in one single cell (Knudson double-hit model; fig. 1). In the case of NF2 disease, one mutated allele is inherited from one parent (germinal mutation) and the probability to observe the second mutation (somatic mutation) in the same Schwann cell (1 out of one million cells) is not so rare, which explains the frequency of multiple schwannomas in NF2 patients. In the case of non-NF2 patients, the probability to have both mutations in the same Schwann cells is extremely rare, which explains the rarity of the disease. It may be postulated that loss of heterozygosity (LOH) can represent the second hit of the remaining allele. So far and using the current techniques of gene screening, mutation of the NF2 gene is found in 60% of sporadic unilateral schwannomas. It is noteworthy that the majority of known diseases linked to TSG inactivation lead to the development of malignant tumors, while the tumors (schwannomas, meningiomas, ependymomas, …) harbored by NF2 patients are benign.

Genetic linkage analysis of a large number of NF2 patients was used to map the NF2 locus that had been located on the 22q12 locus [9]. The protein product of the NF2 gene was named schwannomin or merlin. For the purpose of this chapter, it will be named S/M. This peptide is formed by 595 amino acids and displays a high degree of homology with 4.1 erythrocyte superfamily protein. This superfamily includes the MER protein (moesin, esrin, radixin) that is highly conserved in the mammalians and plays a role in the link between membranous glycoproteins and cytoskeleton actin. Therefore, an important role in the cellular remodeling process has been attributed to MER [10]. Although not extensively understood, both extremities of S/M seem to play distinct roles. The N-terminal part of the protein is a zone of connection with cell surface glycoproteins like glycophorin C, p55, CD44 and intercellular adhesion molecules. S/M also associates with a number of molecules implicated in cell signaling, including sodium-hydrogen exchange regulatory factor (NHE-RF) [11], hepatocyte growth factor-regulated tyrosine kinase substrate (HRS) [8]. Such connection may implicate S/M in various processes of intracellular signal transmission [12]. The role played by the C-terminal part of the protein is less clear because S/M lacks the conventional C-terminal actin-binding domains. However, Xu and Gutmann [13] have shown that S/M can associate with polymerized actin in vitro by virtue of an N-terminal actin-binding domain.

Taken collectively, these data indicate that S/M plays a major role in the stability of the cell membrane, in cell motility, in the intercellular cohesion and in adhesion of the cell to the extracellular matrix [14].

Epigenetic Factors Leading to Alteration of the Neurofibromatosis Type 2 Gene Transcription

Methylation-induced gene silencing is as important as gene mutation or LOH in the progression to cancer. Promoter methylation is an alternative form of gene silencing, which relies on epigenetic factors rather than direct DNA mutations. Addition of methyl groups to the CpG islands silences genes by facilitating the association of methylated DNA with a methyl-binding complex. This methylation ultimately leads to histone deacetylation, which then prevents transcription of the subsequent gene. Thus, gene products are not produced, even though the DNA coding sequence is maintained [15].

Gonzalez-Gomez et al. [16] used a methylation-specific PCR to analyze a series of 44 sporadic and NF2-associated schwannomas for methylation of 12 genes, including tumor suppressor genes (NF2 gene), angiogenesis and invasion inhibitors (thrombospondin-1), DNA repair genes (O6 methylguanine DNA-methyltransferase – MGMT), and detoxification genes. They showed that the majority of tumors (81.8%) displayed methylation of 1 or more genes while control tissue did not display any methylation. The most frequently methylated genes were thrombospondin-1 (36%), p73 (27%), MGMT (20%), and TIMP-3 (18%). TIMP-3 encodes for an extracellular matrix-binding protein. The NF2 gene was aberrantly hypermethylated in 18% of specimens.

Alternative Mechanisms of Action of Schwannomin/Merlin

Schwannomin/Merlin, Cell Cycle and Apoptosis. Nuclear factor kappa B (NF-κB) is a transcription factor that is implicated in cellular transformation, tumor growth, and inhibition of apoptosis.

Kim et al. [17] have shown that S/M is an inhibitor of the serine/threonine kinase which activates NF-κB. This role has been attributed to the N-terminal extremity of S/M.

The ability of a tumor mass to grow is determined by the proportion of cells in an S-state by comparison of the cells in the G0-G1 state of the cell cycle. The percentage of cells that are engaged in a programmed cell death mechanism (apoptosis) is also a key point. Schulze et al. [18] have transduced Schwann cells that displayed a normal S/M activity into a human schwannoma culture using incorporation of the normal NF2 gene in an oncoretroviral vector. Restoration of the normal expression of S/M was shown, and a significant rate of G0-G1 cells with a decrease in S cells was observed on one hand, and on the other a double proportion of apoptotic activity under special condition (unmasked C-term extremity).

HRS strongly interacts with S/M and is a potential inhibitor of 'signal transducers and activators of transcription' (STAT). Cultures of schwannoma cell lines where S/M display some mutations show that S/M is not able to interact with HRS and that contact between HRS and STAT is thereby not possible. Thus, correct interaction between HRS and S/M is necessary in order to obtain inhibition of STAT which is strongly implicated in the cell cycle progression [19].

Schwannomin/Merlin and Interaction with Growth Factors. The platelet-derived growth factor (PDGF) is a growth factor that has been implicated in the growth of numerous tumors in the human. NHE-RF is known to interact with the receptor of PDGF and we have seen that it also interacts with S/M. Recently, Fraenzer et al. [20] have shown that in a model of human schwannoma mutated for the NF2 gene, the correction of the normal activity of the NF2 gene (gene transfection using adenoviral vector) was able to inhibit cell proliferation by early internalization of the PDGF receptor and by inhibition of the MAP kinase activity.

Regulation of Schwannomin/Merlin Activity

S/M forms intra- and intermolecular complexes and its in vitro and in vivo growth-suppressing activity is regulated by its ability to display a closed configuration (fig. 2) [21].

RhoGTPases, including RhoA, Rac1 and Cdc42, constitute a family of Ras-related proteins that are in an active state when bound to GTP and are inactive when bound to GDP. Rho family members have well-established roles in cell-cycle progression. Rac 1 can regulate both the transcription and translation of cyclin D-1, a key regulator of cell-cycle progression. Aberrant activation of Rac-1 might directly influence cell-cycle progression. The Rho family members have distinct effects on remodeling of the actin cytoskeleton. Cdc42 promotes filopodia formation, Rac proteins induce membrane ruffling and Rho proteins contribute to the formation of stress fibers. Strong links between S/M and the function of small GTPases have been demonstrated by Shaw et al. [22] who found that activation of Rac1 or Cdc42 promoted merlin phosphorylation. This phosphorylation inactivates S/M by giving it an open configuration and decoupling S/M to actin, while the hypophosphorylation state is associated with a closed and activated state of S/M. Recent studies have implicated S/M phosphorylation in the regulation of S/M subcellular localization and growth suppression. Merlin is growth inhibitory when hypophosphorylated. P21-activated kinase (PAK), a downstream target of Rac or Cdc42, directly phosphorylates merlin at serine 518. PAK2 phosphorylation impairs the ability of merlin to bind to 2 interacting proteins, CD44 and HRS [23].

CD44, the hyaluronate receptor, can regulate both Rac1 and S/M activity. Several signaling molecules associated with CD44, including the receptor tyrosine kinases erbB2 and erbB3 could promote either Rac1 activation of merlin phosphorylation in a Rac-1 independent fashion [24]. Loss of S/M might influence both downstream targets of Rac 1 signaling as well as Rac1 itself.

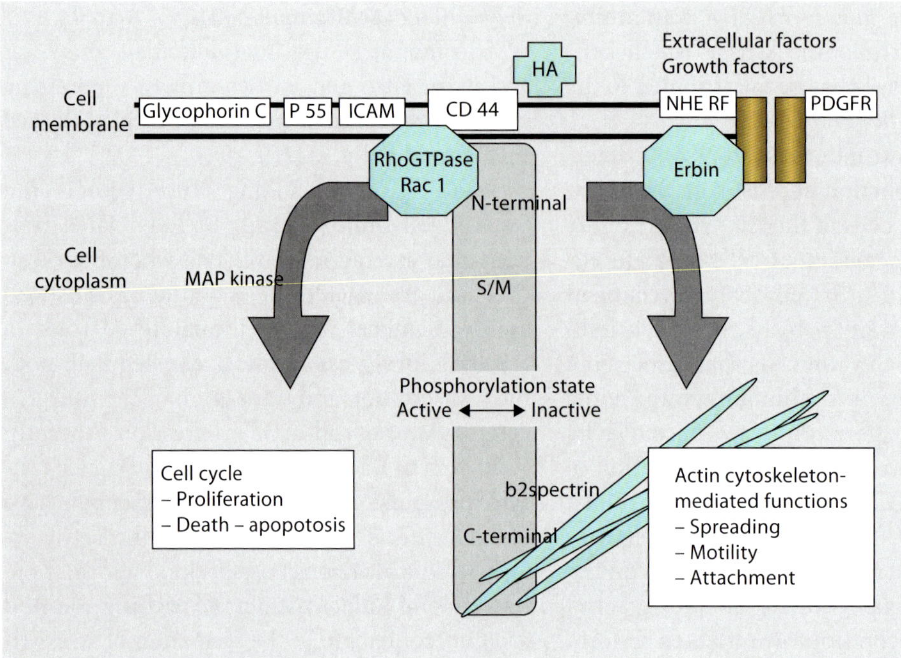

Fig. 2. Connection of S/M with cell membrane glycoprotein and cytoskeleton explains its role in the cell cycle and processes of adhesion, motility and cell-cell interactions. Regulation of the activity of S/M depends on its state of phosphorylation (see text). ICAM = Intercellular adhesion molecule.

Recently, Surace et al. [25] have underlined the importance of the C-terminal portion of S/M by localizing the site of Rac1-dependent site of phosphorylation at an S518 position, close to the C-term extremity. From the RT4 schwannoma cell line, they have shown that mutation for S518 reproduced the phosphorylation state of S/M, which thereby could not inhibit cell growth and motility. Moreover, cell phenotype was dramatically modified, displaying significant changes of cell shape and filopodial elaboration.

Vestibular Schwannomas and Neurofibromatosis Type 2 Gene-Unrelated Actors

Hormonal Factors

An early series [26] of VSs indicated an increased incidence in females (60%) compared to males (40%). More recent observations of early diagnosed tumors using MRI indicated that the female predominance was less marked (55% in the 1,000 operated VSs from Matthies and Samii [27]). It is still noteworthy that pregnancy and delivery may accelerate tumor growth. Moreover, evidence of estrogen and progesterone receptors at the surface of the tumor cells was also found [28]. However, other studies using more sensitive and specific technology found that the concentration of receptors was low and inconsistent and not prevalent in women [29]. Carroll et al. [30] using a PCR technique, observed a lack of estrogen receptor even in pregnant women while 33% of cases displayed progesterone receptors. This work indicated a positive finding of glucocorticoid receptors in all cases.

Growth Factors

Vestibular Schwann cells are a distinct subpopulation of peripheral glia with specific sensitivity to growth factors and extracellular matrix components [31]. In a study that was conducted on Schwann cell cultures of rats, it was shown that progesterone and FGF-2 associated with forskoline increased cell density of Schwann cells from the sciatic nerve, while IGF-1 and GDNF increased the density of vestibular Schwann cells. Intracytoplasmic expression of the vascular endothelial growth factor [32] has been demonstrated with an immunohistochemical technique, and the level of this expression seemed correlated with the tumor growth rate. In another study [33], Schwann cells from the Antoni A zones [34] of schwannomas strongly expressed the epidermal growth factor receptor (EGFr) while normal Schwann tissue did not express this receptor. Actually, it has been shown by Curto et al. [35] in NF2 tumors that failure of downregulation of EGFr with persistent physiological expression of this receptor was the pertinent mechanism instead of EGFr overexpression. The same work showed that there was a clear relationship between S/M and EGFr since S/M had the ability to restrain EGFr into a membrane compartment from which it could neither signal nor be internalized.

From the RN22 schwannoma cell line, Gentry et al. [36] showed a link between the nerve growth factor with p75, which is a member of the superfamily of neurotrophin and TNF receptor superfamily. This link was responsible for a double signal activation pathway, with activation of proapoptotic factors in one arm (activation of c-Jun N-terminal kinase) and activation of an anti-apoptotic cascade by its link to NF-κB.

Using cDNA microarray techniques, Welling et al. [37] showed the overexpression of osteonectin (angiogenic mediator) in 5 out of 7 VSs.

Modification of Expression of the Non-Neurofibromatosis Type 2 Gene

Chromosome Gain. In a recent study using the comparative genomic hybridization technique conducted in a group of 76 VSs, it has been shown that apart from the loss on chromosome 22, gain on copy number on chromosome 9q34 was identified in 10% of cases [38]. This gain is commonly seen in a variety of solid tumors, including colorectal carcinomas and prostate cancer. It is possible to identify a number of interesting genes in this region, including Ral guanine nucleotide dissociation stimulator and Nectrin G2. Products of both genes may influence pathways involving S/M and consequently its role as a tumor suppressor. A potential third genetic hit may be necessary for the development of VS and a gene on 9p may well be a candidate for the site of a third mutational event [38].

Oncogene Activation. Activation of the ras oncogene by GTPase could influence the regulation of S/M expression. In the study from Welling et al. [37], RhoB GTPase gene was overexpressed in 5 out of 7 tumors.

Expression of the Retinoblastoma Gene. The retinoblastoma (Rb) gene is a tumor suppression gene whose inactivation of both alleles gives rise to Rb. This gene plays a role in cell cycle control and apoptosis. The lack of production of the Rb protein has also been identified in several solid tumors and leukemia. Complex interaction of cyclin-dependent kinase (CDK) with pRb provides signals to the gene transcription that is necessary for the progression in the cell cycle [39]. Lasak et al. [40] have compared the differential gene expression between VS ad normal nerve using the cDNA microarray method. In this study, they have shown for the VS specimen a strong deregulation of the gene expression that was involved in the pRb-CDK pathway.

Apopotic Modulation

Survivin is a protein involved in the inhibition of proapoptotic genes. Survivin blocks apoptosis by a direct link to caspases 3 and 7, and abnormal concentration of this protein has been found in several malignant tumors. In a study that used reverse transcriptase PCR, Western blot and immunohistochemistry, Kato et al. [41] showed that several schwannomas expressed this protein. In another study, it was found that the cytoplasmic expression of partners of the Fas-Fas-L system was significantly modified [42]. This system is known to be a major regulator of the apoptotic mechanism.

Conclusion

Among several factors that may contribute to tumorigenesis and growth of VS, loss of S/M function is a major event. Interaction of S/M with CD44 and RhoGTPases is an essential mechanism of regulation of motility and growth of Schwann cells. In 60% of cases of unilateral sporadic VS, mutation of the NF2 gene that leads to the production of an abnormal or inactive S/M is observed. In the remnant cases, it may be assumed that expression of S/M is downregulated by epigenetic factors or by activation of proteolytic cascades mediated by proteases like caspase [43].

An improved knowledge of the pathways of action and regulation of S/M may provide the basics for identifying potential therapeutic targets. This issue is of special importance for future treatments of NF2 patients.

References

1 Neely JG, Britton BH, Greenberg SD: Microscopic characteristics of the acoustic tumor in relationship of its nerve of origin. Laryngoscope 1976;86:984–991.

2 Bridger MW, Farkashidy J: The distribution of neuroglia and schwann cells in the 8th nerve of man. J Laryngol Otol 1980;94:1353–1362.

3 Foncin JF, Sterkers JM, Perre J, Corlieu P: The origin of acoustic neuroma. An ultrastructural study of operated neurinoma incipiens. Ann Otolaryngol Chir Cervicofac 1979;96:11–22.

4 Pirsig W, Eckermeier L, Mueller D: As to the origine of vestibular schwannomas; in House WF (ed): Acoustic Tumors. Vol 1 – diagnosis. Baltimore: University Park Press, 1979, pp 52–55.

5 Boutin P, Guth A, Bouccara D, El Garem H, Rey A, Sterkers O: Intralabyrinthine schwannomas: a report of two cases. Ann Otolaryngol Chir Cervicofac 1998;115:35–41.

6 Tos M, Drozdziewicz D, Thomsen J: Medial acoustic neuromas. A new clinical entity. Arch Otolaryngol Head Neck Surg 1992;118:127–133.

7 Lanser MJ, Sussman SA, Frazer K: Epidemiology, pathogenesis, and genetics of acoustic tumors. Otolaryngol Clin North Am 1992;25:499–520.

8 Seizinger BR, Martuza RL, Gusella JF: Loss of genes on chromosome 22 in tumorigenesis of human acoustic neuroma. Nature 1986;322:644–647.

9 Wertelecki W, Rouleau GA, Superneau DW, Forehand LW, Williams JP, Haines JL, Gusella JF: Neurofibromatosis 2:Clinical and DNA linkage studies of a large kindred. N Engl J Med 1988;319:278–283.

10 Tsukita S, Oioshi K, Sato N, Sagara J, Kawai A: ERM family members as molecular linkers between the cell surface glycoprotein CD44 and actin-based cytosqueletons. J Cell Biol 1994;126:391–401.

11 Murthy A, Gonzalez-Agosti C, Cordero E, Pinney D, Candia C, Solomon F, Gusella J, Ramesh V: NHE-RF, a regulatory cofactor for Na^+-H^+ exchange, is a common interactor for Merlin and ERM (MERM) proteins. J Biol Chem 1998;273:1273–1276.

12 Gutmann DH: The neurofibromatoses : when less is more. Hum Mol Genet 2001;10:747–755.

13 Xu HM, Gutmann DH: Merlin differentially associates with the microtubules and actin cytoskeleton. J Neurosci Res 1998;51:403–415.

14 Gutmann DH, Sherman L, Seftor L, et al: Increased expression of the NF2 tumor suppressor gene product, merlin, impairs cell motility, adhesion and spreading. Hum Mol Genet 1999;8:267–275.

15 Fuks F: DNA methylation and histone modifications: teaming up to silence genes. Curr Opin Genet Dev 2005;15: 490–495.

16 Gonzalez-Gomez P, Bello MJ, Alonso ME, Lomas J, Arjona D, de Campos JM, Vaquero J, Isla A, Lassaletta L, Gutierrez M, Sarasa JL, Rey JA: CpG Island Methylation in sporadic and Neurofibromatosis Type 2-Associated schwannomas. Clin Res Cancer 2003;9:5601–5606.

17 Kim JY, Kim H, Jeun SS, Rha SS, Kim YH, Ko YJ, Won J, Lee KH, Rha HK, Wang YP: Inhibition of NF-kB activation of merlin. Biochem Biophys Res Commun 2002;296:1295–1302.

18 Schulze KM, Hanemann CO, Müller HW, Hanenberg H: Transduction of wild-type merlin into human schwannoma cells decreases schwannoma cell growth and induces apoptosis. Hum Mol Genet 2002;11:69–76.

19 Scoles DR, Nguyen VD, Qin Y, Sun CX, Morrison H, Gutmann DH, Pulst SM: Neurofibromatosis 2 (NF2) tumor suppressor schwannomin and its interacting protein HRS regulate STAT signaling. Hum Mol Genet 2002;11:3179–3189.

20 Fraenzer JT, Pan H, Minimo L, Smith GM, Knauer D, Hung G: Overexpression of the NF2 gene inhibits schwannoma cell proliferation through promoting PDGFR degradation. Int J Oncol 2003;23:1493–1500.

21 Sherman LS, et al: Interdomain binding mediates tumor growth suppression by the NF2 gene product. Oncogene 1997;15:2505–2509.

22 Shaw RJ, Paez JG, Curto M, Yaktine A, Pruitt WM, Saotome I, O'Bryan JP, Gupta V, Ratner N, Der CJ, Jacks T, McClatchey AL: The Nf2 tumor suppressor, merlin, functions in Rac-dependent signaling. Dev Cell 2001;1:63–72.
23 Rong R, Surace EI, Haipek CA, Gutmann DH, Ye K: Serine 518 phosphorylation modulates merlin intramolecular association and binding to critical effectors important for NF2 growth suppression. Oncogene 2004;23:8447–8454.
24 Sherman LS, Gutmann DH, Merlin: Hanging tumor suppression on the Rac. Trends Cell Biol 2001;11: 442–444.
25 Surace EI, Haipek CA, Gutmann DH: Effect of merlin phosphorylation on neurofibromatosis 2 (NF2) gene function. Oncogene 2004;15:580–587.
26 Cushing H: Tumor of the nervus acousticus and the syndrome of the cerebellopontine angle. 1917.
27 Matthies C, Samii M: Management of 1000 vestibular schwannomas: clinical presentation. Neurosurgery 1997;40:1–9.
28 Kazantikul V, Brown WJ: Oestrogen receptors in acoustic neurilemmomas. Surg Neurol 1981;15:105–109.
29 Markwalder TM, Waelti E, Markwalder RV: Estrogen and progesterone receptors in acoustic and spinal neurilemmomas. Clinicopathologic correlations. Surg Neurol 1986;26: 142–148.
30 Carroll RS, Zhang JP, Black PM: Hormone receptors in vestibular schwannomas. Acta neurochir 1997;1139: 188–193.
31 Bartolami S, Auge C, Travo C, Venteo S, Knipper M, Sans A: Vestibular schwann cells are a distinct subpopulation of peripheral glia with specific sensitivity to growth factors and extracellular matrix components. J Neurobiol 2003;57:270–290.
32 Caye-Thomasen P, Baandrup L, Jacobsen GK, Thomsen J, Stangerup SE: Immunohistochemical demonstration of vascular endothelial growth factor in vestibular schwannomas correlates to tumor growth rate. Laryngoscope 2003;113:2129–2134.
33 Sturgis EM, Woll SS, Aydin F, Marrogi AJ, Amedee RG: Epidermal growth factor receptor expression by acoustic neuromas. Laryngoscope 1996;106:457–462.
34 Antoni NRE: Über Rückenmarkstumoren und neurofibroma. Kommissions-Verlag von J.F. Bergmann, Munich, 1920, pp 234–311.
35 Curto M, Chan A, Cole B, McClathey AI: The role of Merlin and the ERM proteins in membrane organization. International workshop on neurofibromatosis type 2, Paris, 2006.
36 Gentry JJ, Casaccia –Bonnefil P, Carter BD: Nerve growth factor activation of nuclear factor kB through its p75 receptor is an anti-apoptotic signal in RN22 schwannoma cells. J Biol Chem 2000;275:7558–7565.
37 Welling DB, Lasak JM, Akhmametyeva E, Ghaheri B, Chang LS: CDNA microarray analysis of vestibular schwannomas. Otol Neurotol 2002;23:736–748: 403–415.
38 Warren C, James LA, Ramsden RT, Wallace A, Baser ME, Varley JM, Evans DG: Identification of recurrent regions of chromosome loss and gain in vestibular schwannomas using comparative genomic hybridization. J Med Genet 2003;40:802–806.
39 Sherr CJ: The Pezcoller lecture : Cancer cell cycle revisited. Cancer Res 2000;60:3689–3695.
40 Lasak JM, Welling B, Akhmametyeva EM, Salloum M, Chang LS: Retinoblastoma-Cyclin-Dependent kinase pathway deregulation in vestibular schwannomas. Laryngoscope 2002; 112:1555–1561.
41 Kato M, Wilmotte R, Belkouch MC, de Tribolet N, Pizzolato G: Survivin in brain tumors : an attractive target for immunotherapy. J Neurooncol 2003;64:71–76.
42 Mawrin C, Kirches E, Dietzmann K, Roessner A, Boltze C: Expression pattern of apoptotic markers in vestibular schwannomas. Pathol Res Pract 2002;198:813–819.
43 Kimura Y, Koga H, Araki N, Mugita N, Fujita N, Takeshima H, Nishi T, Yamashima T, Saido TC, Yamasaki T, Moritake K, Saya H, Nakao M: The involvement of calpain-dependent proteolysis of the tumor suppressor NF2 (merlin) in schwannomas and meningiomas. Nat Med 1998;4: 915–922.

Prof. Pierre-Hugues Roche
Service de Neurochirurgie de l'Hôpital Nord
Assistance Publique-Hôpitaux de Marseille
Chemin des Bourrelly
FR–13915 Marseille Cedex 20 (France)
Tel. +33 4 91 96 86 20, Fax +33 4 91 96 89 15, E-Mail proche@mail.ap-hm.fr

Régis J, Roche P-H (eds): Modern Management of Acoustic Neuroma.
Prog Neurol Surg. Basel, Karger, 2008, vol 21, pp 32–42

Radiobiology, Principle and Technique of Radiosurgery

Ajay Niranjan · John C. Flickinger

Departments of Neurological Surgery and Radiation Oncology, The Center for Image-Guided Neurosurgery, University of Pittsburgh School of Medicine, Pittsburgh, Pa., USA

Abstract

Stereotactic radiosurgery involves the use of precisely directed closed skull single-session radiation to create a desired radiobiologic response within the intracranial target with minimal effects to surrounding structures or tissues. It provided a way for physicians to administer high single doses of radiation to intracranial targets in patients with relative safety. Rapid advances in imaging and computer technologies in the last decade have resulted in development of a variety of different radiosurgery techniques and their wider applications. The Gamma Knife-, proton beam- and LINAC-based radiosurgery devices represent the three main radiosurgery systems. Successful clinical experience with radiosurgery for a diversity of applications has led to a re-examination of radiobiological principles. For radiosurgical doses, the response of the tumor or target tissue and the adjacent normal tissue seems determined predominantly by the supporting vasculature.

Radiosurgery is a multidisciplinary field, which involves coordinated input from neurosurgeons, radiation oncologists, medical physicists, and engineers. The goal of radiosurgery differs from that of the conventional neurosurgery since the target is not physically removed immediately but instead is exposed to a single high dose of radiation, which ultimately translates into a specific (toxic) radiobiological response. The term stereotactic radiosurgery (SRS) is used for stereotactically guided delivery of focused radiation to a defined target volume in a single session. Radiosurgery or SRS can be performed using Gamma Knife, LINAC-based systems or Proton beam-based systems. The term fractionated stereotactic radiosurgery is used when stereotactically guided focused radiation is delivered to the defined target volume in 2–5 sessions. The term stereotactic radiation therapy refers to stereotactically guided delivery of focused radiation to the defined target volume in multiple fractions using relocatable frames.

Prior to the development of radiosurgery, essentially all clinical irradiation of intracranial targets was administered with 1.8- to 3-Gy fractions. Radiation oncology residents were taught that fractionating therapeutic radiation lessens the relative risk of injury to normal tissue compared to essentially all tumors. Radiobiological studies of a few cell culture lines of fast-growing malignant tumors and clinical experience with common fast-growing malignant tumors treated with conventionally fractionated radiotherapy in the clinic helped establish this radiobiological dogma. Increasing the fractionation for radiotherapy of slow-growing benign tumors may not necessarily improve the balance between tumor control and radiation complication. Slow-growing benign tumors are notoriously difficult to study in cell culture or in animal models, and therefore their radiobiology with respect to fractionation is not well defined. SRS allowed clinicians to administer high single-doses of radiation to intracranial targets with relative safety. Radiosurgery led to a new understanding of how different approaches to radiation treatment planning and radiobiology may be modified in the clinic to achieve goals previously thought unreachable.

Radiosurgical Techniques

Radiosurgery was originally devised to treat intracranial lesions by delivering a high dose of ionizing radiation in a single treatment session using multiple beams precisely focused at the target inside the cranium. Rapid advances in imaging and computer technologies in the last decade have resulted in wider applications of radiosurgery. A variety of different radiosurgery techniques have been developed during the past two decades.

Gamma Knife Radiosurgery
The first prototype Gamma Knife was created in 1967 by Leksell and Larsson. In Gamma Knife, the radiation from Co-60 is focused at the center to create a cumulative radiation field. The earlier model originally was referred to as the U-style and contained cobalt sources arranged in hemispherical array. These units present challenging cobalt-60 loading and reloading issues. To eliminate this problem, the B-unit (after Bergen, Norway, the first site) was redesigned so that sources were arranged in an annular configuration. In 1999, the Model C version of the Gamma Knife was introduced. The Model C Gamma Knife unit has an option to use the robotic technology to set various head positions. This obviates the need to set these coordinates manually in a multiple-isocenter plan. The other features of the Model C unit include an integral helmet changer, dedicated helmet installation trolleys, and color-coded collimators and occlusive plugs. In 2005, the fourth generation Leksell Gamma Knife model 4-C was introduced. The model 4-C is equipped with enhancements designed to improve workflow, increase accuracy and provide integrated imaging capabilities. The Leksell Gamma Plan has the ability to co-register images from multiple sources (CT, MR, PET, MEG) and offers digital brain atlas that can be used for functional radiosurgery. The planning information can be viewed on both sides of the treatment couch. The helmet changer and robotic Automatic Positioning System are faster and reduce total treatment time.

Rotating Gamma System
A radiosurgery device called the Rotating Gamma System (RGS) has been developed. The RGS (OUR International Inc., Shenzen, China) utilizes 30, cobalt-60 radiation sources. The radiation sources in the RGS are contained in a revolving hemispherical shell. The secondary collimator is a coaxial hemispheric shell that has six groups of five collimator holes arranged in the same fashion as the radiation sources. By selecting a particular group of collimator holes that can be aligned with the radiation sources, different beam diameters can be achieved. This obviates the need to change helmets manually. The experience with such system is limited.

Charged-Particle Radiosurgery
This radiosurgery system uses either the Bragg-peak method where atomic-charged particles stop within the target volume or, plateau-beam method in which charged particles are cross-fired at the target. The first treatment of a malignant tumor by irradiation with the Bragg-Gray peak was carried out in 1957. Beginning in 1958, proton beam irradiation was used to perform

functional surgery in patients with advanced Parkinson's disease. In 1961, Kjellberg began performing radiosurgery with Bragg-peak, using the 165-MeV proton beam facility in Cambridge, Massachusetts. Although originally constructed for basic scientific research, these cyclotron units were subsequently reengineered for human use. These facilities are only available at a limited number of centers due to high cost of equipment and maintenance.

LINAC Radiosurgery
Linear accelerators are devices where electrons are accelerated to nearly the speed of light and the electron beam is directed to a heavy metal plate. The resulting interactions produce X-rays, which are guided and focused on a biologic target. Linear accelerators (LINACs) were developed simultaneously in the United States as well as in Britain in 1950s and became the preferred devices for conventional fractionated radiotherapy. Pioneering work of many researchers in 1980s led to the gradual modifications of newly redesigned LINACs for use as radiosurgery system. LINAC technologies were modified by incorporating improved guiding (stereotactic) devices and methods to measure accuracy of various components. In LINAC-based radiosurgery, multiple radiation arcs are utilized to crossfire X-rays at a target defined in 3-D space. Most of the presently functioning systems use nondynamic techniques in which the patient couch is set at a fixed angle and the head of the LINAC is moved around the patient firing in an arc. The radiation beams enter the skull through many different points. In dynamic techniques, both the couch and the arc radiation delivery system move to shape the target volume. Different techniques and dose planning software have also been developed to enhance conformity of dose planning and delivery using LINAC-based systems. These include beam shaping and intensity modulation. Newer developments include introduction of jaws, noncircular, mini and microleaf collimators. Single isocenter radiosurgery is now possible with newer LINAC-based systems. The conformal beam can be delivered with the micromultileaf collimation or conformal blocks. Micromultileaf collimation consists of multiple individually motorized tungsten 'leaves' that shape a treatment field. Many LINAC-based systems such as Xknife® (Radionics Inc., Burlington, Mass., USA), Novalis® (BrainLAB, Heimstetten, Germany), the Peacock System® (NOMOS Corp., Sewickley, Pa., USA), and Cyberknife® (Accuray Inc., Sunnyvale, Calif., USA) are commercially available. The Peacock system (NOMOS Corporation, Sewickley, Pa., USA) uses inverse planning and multileaf wedge-generated intensity modulated beams to obtain target conformity. The Cyberknife, combines X-ray beams, computers, imaging, and robotic technology for target localization, and radiation delivery. This system utilizes a 6-MeV LINAC attached to a six-axis robotic manipulator. The robot positions the LINAC at different beam positions, always aiming the center of the radiation beam at the target. A stereotactic frame is not used for targeting. Before the radiation is delivered from any position, the patient's movements are tracked using an integrated X-ray image processing system, which consists of two orthogonal diagnostic X-ray cameras and an optical tracking system. During Cyberknife treatment, the image processing system acquires X-ray images of the patient's body multiple times throughout the treatment, and the software compares the actual images with the images in a database to determine the direction and amount of any head motion. The information regarding the new location is delivered to the robot, which corrects for the motion and then delivers radiation.

Tomotherapy
Tomotherapy, literally 'slice' therapy, is a new form of radiation therapy that combines the precision of a computed tomography (CT) scan with the radiation treatment. Unlike traditional radiation therapy systems which have beams

projecting onto the tumor from a few different directions, tomotherapy rotates the beam source around the patient, thus allowing the beam to enter the patient from many different angles in succession. The intensity of the beam can be modulated through the use of a multi-leaf collimator system. The inclusion of CT imaging technology within the tomotherapy device allows for precise localization of the tumor before and during treatment.

Image-Guided Radiotherapy
The emphasis on focused radiation delivery using volumetric imaging and 3-D conformal planning and the understanding of set-up errors and patient or organ movement during treatment have ushered in the development of clinical process and techniques collectively known as image guided radiation therapy. The intensity of the beam is modulated through the use of a multi-leaf collimator system, thus further improving the precision of the treatment. Several manufacturers currently offer image guided radiation therapy using LINAC technology that can perform both radiosurgery in one session and radiotherapy. Trilogy® (Varian Medical Systems, Inc.) radiosurgery system incorporates a low-dose, high-resolution X-ray imager that facilitates accurate patient positioning. The synergyS® (Elekta, Inc.) uses a cone beam CT to eliminate setup errors.

Radiosurgery Technique for Vestibular Schwannomas

Vestibular schwannoma SRS using the Gamma Knife was first performed by Leksell in 1969. The goals of vestibular schwannoma radiosurgery are to prevent tumor growth, and to preserve cochlear and other cranial nerve function. The long-term results have established radiosurgery as an important minimally invasive alternative to microsurgery for small- to moderate-sized vestibular schwannomas.

Pre-Radiosurgery Evaluation
Patients with vestibular schwannomas are evaluated with high-resolution MRI (CT is performed for those who cannot undergo MRI scans) and audiological tests that include pure tone average (PTA) and speech discrimination score (SDS) measurements. Hearing is graded using the Gardner-Robertson modification of the Silverstein and Norell classification and/or the American Academy of Otolaryngology-Head and Neck Surgery guidelines. 'Serviceable' hearing (class I and II) is defined as a PTA or speech reception threshold (stereotactic radiation therapy) lower than 50 dB and SDS better than 50%. The facial nerve function is assessed according to the House-Brackmann grading system.

Radiosurgery Technique
Radiosurgery can be performed using the Gamma Knife, modified LINACs or the proton beam. Although the concept is similar, the specific technical details of head immobilization, imaging, dose planning and dose delivery differ in these three modalities. In Gamma Knife radiosurgery, the procedure begins with application of an MRI-compatible Leksell stereotactic frame (model G, Elekta Instruments, Atlanta, Ga., USA) to the patient's head under local anesthetic scalp infiltration (5% marcaine and 1% xylocaine), supplemented by mild intravenous sedation. High-resolution MR images are acquired with a fiducial system attached to the stereotactic frame. For vestibular schwannoma radiosurgery, a 3-D volume acquisition MRI using a gradient pulse sequence (divided into 1- or 1.5-mm-thick 28–36 axial slices) is performed in order to cover the entire lesion and surrounding critical structures. A T_2-weighted 3-D volume sequence is performed to visualize cranial nerves and inner ear structures (cochlea and semicircular canals). Centers using LINAC-based systems may use mask immobilization of the patients' head along with image guidance and typically deliver the radiation dose in 3 or

more stages. CT is used for planning but may be fused to MRI scans.

Radiosurgical Dose Planning

Dose planning is the most important aspect of radiosurgery. Conformal coverage of the tumor and preservation of facial, cochlear and trigeminal nerve function is given priority during dose planning. For large tumors, preservation of brainstem function is also a consideration. A conformal radiosurgery plan is necessary for hearing and facial nerve preservation. Highlights of Gamma Knife vestibular schwannoma radiosurgery planning include outlining of tumor volume, use of multiple isocenters, beam weighting, and use of plug patterns. Precise 3-D conformality between treatment and tumor volumes is needed to avoid radiation-related complications. This degree of conformality can be achieved through complex multi-isocenter planning. Vestibular schwannoma planning is usually performed using a combination of small-beam diameter (4- and 8-mm) collimators. For large tumors, 14-mm collimators are also used. A series of 4 mm isocenters are used to create a tapered isodose plan to conform to the intracanalicular portion of the tumor. Success of vestibular schwannoma radiosurgery depends upon high conformality to the tumor margin. Because the facial and the cochlear nerve complex generally courses along the anterior margin and anterior-inferior side of the tumor, the dose plan should be highly conformal in this region.

Dose Prescription

After optimizing the plan, a maximum dose to the target is determined. The treatment isodose, maximum dose, and dose to the margin are jointly decided by a neurosurgeon, radiation oncologist, medical physicist and, in some centers, a neurotologist after considering the goal of radiosurgery in an individual patient and the tolerance of the surrounding structures. In Gamma Knife radiosurgery, a dose of 12–13 Gy is typically prescribed to the 50% (or other) isodose line, that conforms to the tumor margin. Dose prescription for vestibular schwannomas has changed significantly over the past 10 years. A margin dose of 12–13 Gy is associated with a low complication rate and yet maintains a high rate of tumor control. After prescribing the margin dose, the fall off on cochlea, semicircular canal, and brainstem are checked to keep them below tolerance level. For LINAC-based treatments using a frameless system, total dose may be divided into 3–5 delivery sessions, typically prescribed to the 80% isodose line.

Dose Delivery

Gamma Knife radiosurgery is performed with a 201-source, cobalt-60 unit, (model B or model C, Elekta Instruments, Atlanta, Ga., USA) where the patient's head and stereotactic frame are immobilized within the appropriate collimator helmet at a calculated target coordinate. Dose delivery is accomplished in a single session by positioning the head serially for each subsequent isocenter until a fully conformal field encompasses the tumor volume. Radiosurgery using modified LINACs is typically performed with micro-multileaf collimators or cone system. Cyberknife stereotactic radiotherapy treatments use a robotically directed LINAC. Cyclotron facilities use a specially modulated proton beam to deliver energy to the target.

Postoperative Care

There is no consensus on the use of corticosteroids on the day of radiosurgery. Some physicians do not use steroids at all before, during or after radiosurgery. At some centers patients receive an intravenous dose of 40 mg of methylprednisolone at the onset or conclusion of the procedure. At others centers, 6 mg of dexamethasone is given immediately before dose delivery, which is repeated every 3 h for the duration of the treatment. The stereotactic frame is removed immediately after radiosurgery. Patients are observed for few hours in the same day surgery unit and are usually discharged within 24 h.

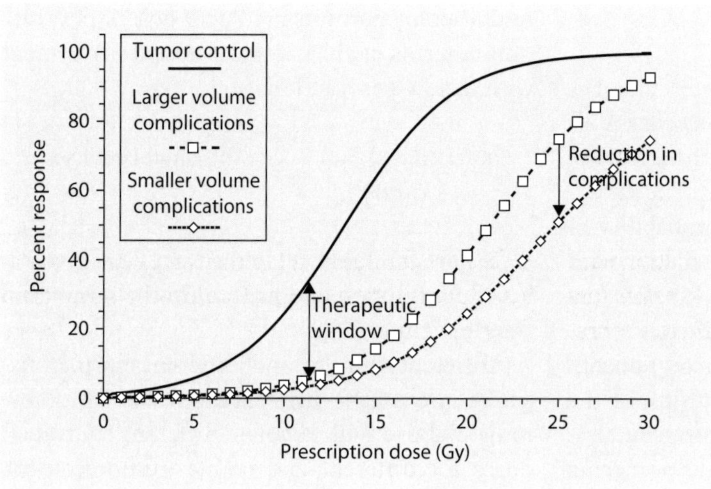

Fig. 1. Theoretical sigmoid dose-response curves for tumor control with separate curves for complications with different treatment volumes. The two complication curves for radiation to a target with either a 15-mm margin and with no margin show how radiosurgery with no margin reduces complications for the same treatment dose (second arrow at 20 Gy pointing downwards). The complication curves shown were estimated from the RTOG radiosurgery dose-escalation data [11] for brain metastases <2 cm in diameter (lower curve) and 3–4 cm in diameter (middle curve). Since more normal tissue would be irradiated when treating with a margin than treating a larger tumor, the middle curve most likely underestimates the complication risk.

Postradiosurgery Evaluations

After radiosurgery, all patients are followed-up with serial gadolinium-enhanced MRI scans, which are generally requested following a schedule such as at 6-months, 12 months, 2, 4, 8, and 16 years. All patients who have some preserved hearing are advised to obtain audiological tests (PTA and SDS) near the time of their MRI follow-up.

Radiobiology

Optimizing any clinical intervention (radiation, drug therapy, or surgery) requires equal attention to maximizing desired outcomes (tumor cure, vascular malformation obliteration, etc.) and minimizing undesired outcomes (complications) from the intervention (radiation injury, operative morbidity, etc). The relationship of dose to both desired and undesired outcomes can be represented by a pair of sigmoid dose-response curves for the desired outcome (tumor control or arteriovenous malformation, AVM, obliteration) and complications, as shown in figure 1. The key radiobiological principle exploited in radiosurgery is that small volumes of normal tissue can withstand high-doses of radiation with dramatically lower complication risks than larger volumes of normal tissue. Radiosurgery plans minimize target volumes with highly conformal plans with no extra margin of normal tissue around the target. Standard, nonstereotactic radiotherapy plans routinely add 5–15 mm margins of normal tissue around the target volume to allow for positioning error. Reducing the volume of tissue irradiated shifts dose-response curve for complications down and to the right, increasing the separation between cure and complication probability. The separation between cure and complications, referred to as the therapeutic window, is increased by reducing the volume of normal tissue irradiated. Understanding the underlying radiobiological principles affecting the desired radiation effects (tumor cure, AVM obliteration, etc.) and complications is vital to optimizing radiosurgery outcomes.

The Linear-Quadratic Formula

The linear-quadratic formula is presently the standard way to mathematically represent the effect of radiotherapy to account for the effects of different fractionation schemes [1–6]. The linear-quadratic formula represents the probability of cell survival after a dose of ionizing radiation with a combination of single-hit or linear kinetics (the alpha component) and double-hit kinetics represented by a quadratic term (the β-component). Conceptually, it can be helpful to think of the α-component as representing irreversible, immediate double-stranded DNA breaks occurring with each fraction of radiation administered. As the linear component, alpha cell killing depends on the total dose administered and not on the dose per fraction. β-Cell killing could be thought of as multiple single-fraction DNA breaks occurring after each fraction of radiation. The chance that this component leads to cell death relates to the square of the dose per fraction administered. For single-fraction irradiation, the linear-quadratic formula represents the probability of a desired or undesired response (cure of a tumor or normal tissue injury) by the following probabilistic (probit) double-exponential equation:

$$P(\text{response}) = \text{EXP}[-k \times \text{EXP}(-\alpha \times \text{dose} - \beta \times \text{dose}^2)] \quad (1)$$

Where P(response) is the probability of cure or complications, EXP represents the number e (2.7183, commonly used in natural logarithms) raised exponentially to the power of the terms that follow, k represents the number of clonogens in the target tissue, while α and β are coefficients for the respective linear and quadratic coefficients.

The value of the α-coefficient divided by the β-coefficient (the α/β ratio) characterizes how a tissue or tumor is affected by different fractionation schemes. It is used in the following formula to equate the effect of a course of fractionated radiotherapy administered with dose X per fraction in terms of an equivalent dose for treatment with dose Y per fractions.

$$[\text{total dose(x)}] \times [1 + X/(\alpha/\beta)] = [\text{total dose(y)}] \times [1 + Y/(\alpha/\beta)] \quad (2)$$

Where total dose(y) is the total dose given at Y Gy per fraction and is equal to the number of fractions times Y.

Different tumors and different normal tissue reactions have different α/β ratios. Thus, formula 2 above will calculate different equivalent doses for different end points (tumor control, optic nerve injury, edema response, etc.). Studies of fractionated radiotherapy in the clinic and in animal models found that most late-responding tissues such as brain or spinal cord have α/β ratios around 2. Faster responding normal tissues such as skin or mucosal erythematous reactions have α/β values of 5–8, while most malignant tumors have values closer to 10 [1, 4]. Small radiation dose fractions cause proportionally less injury to tissues with low α/β ratios than tissues or tumors with higher α/β ratios.

Tumors do not always have a higher α/β ratio than normal tissue, so increasing fractionation does not always reduces radiation injury to normal tissue compared to tumors. Some malignant tumors such as melanoma or prostate cancer (or at least some strains of them) have lower α/β ratios than surrounding normal tissues supporting the use of larger dose fractions for treatment [5].

Equations 1 and 2 above do not account for the effects of time, which allows for repopulation and repair. Time effects should be negligible for central nervous system tissue and most benign tumors in normal circumstances. A time-dependent repopulation term should be added for protracted fractionated treatment of fast-growing malignant tumors. Table 1 shows the fractionated radiotherapy equivalent doses for single-fraction radiosurgery predicted using the linear-quadratic formula.

Table 1. Radiobiologically equivalent dose (normalized total dose) for fractionated radiotherapy with 2-Gy fractions from single-fraction radiosurgery according to the linear-quadratic equation using different values of α/β (and no time correction)

Single-fraction dose Gy	2 Gy/fraction equivalent dose, Gy		
	late-reacting tissue, α/β = 2	late response with α/β = 0	early-reacting tissue, α/β = 10
4	6	8	4.7
6	12	18	8.0
8	20	32	12.0
10	30	50	16.7
12	42	72	22.0
14	56	98	28.0
16	72	128	34.7
18	90	162	42.0
20	110	200	50.0
22	132	242	58.7
24	156	288	68.0

Radiosurgical Data and the Linear-Quadratic Formula

The linear-quadratic formula reasonably fits data from the laboratory and the clinic for extrapolating from one course of fractionated radiotherapy to another with different-sized dose fractions, as long as the dose fractions stay in the range of 1–8 Gy. The reliability of extrapolating from conventional radiotherapy with 1.8–2.0 Gy fractions to the high doses of single-fraction irradiation used in radiosurgery is questionable. Table 1 gives the predicted equivalent fractionated radiotherapy doses with 2-Gy fractions (NTD_2) using α/β values of 10 early-reacting tissues and 2 for late-reacting tissue (which is the accepted value for brain tissue) for single fraction doses. The second column shows dose-equivalent calculations using an α/β value of zero (specifically, α = 0), making it a quadratic exponential formula rather than a true linear-quadratic formula. The equivalent value using an α/β value of zero is given by the formula below:

$$\text{Equivalent dose}(\alpha/\beta = 0) \text{ for 2-Gy fractions} = 1/2\,(\text{single fraction dose})^2 \quad (3)$$

Using an α/β value of zero does not fit the theoretical basis of the linear quadratic formula, which presupposes some contribution with single-hit kinetics (the α-component).

Optic Nerve Tolerance Doses in Radiosurgery

An early analysis of optic nerve complications in a combined Harvard/University of Pittsburgh study of radiosurgery complications, recommended 8 Gy as a safe dose limit for the optic nerves/chiasm [7]. The lowest optic chiasm dose at which optic neuropathy developed in that study was 9.7 Gy in that study. According to table 1, the linear-quadratic formula predicts that a 10-Gy single-fraction dose to the optic chiasm

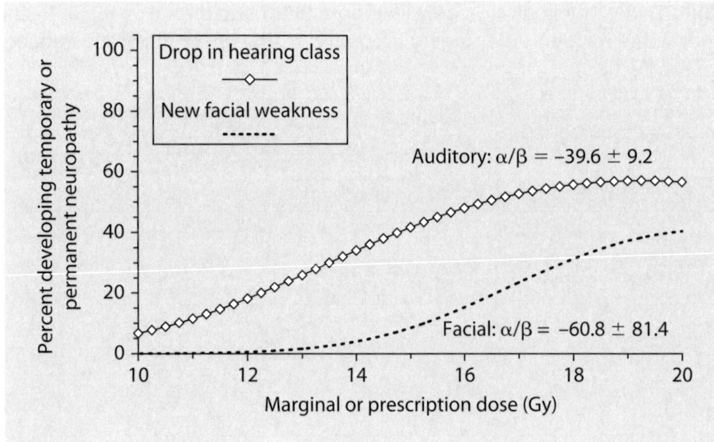

Fig. 2. Linear-quadratic (probit) dose-response curves for the development of auditory and facial neuropathies according to marginal (minimum tumor) dose. These curves and their corresponding α/β ratio values were derived from nonlinear regression analysis of 218 acoustic neuroma patients who underwent radiosurgery at the University of Pittsburgh from 1987 to 1997 with more than 2 years of follow-up.

should have the equivalent effect of 32 or 50 Gy at 2 Gy per fraction for α/β = 0 or 2, respectively. With an α/β value of zero, the equivalent dose at 2 Gy per fraction for the 9.7-Gy radiosurgery dose that caused optic neuropathy would have been 47 Gy. From clinical experience with conventional fractionated radiotherapy of pituitary adenomas, the risk of optic neuropathy for 46–48 Gy at 2 Gy per fraction should be approximately 1/300 or less [8]. This suggests that the equivalent effect for high-dose single fractions is greater than that predicted by the linear-quadratic formula, even when an α/β value of zero is used (which stretches the theoretical basis of the formula).

Dose-Response Analysis for Cranial Neuropathies after Acoustic Neuroma Radiosurgery

The linear-quadratic formula runs into problems calculating α/β ratios from single-fraction dose-response data from radiosurgery. We analyzed 218 acoustic neuroma patients who underwent radiosurgery at the University of Pittsburgh from 1987 to 1997 with more than 2 years of follow-up. This analysis assumed that the dose to the facial, and auditory nerves matched the marginal doses prescribed at the time of radiosurgery, since these nerves normally lie along the capsule of the tumor. This assumption is not as reliable for the trigeminal nerve, which may not lie up against smaller tumors. We found small negative β-coefficients for facial and auditory neuropathy, with best-fitting α/β ratios in the range of –30 to –55 (fig. 2; table 2). This does not match with the expected value of α/β = 2. The negative values for the α/β ratios which mathematically describe the best-fitting dose-response curves for these data contradict the theoretical rationale for the linear-quadratic formula.

We found similar difficulty fitting linear-quadratic dose-response curves to data from radiosurgery of AVMs [9, 10]. As shown in table 2, we also found negative α/β ratios for the endpoints of postradiosurgery normal tissue injury imaging changes and for AVM obliteration.

Comparison of Postradiosurgery Injury Reactions for AVM and Meningioma

As a way to investigate differences in normal tissue injury reactions between different targets, we analyzed postradiosurgery imaging changes (symptomatic or asymptomatic edema) that developed in 27/307 AVM patients compared to 14/291 meningioma patients with 2 or more years

Table 2. Estimation of α/β ratios for different endpoints from University of Pittsburgh acoustic schwannoma radiosurgery and AVM radiosurgery

End point	Number and type of patients	α/β ratio
Hearing change	57/138 acoustics with hearing	-39.6 ± 9.2
Facial neuropathy	31/218 acoustic schwannomas	-60.8 ± 81.4
Postradiosurgery imaging changes	87/307 AVM patients	-29.7 ± 2.4
In-field AVM obliteration	293/355 AVM patients	-49.3 ± 5.3

Table 3. Multivariate logistic regression modeling comparison of postradiosurgery imaging changes (symptomatic or asymptomatic edema) after radiosurgery in 307 AVM patients and 291 meningioma patients with 2 or more years of follow-up

Variable	p value	Odds ratio	95% confidence interval
AVM versus meningioma	<0.0001	7.502	3.43–16.40
Marginal dose[a]	0.0143	2.457 per Gy	1.197–5.043
Marginal dose squared[a]	0.0148	0.9789 per Gy^2	0.9624–0.9958
Volume	<0.0001	1.142 per ml	1.217–3.431

[a]Approximated value of $\alpha/\beta = -42.21 \pm 17.22$.

of follow-up. Table 3 shows a multivariate logistic regression comparison of postradiosurgery imaging changes for AVM versus meningioma controlling for the effects of dose (in a linear quadratic expression with marginal dose and marginal dose squared) and for treatment volume. Postradiosurgery imaging changes were significantly likely ($p < 0.0001$) in the AVM patients by a factor of 7.5 (95% confidence interval: 3.4–16.4). The ratio of the regression coefficients for marginal dose and marginal dose squared gave an approximate alpha/beta ratio of -42.2 ± 17.2.

This comparison of postradiosurgery imaging changes for AVM versus meningioma radiosurgery target volumes demonstrate that the target tissue affects the chance of developing a radiation injury reaction. In contrast, normal tissue complication probability models predict radiation injury based only on the dose of radiation received by the tissue or organs surrounding the tumor/target and ignore the effects of the target tissue.

Radiosurgery of Brain Metastases

The RTOG Radiosurgery Dose-Escalation Study (95–05) established tolerance doses for radiosurgery of recurrent brain metastases and high-grade gliomas [11]. 156 patients with brain metastases or primary tumors (not involving brainstem) that progressed after conventional radiotherapy were prospectively treated following a dose-escalation protocol [11]. Starting with initial doses of 18, 15, and 12 Gy for diameters ≤20, 21–30, and 31–40 mm, respectively, they escalated prescription doses in

3-Gy intervals until toxicity was seen in over 30% of patients. The recommended tolerance doses from that protocol were 24, 18, and 15 Gy for diameters of ≤20, 21–30, and 31–40 mm, respectively.

Another interesting finding from the treatment of brain metastases is that tumor control rates are similar for all different types of brain metastases that would be expected to differ because of different α/β ratios. This would support laboratory studies that suggest that the radiation response for the high-dose single fractions used in radiosurgery is predominantly related to the supporting endothelial cells [12]. Pathology studies of benign and malignant tumors treated by radiosurgery also support a vascular response [13].

Conclusions

Radiobiological analysis of clinical data from radiosurgery leads to the following conclusions: (1) The linear-quadratic equation cannot reliably represent equivalent radiation effects when extrapolating from conventional fractionation (1.5–4 Gy per fraction) to high-dose (12–25 Gy) single fractions for radiosurgery. (2) Mathematical models of radiation injury probability need to take into account that the target/tumor tissue's radiation response may affect the reaction of the surrounding normal tissue. (3) The predominant radiation response of a radiosurgical target is mediated through the target or tumor vasculature.

References

1 Barendsen GW: Dose fractionation, dose rate and iso-effect relationships for normal tissue responses. Int J Radiat Oncol Biol Phys 1982;8:1981–1997.
2 Dale RG: The application of the linear-quadratic dose-effect equation to fractionated and protracted radiotherapy. Br J Radiol 1985;58:515–528.
3 Fowler JF: The linear-quadratic formula and progress in fractionated radiotherapy. Br J Radiol 1989;62:679–694.
4 Hall EJ, Brenner DJ: The radiobiology of radiosurgery: rationale for different treatment regimes for AVMs and malignancies. Int J Radiat Oncol Biol Phys 1993;25:381–385.
5 Brenner DJ, Hall EJ: Fractionation and protraction for radiotherapy of prostate cancer. Int J Radiat Oncol Biol Phys 1999;43:1095–1101.
6 Flickinger JC, Kalend A: Use of normalized total dose to represent the biological effect of fractionated radiotherapy. Radiother Oncol 1990;17: 339–347.
7 Tishler RB, Loeffler JS, Lunsford LD, Duma C, Alexander E III, Kooy HM, Flickinger JC: Tolerance of cranial nerves of the cavernous sinus to radiosurgery. Int J Radiat Oncol Biol Phys 1993;27:215–221.
8 Flickinger JC, Rush SC: Linear accelerator radiotherapy of pituitary adenomas; in Landolt AM, Vance, Reilly (eds): Pituitary Adenomas – Biology, Diagnosis and Treatment. Edinburgh, Churchill Livingstone, 1996, pp 475–483.
9 Flickinger JF, Kondziolka D, Maitz AH, Lunsford LD: An analysis of the dose-response for arteriovenous malformation radiosurgery and other factors affecting obliteration. Radiother Oncol 2002;63:347–354.
10 Flickinger JC, Kondziolka D, Lunsford LD, Kassam A, Phuong LK, Liscak R, Pollock BE: Development of a model to predict permanent symptomatic post-radiosurgery injury for arteriovenous malformation patients. Int J Radiat Oncol Biol Phys 2000;46:1143–1148.
11 Shaw E, Scott C, Souhami L, Dinapoli R, Kline R, Loeffler J, Farnan N: Single dose radiosurgical treatment of recurrent previously irradiated primary brain tumors and brain metastases: final report of RTOG protocol 90–05. Int J Radiat Oncol Biol Phys 2000; 47:291–298.
12 Garcia-Barros M, Paris F, Cordon-Cardo C, Lyden D, Rafii S, Haimovitz-Friedman A, Fuks Z, Kolesnick R: Tumor response to radiotherapy regulated by endothelial cell apoptosis. Science 2003;300:1155–1159.
13 Szeifert GT, Massager N, DeVriendt D, David P, De Smedt F, Rorive S, Salmon I, Brotchi J, Levivier M: Observations of intracranial neoplasms treated with Gamma Knife radiosurgery. J Neurosurg 2002;97:623–626.

Ajay Niranjan, MBBS, MCh
Neurological Surgery B400, 200 Lothrop Street, Pittsburgh, PA 15213 (USA)
Tel. +1 412 647 9699, Fax +1 412 647 8447, E-Mail niranjana@upmc.edu

Régis J, Roche P-H (eds): Modern Management of Acoustic Neuroma.
Prog Neurol Surg. Basel, Karger, 2008, vol 21, pp 43–53

Cerebellopontine Cistern: Microanatomy Applied to Vestibular Schwannomas

Emmanuel Lescanne[a,b] · Patrick François[a,c] · Stéphane Velut[a,c]

[a]Laboratoire d'Anatomie de la Faculté de Médecine, Université de Tours, [b]Service d'ORL et Chirurgie Cervico-Faciale et [c]Service de Neurochirurgie, Hôpital Bretonneau, CHRU de Tours, Tours, France

Abstract

The microanatomy of the cerebellopontine cistern (CPC) is of interest to many surgeons and has been the subject of controversial works especially concerning the study of the subarachnoid space in the internal acoustic meatus (IAM). The CPC lies in the cerebellopontine angle between the brainstem, cerebellum and petrous bone. It contains in its upper part the trigeminal nerve with the superior petrosal vein. The cochleovestibulofacial bundle occupies the middle portion and lies between the pontomedullary sulcus and the IAM. The glossopharyngeal, vagus and accessory nerves are located in the inferior part of the cerebellopontine angle close to the vertebral artery and the posteroinferior cerebellar artery. The acousticofacial cistern is a lateral extension of the CPC in the IAM. The anatomy of the meningeal layers within the IAM is discussed especially concerning 'the arachnoidal cleavage plane' in acoustic neuroma surgery.

Full comprehension of the development of vestibular tumors and their relations to the neighboring nerves (the facial, cochlear, trigeminal, glossopharyngeal, vagus and accessory nerves) requires a perfect understanding of the anatomy of the arachnoid of the cerebellopontine angle. Similarly, effective surgical treatment of these tumors also implies a perfect understanding of the morphology of this meninx. A solid comprehension of how it behaves when a vestibular tumor arises can help the surgeon refine his or her operating technique.

Thus, it seems more appropriate to describe the poorly understood and controversial relationships of the arachnoid than to present a detailed description of the anatomical elements comprising the cerebellopontine angle, which are generally well known. The controversy that surrounds the relationships of the arachnoid is due to the difficulties encountered in studying this extremely fragile meninx.

The Different Methods Used to Study the Cisterns of the Brain in the Literature

Since the early days of neurosurgery, numerous studies in the neurosciences have been devoted to the microanatomy of the cisterns of the brain. As Vinas et al. [1] have suggested, the study of the subarachnoid spaces can be divided into two main periods: the anatomical period and the radiological period. The different techniques which were used most often tried to avoid collapsing the cisterns rather than conserving the integrity of the arachnoid. Since the end of the 20th century, the microneurosurgical period has heralded a new requirement for anatomical descriptions, notably the conservation of the arachnoid, thus reflecting its uncontested anatomical and surgical importance.

Communication between the ventricular system and the subarachnoid spaces was demonstrated in the 19th century. In order to accomplish this, Magendie [2] injected India ink, and Lushka stained gelatine [3]. In 1875, Key and Retzius [4] injected Berlin blue-colored jelly into the ventricular system and the subarachnoid space through the suboccipital and spinal routes. They recorded their dissections in extremely delicate and detailed drawings. At the beginning of the 20th century, Locke and Naffziger [5] first published their work on this subject. After rinsing the ventricles and the subarachnoid spaces in acetone, they injected a mixture of celloidine and camphor diluted in acetone through the ventricular and suboccipital route. This mixture colored the various spaces that they studied differently. The specimen was then emerged in cold water for 24 h before it was corroded with hydrochloric acid. After corroding the soft tissues of the face, neck, bones and the dura mater, the brain was softened by using a solution of 0.5% pancreatine at 40°C. Finally, it was completely dissolved by a stream of water under pressure. This technique provided the authors with a description of the subarachnoid spaces and the ventricles thanks to the 'negative' mold they obtained. In 1956, Liliequist [6] ushered in the radiological period by comparing anatomical descriptions to the new radiological data. He insisted on the difficulty he had in describing the arachnoid because mere cerebral extraction allowed the cerebrospinal fluid (CSF) to escape resulting in the collapse of the subarachnoid spaces. Consequently, he recommended that the spaces be injected with resin or barium gelatine prior to cerebral extraction. Most often, these injections were performed at the level of the cerebellomedullary cistern. For the purposes of radiological study, the brain was extracted according to the conventional method. Then, after ablation of the falx cerebi, the brain was immersed in a 10% formaldehyde solution and a radiography was taken using different incidences. When resin injections were used, the brain was dissolved with caustic soda. These techniques provided an excellent study of the cisterns themselves and their communications but the price paid was loss of the fine morphology of the arachnoid and the vasculonervous contents of these spaces. Liliequist's publication inaugurated the detailed description of the subarachnoid spaces and preceded the more detailed descriptions published by Yasargil which remain a benchmark even today.

Yasargil and Konstantin's first study in 1976 concerned skull base cisterns [7] and was based on 1,500 dissections using optic magnification. He described the cisterns by using in vivo 'microdissections' during the treatment of arterial aneurysms, arteriovenous malformations, meningiomas of the skull base, craniopharyngiomas and neuromas. Illustrated with 4 drawings, this pioneering article inspired a number of didactic chapters in numerous works dealing with the microsurgery of acoustic neuromas. In a second and even more extensive publication in 1984, additional observations were based on 4,200 intracranial interventions and 200 dissections performed on cadavers using optic magnification [8]. The anatomical description of the subarachnoid cisterns was illustrated with 20 personal drawings, 46 perioperative photographs and 6 photographs from cadaver dissections. Yasargil chose to rely on his more 'physiological' surgical findings since the anatomical techniques using cadavers did not allow the arachnoid to be integrally conserved. Nonetheless, he recognized that there are forcibly variations between different individuals and additional anatomical modifications related to local changes induced by disease. Accordingly, he suggested that a complementary radiologic study was required in order to describe the cisterns which are surgically inaccessible, and more recently he recommended a complementary neuropathological study to corroborate his descriptions [9].

Matsuno and Rhoton based their publication [10] on studies using optic magnification in 15 cadavers in whom they injected colored latex via both the arterial and venous routes. The author removed the portion of the cranium surrounding the posterior fossa and was able to avoid disrupting the arachnoid by using an operating microscope. His descriptions were illustrated with 7 personal drawings and 51 photographs which were underlined by hand and obviously retouched. Using 20 fixed or unfixed injected brains, Vinas et al. [1, 11, 12] added to the exhaustive description of the arachnoid of the skull base cisterns. He used the so-called immersion technique: the injection of air into the subarachnoid spaces of a brain which had been removed with the dura mater left intact, then immersed in Ringer's solution. Thus, he was able to perform dissections under optic magnification in water, a technique which provided more physiological conditions. He added a drawing to his description which was illustrated with black and white photos since underwater photography can change the appearance of objects due to the phenomenon of diffraction. The technique used by Velut [13] was developed in preparation for his future anatomic studies [14–16] and consisted in prolonged softening of the bony components with hydrogen peroxide in order to remove the base or the vault of the skull without any traction on the meningeal layers. The microanatomic descriptions of the different cisterns, which were documented with photographs, were possible because the arachnoid was left completely intact.

Complementing these anatomical studies, neuroendoscopic anatomical studies on injected specimens have been added providing a view of the cisterns and their contents [17, 18]. These very 'physiological' descriptions supply us with additional details on the vascularization of the cranial nerves and the arachnoid trabeculations of the deep layer.

The Cerebellopontine Cistern and Its Contents

The cerebellopontine cistern (CPC) occupies the space commonly called the 'cerebellopontine angle'. When the superficial sheath of the prepontic arachnoid is opened ventrally, one sees that the CPC communicates freely with the prepontic and premedullary cisterns without any interposition or arachnoid partition. Medially, the caudal portion of the CPC communicates with the premedullary cistern. At his level, a partition is sometimes present when the vertebral artery makes a loop. In that case, arachnoid rows join the artery to the pial surface of the medulla oblongata and constitute a partial limit between these two cisterns. The dimension of the CPC is related to the abundance of its vascular and nervous contents.

The Trigeminal Nerve

The trigeminal nerve (V) is located in the rostral and ventral portion of the CPC. The arachnoid covering its dorsal surface is continuous with the sheath lining the rostral surface of the cerebellum. This sheath constitutes the superior limit of the superior cerebellar cistern. The nerve is surrounded by an arachnoid sheath up to the rostral border of the trigeminal ganglion, thus limiting the trigeminal cistern. The superior petrous vein goes through this sheath covering the nerve laterally. This vein is located in the vertical axis of the trigeminal nerve although it is occasionally located at the same level or behind the porus.

The Cochleovestibulofacial Bundle

The cochleovestibulofacial bundle (VII–VIII; figure 1) occupies the middle portion of the CPC. It is termed the cochleovestibulofacial bundle or complex because the nerves exchange their fibers at that point during their course.

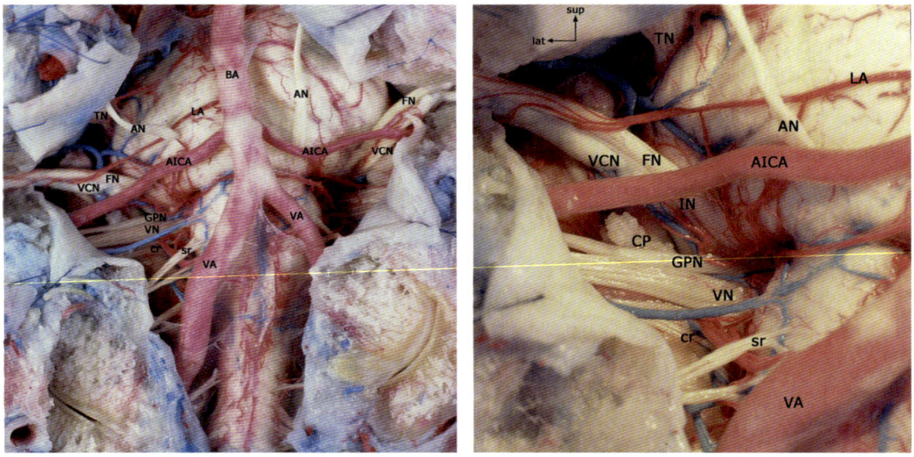

Fig. 1. Photographs showing anterior overview of the brain stem and a magnification on the right CPC after opening the superficial layer of arachnoid. Note the right labyrinthine artery arising from the basilar artery. AICA = Anteroinferior cerebellar artery; AN = abducens nerve; cr = cranial root of the accessory nerve; BA = basilar artery; CP = choroid plexus; FN = facial nerve; GPN = glossopharyngeal nerve; IN = nervus intermedius; LA = labyrinthine artery; sr = spinal root of the accessory nerve; TN = trigeminal nerve; VA = vertebral artery; VCN = vestibulocochlear nerve; VN = vagus nerve.

Facial Nerve (VII)

The facial nerve exits through the pontomedullary groove, goes through the CPC and attains the rostral portion of the porus near its dorsal edge. It has a tubular shape during its entire intracranial pathway. Beginning at its origin, it is in a close relation to the nervus intermedius (or Wrisberg's nerve). This much thinner nerve penetrates the pontomedullary groove at a point slightly more lateral and caudal.

Vestibulocochlear Nerve (VIII)

The vestibulocochlear nerve is larger than the facial nerve. It exits the porus from its dorsocaudal border. It is shaped like a gutter which is initially ventrorostrally concave to the internal acoustic meatus (IAM) before becoming dorsorostral at its pontomedullary termination. The vestibular and cochlear fibers penetrate into the brainstem at the level of the pontomedullary groove, more lateral and caudal than the facial nerve and the nervus intermedius. The vestibulocochlear nerve penetrates medial to the choroid plexus of the fourth ventricle, lateral to the flocculus and caudal to the origin of the glossopharyngeal nerve. Both the facial nerve and the nervus intermedius circulate freely in the cistern without any interposition of the arachnoid trabeculations.

Glossopharyngeal, Vagus and Willis' Accessory Nerves

The glossopharyngeal (IX) vagus (X) and accessory (XI) nerves are located in the dorsocaudal portion of the CPC. The arachnoid sheath covers the pial surface of the medulla oblongata, the vertebral artery and the posteroinferior cerebellar artery. Sometimes, they are attached to it by arachnoid trabeculations.

Vascularization

The CPC communicates medially with the prepontic cistern. The basilary and anteroinferior cerebellar arteries as well as the abducens nerve also continue their course here (figure 1). At this point, these components are intimately attached to the ventral surface of the pons and covered by Liliequist's membrane. The arterial supply to the vestibulocochlear bundle is extremely variable, most often coming from the anteroinferior cerebellar artery (AICA) which branches from the basilar artery. Beginning at its origin, the AICA goes around the pons directly at the level of the pontomedullary groove or a few millimeters above it. Afterwards, it comes in contact with the facial vestibulocochlear bundle at its middle third. Its course goes around the nerve or pushes it against the pons or the porus. The term 'cerebello-acoustico-facial system' comes from the multitude of collaterals seen during its course. Its relationship to adjacent nervous structures is variable since it can go around the brainstem in different manners: either travelling above the vestibulocochlear nerve, between it and the facial nerve or even above the facial nerve. At these different levels, the AICA makes a ventrally convex loop adjacent to the IAM which it sometimes penetrates. Afterwards, it distances itself from the nervous pedicle and arrives in the cerebellum. At that point, the labyrinthine artery, which comes from the AICA, provides the entire vascularization for the components of the IAM. Very infrequently, it comes directly from the basilar artery just above the facial nerve. Complementing this principal source of vascularization, thin arterioles perforate the arachnoid sheath after having followed a variable course inside the IAM and constitute an arteriolar network which anastomoses with the cerebello-labyrinthine system of the middle meningeal system.

The superior petrous vein is the veritable drainage vein for the CPC. It comes from a poorly systematized, dense and anastomatic venous network where the anterior cerebellar vein, the vein from the middle cerebellar pedoncle and the pontotrigeminal vein converge. The superior petrous vein is most often unique (and termed Dandy's vein) and perforates the arachnoid before it goes into the superior petrous sinus. When it is double, the superior ventral petrous vein drains the pontotrigeminal territory while the superior dorsal petrous vein drains the cerebellar territory.

The Acousticofacial Cistern

At the interior of the IAM, an invagination of the dural and arachnoidal meninges extends the CPC laterally thus limiting a subarachnoid space for the intrameatal portion of the cochleovestibulofacial bundle: the acousticofacial cistern.

Contents

The IAM is a cylindrical bony canal located on the medial surface of the petrous portion of the temporal bone, just in front of its middle portion. Medially, it opens into the CPC through the internal porus acousticus or porus. Through this aperture, the IAM allows the cochleovestibulofacial neurovascular complex to pass and travel laterally up to the fundus in a meningeal envelope. It travels in a transversal direction, slightly oblique laterally and ventraly. The fundus corresponds to the medial surface of the vestibule and the tractus spiral of the cochlear area at the base of the columella. It is divided into two levels by the transverse crest (falciform crest).

At the lower level, the branches of the saccular nerve go through the inferior area vestibularis. The foramen singulare (or Morgagni's foramen) is located on the dorsal wall of the meatus, near the floor and gives way to the posterior ampullar nerve. Thc cochlear area, which is in front of it, extends beyond the ventral wall of the meatus. It is perforated by two columns of orifices which allow the fibers, which make up the cochlear nerve, to pass through. These two areas are separated by a truncated vertical crest.

The upper level is narrower and separated by the vertical crest ('Bill's bar') which forms the posterior wall of the origin of the facial canal (called the Fallopian aqueduct). This aqueduct is frankly oblique in a rostrodorsal direction and separates the superior vestibular area from the area of the facial nerve. The superior vestibular area contains a number of superimposed orifices: the anterior ampullar (superior), the lateral and the utricular which give way to the nerves having the same name and make up the superior vestibular nerve. Thus, at the fundus of the meatus, the facial nerve is above the superior vestibular nerve.

By dissecting the normal bony constituents, we have been able to measure the distances which can be useful for locating the IAM. The distance separating the squamous portion of the porus acousticus on a line passing through the vertical crest is between 27 and 28.5 mm. On this line, the axis of the IAM makes a 50–60° angle with the plane of the anterior semicircular canal. The length of the IAM, measured along a line connecting the vertical crest with the porus acousticus, is between 11 and 13 mm. Measurements obtained with computed axial tomography [20] give quite different results compared to these anatomical measurements; they demonstrate important variations between different individuals. The average length of the IAM on a line drawn on the floor ranges between 9.5 and 22 mm (average: 14.9 ± 2.9; median: 15). The average thickness of the roof is 3.4 mm but ranges from 1.5 to 6.5 mm according to the degree of pneumatization of the pars petrosa. At the level of the porus, the average thickness of the roof is 5 mm with a range of 3.5–7 mm. The average axial diameter of the porus is 4.5 mm (range: 2.5–6); the average frontal diameter is 5 mm (range: 3.5–6.5) [21]. The principal structures found in the acoustic meatus are neurovascular. They are surrounded by a meningeal envelope in which CSF circulates.

The Facial and Intermedius Nerves

The facial nerve transports branchiomotor neurofibers originating in the facial nucleus which go to the cutaneous muscles of the face and neck as well as the visceromotor neurofibers originating in the parasympathetic nucleus of the facial nerve, which innervate the lachrymal, nasal and palatine glands. It exits from the middle portion of the pontomedullary groove above the retro-olivary area of the lateral funiculus of the medulla oblongata, in front of the mixed IXth, Xth and XIth nerves.

The nervus intermedius is sensory and thinner than the facial nerve. It transports the sensory neurofibers for the external acoustic meatus, the sensory neurofibers for the anterior two thirds of the tongue and the visceromotor neurofibers going to the submandibular and sublingual glands. It penetrates into the pontomedullary groove slightly behind and lateral to it. While travelling through the IAM, the facial nerve goes towards its ventral and rostral portion before entering into the facial canal at the fundus of the meatus. The nervus intermedius, which is in close contact with the facial nerve, undergoes a torsion which results in a change in position; from dorsocaudal at the level of the porus. It becomes rostral to the facial nerve at the fundus. At this level, the two nerves come into intimate contact with one another before they merge. While it travels through the first portion of its own canal, the facial nerve turns upward and ventrally in the floor of the middle cerebral fossa where it continues in an intervestibulocochlear gorge. This portion, the highest in the facial canal, joins with the second portion of the facial nerve at the level of the fossa of the geniculate ganglion. The vast majority of the cell bodies of both the sensitive and sensorial fibers of the facial nerve are contained in the geniculate ganglion. These ganglion cells are also found at the intrameatal fusion point of the facial and intermedius nerves [22].

The Cochleovestibular Nerve

The cochleovestibular nerve constitutes the peripheral portion or first neuron of the vestibulocochlear pathways. The cell bodies of the neurons of the vestibular root are located in the vestibular ganglion while those of the cochlear root are located in the spiral ganglion. The cochlear and vestibular roots exit the porus and travel towards the CPC which they penetrate at the level of the pontomedullary groove. The three principal roots, grouped together in the form of multifasciculated nerves, become individualized at the fundus. At the porus, only one nerve is individualized, the cochleovestibular nerve, which changes shape during the course of its intrameatal pathway where the fibers of each nerve become grouped together. This cochleovestibular nerve forms a C-shaped gutter with a ventrorostral concavity in which both the facial and intermedius nerves are lodged. The dense and compact cochlear fibers are located ventrally, while the less dense vestibular fibers are grouped together dorsally and caudally [23].

The root of the superior vestibular nerve exits the fundus at the superior vestibular area. The root is composed of the merging of the utricular nerve and the nerves coming from the ampullar crests of the anterior (superior) and lateral (external) semicircular canals. The superior vestibular nerve takes up a dorsal position with respect to the facial nerve from which it is separated at its origin by the vertical crest ('Bill's bar'). The inferior vestibular root, comprised by fibers coming from the saccular nerve, enter the meatus through the inferior vestibular area. It subsequently takes up a caudal position with respect to the superior vestibular nerve with which it merges, thus producing one single vestibular nerve in the meatus. After leaving the singular foramen, the posterior ampullar nerve joins with the inferior vestibular root. This nerve is composed of fibers coming from the posterior ampullar crest.

At its real origin, at the level of the vestibular ganglion, the vestibular nerve resembles a slight transverse bulge which is striated superficially. Located at the fundus, this vestibular ganglion is in fact composed of the merging of the superior vestibular ganglion (called Scarpa's ganglion) and the inferior vestibular ganglion (called Boetcher's ganglion) containing the cell bodies of the neurons of the vestibular root. The cochlear root is constituted by fibers which exit the tractus spiral in the cochlear area. It constitutes the most voluminous element of the cochleovestibular nerve travelling at the ventral and caudal portions of the meatus under the facial nerve. Anastomoses between the different roots are easily recognized; they are vestibulofacial and resemble thin fibers at the level of the porus or a veritable felting near the fundus. They are also vestibulocochlear in the form of a thin, taut root between the utricular nerve and the origin of the cochlear root (or Voit's nerve).

Vascularization
The labyrinthine artery (internal auditory artery) most often comes from the AICA. Its origin is either located before or at the level of its loop which can penetrate at a variable distance into the meatus. More rarely, it comes from the PICA or another accessory cerebellar artery. Only exceptionally does it come directly from the basilar artery. The labyrinthine artery can be unique (51%) or composed of two (45%) or even three roots (4%) [24] thus creating a veritable arterial system in the I.A.M. [25]. Accompanied by the sub-arcuata artery, they enter at the level of the porus and ramify into a multitude of small cochlear, vestibular and vestibulocochlear arterioles supplying the membranous labyrinth and nerves. Its anastomoses with the middle meningeal artery greatly enhance this arteriolar network. The venous network, which is complex and variable, is poorly systematized. The labyrinthine vein drains the meatus and its envelopes before entering the superior petrous sinus.

The Meninges of the Internal Acoustic Meatus
The meningeal sheaths invaginate inside the acoustic meatus, thus allowing the CSF to circulate around the cochleovestibulofacial bundle within an arachnoidal sleeve which constitutes a veritable lateral extension of the subarachnoid spaces (fig. 2, 3). The precise limits of this

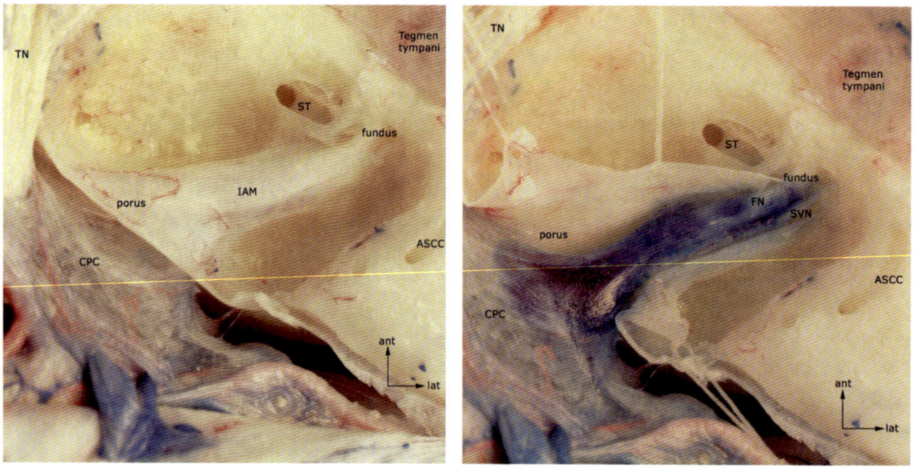

Fig. 2. Photographs showing superior view of the same right-side IAM after removal of its bone roof. After opening the sheath made of dura mater, the arachnoidal membrane is colored with toluidine blue. The external layer of the CPC invaginated into the porus and sheathed the entire vestibulocochleofacial complex in a single arachnoidal sheath. Close to the fundus, the arachnoidal membrane covered the vestibular ganglion. ASCC = Superior semi-circular canal; ST = scala tympani; SVN = superior vestibular nerve.

'acousticofacial' cistern inside the IAM and its relationship to each one of the vasculonervous elements are henceforth readily visible with magnetic resonance imagery. Techniques involving bone softening have enabled us to acquire a detailed description of this anatomy [16].

The Dura Mater

The sheath of the dura which invaginates in the IAM at the porus extends the dura mater which is very close to the medial surface of the petrous portion of the temporal bone. It forms a thick and dense conjunctival tunic intimately adherent to the bony walls of the meatus, resembling a periosteal sheath. The dura mater covering the porus becomes progressively thinner towards the fundus where it covers the transverse crest and the vertical crest as well as the cochlear and vestibular areas. It continues to the level of the facial canal and envelops the geniculate ganglion. It is still present at the level of the tympanic portion of the facial canal as well as in the singular foramen, where it allows the posterior ampullar nerve to pass through.

The Arachnoid

When the dura mater of the meatus is opened, we can see that the arachnoidal layer which limits the CPC invaginates in the acoustic meatus at the porus and that microvessels perforate the arachnoidal layer. These arterioles and venules participate in the vascularization of the cochleovestibulofacial bundle and create an anastomotic network between the meningeal and cerebral and labyrinthine circulation. Near the fundus, the arachnoidal sleeve continues laterally and covers the facial nerve and the emergence of the cochlear nerve from the front and the vestibular ganglion from behind.

The Intrameatal Development of Vestibular Schwannomas

Classic Data

According to Liliequist [6], the arachnoidal diverticule surrounding the facial and vestibulocochlear

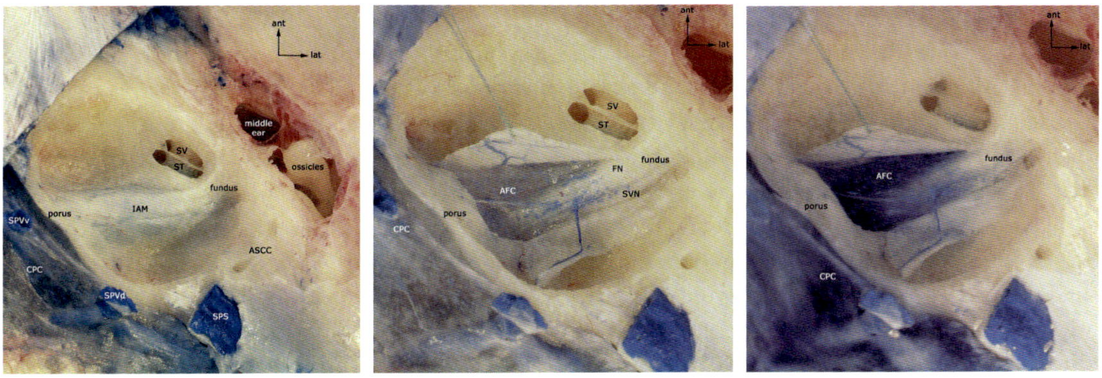

Fig. 3. Photographs showing superior view of the same right-side IAM after removal of its bone roof. The external layer of the CPC invaginated into the porus and sheathed the IAM content in a single arachnoidal sheath. Close to the fundus, the arachnoidal membrane covered a swollen zone corresponding to the vestibular ganglion. A bone bridge was preserved at the porus. The toluidine blue injected into the CSF (B) of the CPC was also visible inside the IAM. This acousticofacial cistern (AFC) extended from the porus to the lateral part of the fundus and embedded the entire vestibulocochleofacial complex, including the vestibular ganglion. SPS = superior petrosal sinus; SV = scala vestibule; SPVd = dorsal part of the superior petrosal; vein SPVv = ventral part of the superior petrosal vein.

nerves in the porus of the IAM usually continues over a short distance into the meatus. Air encephalography has shown that it sometimes continues into the IAM or stops at the porus [26]. Endoscopy has confirmed the existence of a prolongation lateral to the CPC inside the IAM, but has provided no additional details [17]. Matsuno and Rhoton [10] have described the extension of the superficial arachnoidal layer into the IAM covering the nerves during their intrameatal pathway but did not indicate where it stopped.

Only a few descriptions of the surgical anatomy of the arachnoidal sheath in the IAM have been published, in particular those by House [27] and by Perneczky [28], for the most part in acoustic neuroma surgery. Its importance was underlined by French oto-neurological surgery teams as early as 1970 [29] and has been further detailed by Yasargil et al. [30]. Indeed, this last-mentioned researcher was the first, at the onset of the microneurosurgical era, to emphasize the 'arachnoidal cleavage plane' in order to guarantee atraumatic surgery and an uncomplicated neurological outcome. Acoustic neuromas develop in the IAM, at the level of the vestibular ganglion [31]. According to Yasargil et al. [9, 30] the vestibular ganglion is described as extra-arachnoidal, in other words outside the arachnoidal sleeve covering the facial and cochlear nerves in the meatus. During tumor growth, the arachnoidal layer limiting the CPC is pushed medially to form an arachnoid duplication (or even a triplication) before arriving at the adjacent cisterns. This superposition of layers creates a cleavage plane which circumvents the disastrous consequences of a dissection between the arachnoid and the tumor capsule or between the arachnoid and the pia mater. This description remains a major reference and is still found in numerous textbooks on surgical technique [32–38].

Recent Data and Surgical Perspectives

Recent anatomic and histologic studies using bone softening techniques [16] have demonstrated the consistency in the arachnoidal relationships of the cochleovestibulofacial bundle.

The arachnoidal layer doubles the dura mater of the meatus along its entire length. As a result, the vestibular and cochlear nerve fibers penetrate the arachnoid very early, as soon as they enter into the meatus. This fixes the position of the vestibular ganglion in the subarachnoid space. Neuromas which arise at this level are thus all contained in the acousticofacial cistern. Consequently, the surgical importance of the arachnoidal layer is not supported by the theory of arachnoidal wrapping during the extrameatal growth of a tumor arising in an extra-arachnoidal location.

The controversy concerning this description [9] has been summarized by Pellet and Roche [39]. They maintain that when the dura mater is opened along the posterior surface of the petrous bone and the tumor is approached just where it exits the IAM, one invariably discovers an arachnoidal ring surrounding the base of the bud inside the canal. This ring is the reflection zone where the arachnoid, which lines the tumor over its hemispheric convexity, covers it like a bursa. In extra-meatal schwannomas, the tumor pulp and the nerves are not covered by any arachnoidal plane in the IAM, 'as if' the arachnoid of the meatus had been driven back from the fundus towards the porus. According to Pellet and Roche [39], the fact that the arachnoid surrounding the tumor and the nerves in the canal has to be torn to attain a schwannoma which is located inside the canal, proves that it is manifestly intra-arachnoidal. In addition, they state that the tumor is always clearly adherent to the periphery of the porus when it first appears in the CPC. They add that the arachnoidal ring is located precisely at that level, 'as if' its adherences had sectioned the armhole of the arachnoidal sleeve inside the canal and 'as if' the arachnoid of the posterior fossa had quite naturally proliferated in order to seal off the orifice which had become completely opened along its entire length. As the tumor continued to grow, it could have wrapped itself in this arachnoid and continued into the extra-arachnoidal space. A question remains: what happens to the canal's arachnoidal sleeve? It may undergo atrophy due to tumor growth inside the canal, absence of communication with the subarachnoid spaces and absence of CSF. Indeed, when the nerves and the tumor are dissected within the IAM, the surgeon often lacerates thin trabeculations which may correspond to these arachnoidal remains. For Pellet, all these postulates are capable of reconciling the anatomic [16] with perioperative findings [30]. Finally, according to Pellet and Roche [39], in the CPC schwannomas are surrounded by an arachnoidal layer which generally separates them from the nerves after their exit from the canal, providing that these nerves remain on the periphery and have not become wrapped inside the tumor. Even when very large schwannomas are present, the facial nerve is thus placed on the tumor borders and may be cleaved in the CPC. Large tumors often encompass the vestibulocochlear nerve which can only be clearly individualized where it exits the brainstem, just before it enters the tumor, thus constituting a kind of pedicle. Nerves which are not invaded and merely pushed towards the periphery are often fairly easy to cleave provided that the tumor has been neatly hollowed out, the dissection has been carefully performed and that the tumor mass has been removed by following the axis of the nerves, without exerting any lateral traction.

References

1 Vinas FC, Fandino R, Dujovny M, Chavez V: Microsurgical anatomy of the supraratentorial arachnoidal trabecular membranes and cisterns. Neurol Res 1994;16:417–424.

2 Magendie F: Recherches physiologiques et cliniques sur le liquide cephalorachidien ou cerebrospinal. Mequignon-Marvis Paris, 1842.

3 Lushka H: Die anatomie des menschlichen kopfes. Tubingen 1867. Cité par Yasargil MG. Subarachnoid cisterns; in Yasargil MG (ed): Microneurosurgery. New York: Geng Thieme Verlag, 1984, vol 1, pp 5–53.

4 Key A, Retzius G: Studien in der anatomie der nerversistems und des bindegewebes. Surgeon General's Office Library. Stockholm: Samson & Wallin, 1875.
5 Locke CE, Naffziger CH: The cerebral subarachnoid system. Arch Neurol Psy 1924;12:411–418.
6 Liliequist B: The anatomy of the subarachnoid cisterns. Acta Radiol 1956;46:61–71.
7 Yaşargil MG, Konstantin K: Anatomical observations of the subarchnoid cisterns of the brain during surgery. J Neurosurg 1976;44:298–302.
8 Yaşargil MG: Microsurgical anatomy of the basal cisterns and vessels of the brain, diagnostic studies, general operatives techniques and pathological considerations of the intracranial anevrysm; in Microsurgery, Georg Thieme, Stuttgart, 1984, Vol 1.
9 Yaşargil MG, Lescanne E, Velut S, Lefrancq T, Destrieux C: The internal acoustic meatus. J Neurosurg 2002;97:1014–1017.
10 Matsuno H, Rhoton AL: Microsurgical anatomy of the posterior fossa cistern. Neurosurgery 1988;23:58–80.
11 Vinas FC, Dujovny M, Fandino R, Chavez V: Microsurgical anatomy of the infratentorial trabecular membranes and subarachnoid cisterns. Neurol Res 1996;18:117–125.
12 Vinas FC, Fandino R, Dujovny M, Chavez V: Microsurgical anatomy of the arachnoidal trabecular membranes and cisterns at the level of the tentorium. Neurol Res 1996;18:305–312.
13 Velut S: L'arachnoïde des citernes basales de l'encéphale Thèse d'Université, Amiens, 1991.
14 Destrieux C, Velut S, Kakou MK, Lefrancq T, Arbeille B, Santini JJ: A new concept in Dorello's canal microanatomy: the petroclival venou confluence. J Neurosurg 1997;87:67–72.
15 Destrieux C, Kakou MK, Velut S, Lefrancq T, Jan M: Microanatomy of the hypophyseal boundaries. J Neurosurg 1998;88:743–752.
16 Lescanne E, Velut S, Lefrancq T, Destrieux C: The internal acoustic meatus and its meningeal layers: a microanatomical study. J Neurosurg 2002;97:1191–1197.
17 Fukushima T: Endoscopy of Meckel's cavum, cisterna magna and cerebellopontine angle. J Neurosurg 1978;48:302–306.
18 Matula C, Tschabitscher M, Kitz K, Reinprecht A, Koos WT: Neuroanatomical details under endoscopical view – Relevant for radiosurgery? Acta Neurochir 1995;(suppl 63):1–4.
19 Lescanne E, Velut S, Destrieux C, Pollak A, Robier A: Méat acoustique interne (MAI); in Société Française d'Oto-rhino-laryngologie et Chirurgie de la Face et du Cou (ed): Le neurinome de l'acoustique. 2001, pp 25–35.
20 Driscoll CL, Jackler RK, Pitts LH, Banthia V: Is the entire fundus of the internal auditory canal visible during the middle fossa approach for acoustic neuroma? Am J Otol 2000;21:382–388.
21 Pialoux P, Freyss G, Narcy P, Saint-Macary M, Davaine F: Contribution à l'anatomie stéréotaxique du conduit auditif interne. Ann Otol Laryngol 90;7–8 (Paris) 409–422.
22 Gacek RR: On the duality of the facial nerve ganglion. Laryngoscope 1998;108:1077–1086.
23 Schefter RP, Harner SG: Histologic study of the vestibulocochlear nerve. Ann Otol Rhinol Laryngol 1986;95:146–150.
24 Mazzoni A: Internal auditory canal: Arterial relationship at the porus acusticus. Ann Otol Rhinol Laryngol 1969;68:798–814.
25 Fisch U: Anatomie chirurgicale du système artériel du conduit auditif interne. Rev Layngol Otol Rhinol 1968;11–12, 659–671.
26 Portmann M, Sterkers JM, Charachon R, Chouard CH: Le conduit auditif interne (anatomie, pathologie, chirurgie). Lib Arnette (ed), Paris, 1973, p 296.
27 House WF: Acoustic neuroma. Arch Otolaryngol 1968;88:576–715.
28 Perneczky A: Blood Supply of acoustic neuromas. Acta neurochirugica 1980;52:209–218.
29 Pertuiset et coll: Les neurinomes de l'acoustique développés dans l'angle ponto-cérébelleux. Neurochirurgie 1970;(suppl 1):1–140.
30 Yaşargil MG, Smith RD, Gasser JC: Microsurgical approach to acoustic neuromas; in Springer-Verlag (ed): Advances and technical standards in neurosurgery, Wien New York, 1977, Vol 4, pp 94–128.
31 Sterkers JM, Perre J, Vial P, Foncin JF: The origin of acoustic neuromas. Acta Otolaryngol (Stockh) 1987;103:427–431.
32 Tarlov E: Total one-stage suboccipital microsurgical removal of acoustic neuromas of all sizes: with emphasis on arachnoid planes and on saving the facial nerve. Surg Clin North Am 1980;60:565–591.
33 Pellet W, Cannoni M, Pech A: Oto-Neuro-Chirurgie, Springer-Verlag Berlin, 1989, pp 21–29.
34 Sterkers JM: Chirurgie du neurinome de l'acoustique. Paris: Arnette, 1991, pp 20–22.
35 Rosenwasser RH, Bucheit WA: Acoustic neuromas. Suboccipital approach; in Apuzzo MJL (ed): Brain Surgery. New York: Churchill Livingstone, 1993, pp 1743–1772.
36 Portmann M, Richards AES, Sterkers JM: Rhino-Otological Microsurgery of the Skull Base. Edinburgh: Churchill Livingstone, 1995, p 198.
37 Ramsden RT: Vestibular schwanomma, otology; in Kerr AG, Booth JB (eds): Scott-Brown's Otolaryngology, ed 6. Oxford: Butterworth-Heinemann, 1997, p 4.
38 Sanna M, Caylan R: Atlas of Acoustic Neurinoma Microsurgery. New York: Thieme, 1998, pp 18, 56, 58.
39 Pellet W, Roche PH: Microsurgery of vestibular schwannoma: persisting questions Neurochirurgie 2004;50:195–243.

Stéphane Velut, MD, PhD
Laboratoire d'Anatomie de la Faculté de Médecine, Université de Tours
10, bvd Tonnellé, BP 3223
FR–37032 Tours Cedex 1 (France)
Tel. +33 247 366 086, Fax +83 247 366 207, E-Mail velut@med.univ-tours.fr

Régis J, Roche P-H (eds): Modern Management of Acoustic Neuroma.
Prog Neurol Surg. Basel, Karger, 2008, vol 21, pp 54–64

Radiosurgery: Operative Technique, Pitfalls and Tips

Jean Régis · Manabu Tamura · David Wikler · Denis Porcheron · Olivier Levrier

Service de Neurochirurgie Fonctionnelle et Stéréotaxique, Hôpital d'Adulte de la Timone, Marseille, France

Abstract

Rationale: From frame placement to dose administration, each step of the procedure must be optimized in every detail for better preservation of global precision, accuracy, safety and efficacy. **Methods:** Quality control for resolution, accuracy and acquisition parameter optimization of both computed tomography (CT) scanners and magnetic resonance imaging (MRI) must be performed. Inaccuracies should then be quantified through systematic combination of MRI and CT in the radiosurgery planning system. Topography of petrous structures such as cochlea, vestibulum and facial nerve canal should be visible on the CT scan. T_1-weighted volumetric MRI pulse sequences (3DT1) show a contrast-enhanced signal that is useful for both the pons interface delineation in Koos III cases, and the canal ending. High-resolution CISS T_2-weighted volumetric pulse sequences (3DT2) allow direct nerve visualization and give superior stereotactic definition attributable to their better resolution minimizing partial volume effects and to their lower magnetic susceptibility minimizing distortions. The 3DT2 pulse sequences with contrast injection, show improved distinction between the pons and the nerves due to signal differences within the schwannomas. Fat saturation pulse sequences are of interest in postmicrosurgery conditions. The previous technical requirements and the dose planning elaboration will be balanced depending on the lesion volume staging (Koos), treatment history (microsurgery), clinical condition (hearing quality), pathological context (NF2) or age of the patient. The recommended marginal dose is 11–12 Gy. Tumor volume delineation allows the calculation of conformity, selectivity and gradient indexes. These global indexes must be weighted according to the relationship to critical structures and functional status of the patient. **Conclusions:** As an exclusively image-guided surgical method, radiosurgery requires special attention in the choice of imaging modalities and their acquisition parameters need extreme care. Technical nuances during the elaboration of the dose planning itself will directly influence both the toxicity risk and the chance of cure.

In contrast to radiotherapy where the attempt to spare normal tissue is based on the search of a biological differential effect related to fractionation, in radiosurgery a high dose is delivered in a single session and the safety is based on a topological differential effect. Thus, accuracy and precision in radiosurgery turns out to be particularly important. Very high spatial accuracy is required for both imaging and dose planning particularly in vestibular schwannomas (VSs) due to their close contact to highly functional and fragile surrounding structures. The Gamma Knife with its fixed 201 sources provides us with an excellent fall off of dose. However, in order to achieve a highly accurate and precise radiosurgical treatment the precision and accuracy of the radiosurgical instrument is crucial but not sufficient. Each step of the procedure needs to be secured in order to guarantee safety, and quality control will play a major role to ascertain this safety. As a purely image-guided surgery, where immediate control of the effect of the procedure is not possible, radiosurgery requires a very strict quality control of the whole procedure, especially of the imaging part.

Frame Application

The majority of the neurosurgeons still consider frameless procedures as insufficiently precise and accurate for single-dose radiation therapy especially in VSs, where the sparing of the surrounding structures requires high selectivity of the dose delivery. Modern pain management strategies enable to minimize the pain and discomfort related to the frame application procedure. Frame application must guarantee a reliable fixation of the frame to the head with no possible movement of the frame on the head. Frame fixation must be done taking into account both the constraints related to the imaging and the constraints related to the radiosurgery technique.

Imaging

As an exclusively image-guided surgical method, radiosurgery requires special attention in the choice of imaging modalities and their acquisition parameters need extreme care. Quality control for resolution and accuracy of computed tomography (CT) scanners must be performed. Magnetic resonance imaging (MRI) distortions should be limited through magnetic field homogeneity adjustment (shimming) and acquisition parameter optimization. These inaccuracies should then be quantified through systematic combination of MRI and CT in the radiosurgery planning system. MRI pulse sequence selection criteria are defined by their ability to delineate tumor contrast enhancement and to image cranial nerves' and vessels' relative arrangement in the cistern and canal. The topography of intrapetrous neuro-otologic structures such as the cochlea, labyrinth and facial nerve canal should be visible. The exact definition of the lesion's actual extension at the fundus of the internal auditory canal (IAC) may require specific technical solutions. The previous technical requirements will be balanced depending on the lesion volume staging (Koos), treatment history (microsurgery), clinical condition (hearing quality), pathological context (neurofibromatosis type 2) or age of the patient.

T_1-weighted volumetric MRI pulse sequences (3DT1) show a contrast-enhanced signal that is useful for both the pons interface delineation in Koos III cases and the lateral part of the IAC in Ohata A and B. On the other hand, 3DT1 introduces inaccuracies from magnetic susceptibility distortions and partial volume effects. High-resolution constructive interference in steady state (CISS) T_2-weighted volumetric pulse sequences (3DT2) give superior stereotactic definition attributable to their better resolution (0.5 mm) minimizing partial volume effects and to their lower magnetic susceptibility minimizing distortions. Thus, 3DT2 allows direct nerve visualization. Moreover, this pulse sequence with contrast injection shows improved distinction between the pons and the nerves due to signal differences within the schwannomas. Fat saturation pulse sequences are of interest in postmicrosurgery conditions.

Radiology phase quality is critical and its complexity requires high commitment to obtain satisfactory clinical results. It appears to us that sole 3DT1 MRI modality does not conform with minimum security criteria.

Identification of Anatomical Structures

Precise identification of the critical structures surrounding the tumor, in additionally to a good imaging requires a good knowledge of the regional anatomy.

The facial nerve (VIIth nerve) includes the VIIth motor nerve and the VIIbis, which is a sensitive, sensory and secretory nerve. The motor cortex projects corticospinal tract toward the contralateral motor nucleus of the VIIth nerve only for the motor fibers of the inferior half of the face and both the ipsi and contralateral motor nucleus for the superior half of the face. Thus, a supranuclear injury spares the superior facial motor function at the opposite of a peripheral injury. After turning around the VIth nerve nucleus, the fibers of the VIIth nerve appear in the pontomedullary fissure anterior to the VIIIth and posterior to the VIth nerve. The VIIbis is formed by general somatic sensory, vegetative, special visceral afferent sensory, secretory fibers projecting on their spinal, solitary, lacrimal and superior salivary nuclei, respectively. The VIIth nerve runs through the cerebellopontine cistern transversally with a slight cranial and ventral course toward the IAC and reaches the first portion of the Faloppian canal once the vertical crest (Bill's barr) of the upper fundus has been crossed (fig. 1). The motor fibers cover the sensitive fibers. The course of the VIIth nerve in the petrous bone is separated into 3 segments. The first portion (labyrinthine) runs over the internal ear and after 3–4 mm ends in the geniculate ganglion after a 75° curve backward. The second portion (tympanic) is 12–13 mm long and mesial to the middle ear cavity above the promontory and under the loop of the lateral semicircular canal; it ends with a 90–120° downward curvature. The third portion (mastoid segment) is 15–20 mm long, runs vertically into the mastoid air cells toward the stylomastoid foramen and then splits into a superior and inferior branch at the level of the parotid gland.

The sensory fibers (Ramsay-Hunt skin area) running to the spinal nucleus of the trigeminal nerve and the gustatory fibers (from the anterior two thirds of the tongue) running to the solitary nucleus, reach the geniculate ganglion by the way of the lingual nerve and chorda tympani which joins the Faloppian canal at the level of its third portion. The vegetative fibers from the lacrimal and superior salivary nuclei leave the geniculate ganglion and course either toward the sphenopalatin ganglion (by the way of the great superficial petrous nerve and then the pterygoid nerve) or toward the submandibular nerve (by the way of the lingual nerve and chorda tympani).

The VIIIth nerve arises at the lateral end of the canal from the fusion of the cochlear (itself arising at the level of the modiolus), superior vestibular (utricular nerve) and inferior vestibular (saccular nerve) nerves.

Classically, in the lateral part of the IAC the VIIth and VIIbis nerves are located in the anterosuperior quadrant, the cochlear in the anteroinferior quadrant, the vestibular superior in the posterosuperior quadrant and the vestibular inferior in the posteroinferior quadrant. Around the middle of the auditory canal, these three nerves merge into a single stem. The Schwannomas usually arise from the vestibular nerve (more frequently from the inferior one) in the Scarpa ganglion (vestibular ganglion) region close to the Obersteiner-Redlich area. The VIIIth nerve goes through the cerebellopontine cistern downward and backward to the pontomedullary fissure and reaches the brain stem posteriorly to the VIIth nerve.

Fibers reach the cochlear dorsal and ventral nuclei close to the inferior cerebellar peduncle. After going through the midline, the cochlear path follows to the inferior colliculus by the way of the lateral lemniscus pathway. The vestibular fibers run to the vestibular nucleus at the level of the floor of the IVth ventricle. The anteroinferior cerebellar artery gives to the VIIth nerve a part of its vasculature. The petrous branch of the middle meningeal artery, the stylomastoid artery and the retroauricular one also supply the VIIth nerve. More rarely, schwannomas can rise from the cochlea [1, 2] or the vestibule labyrinth [3].

Stereotactic Imaging

We consider the pertinence and quality of the stereotactic imaging as key factors in the strategy of complication avoidance. No single imaging is sufficient for the elaboration of a high-resolution

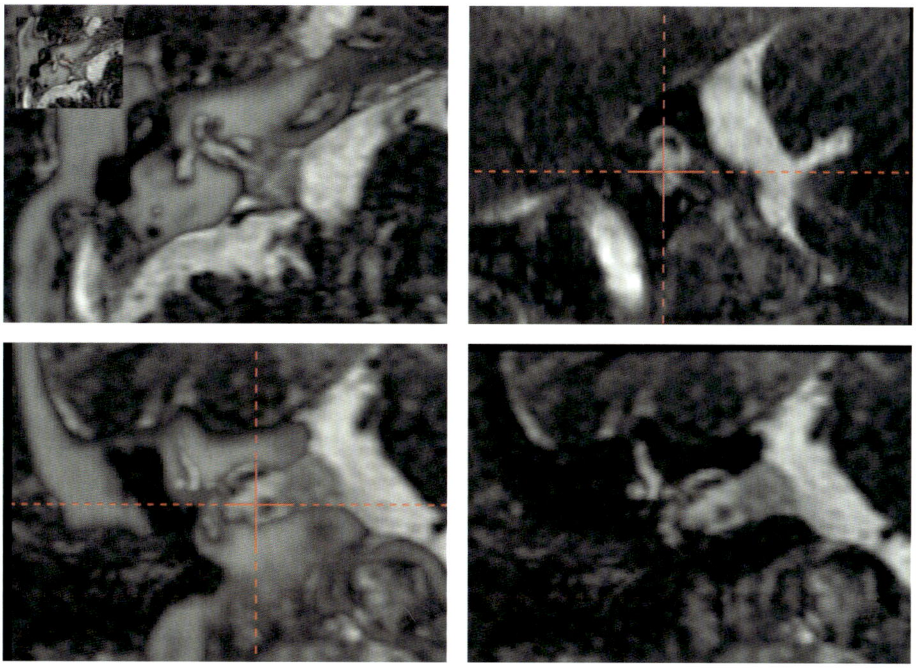

Fig. 1. Perioperative radiological stereotactic anatomy in a case of a Koos II VS on the right side. Nerves in the canal are visualized in axial view fusing the injected CISS and the bony window of the CT scan (**a**), sagittal view of the CISS (**b**), coronal view fusing the bony window of the CT scan and the injected CISS (**c**) or only the injected CISS (**d**). The cochlear nerve is well visualized in the canal entering the modiulus (**a**) or at the level of the cross in sagittal (**b**) or coronal (**c**) view. On coronal (**c** or **d**) and sagittal (**b**) planes, the facial motor nerve is easily identified at the anterior superior part of the canal. At the posterior part of the canal, the vestibular superior and vestibular inferior nerves are directly visualized.

dose planning as long as each modality has its own limitations. A basic idea is to always rely on both the high quality of the MRI and the high resolution and low distortion rate of the CT scan.

In our institution, MR investigation always includes several sequences. High-resolution 0.5-mm^3 3-D T_2-weighted axial sequences like the CISS are performed with and without contrast (constructive interference in steady-state three-dimensional MR, Siemens Magnetom 1.5 T, Erlangen, Germany; FOV 250 mm, TR 15.7 ms, TE 7.85 ms, angle 70%, 64 slices). Similar sequences have been developed by other manufacturers.

The noninjected CISS have the following advantages (fig. 1): (1) high resolution (0.5-mm cubic pixel size); (2) spin echo sequence with few distortion; (3) good visualization of the limit between the cerebrospinal fluid (CSF) and the tumor in the cistern [4]; (4) good visualization of the nerves in the cistern [4, 5] especially in small lesions (Koos I or II).

The noninjected CISS have the following disadvantages: (1) no visualization of the limit between the nerve and the tumor when two structures are in close contact; (2) no visualization between the tumor and the bone of the auditory canal.

Thus the injection of gadolinium corrects these limits. With contrast, the relationship between the tumor and the nerves is dramatically

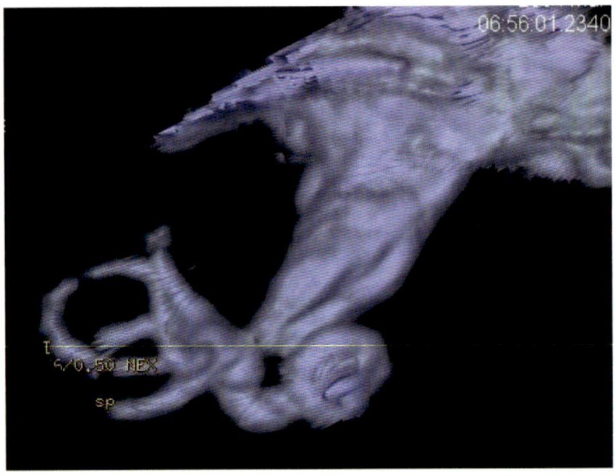

Fig. 2. 3-D reconstruction of a CISS sequence after injection (view from above forward right). The cochlea and vestibule are seen first. The tumor in the canal presents the imprint of the VIIth nerve on its anterosuperior aspect.

improved. The limit of the intracanalicular portion is perfectly visualized. However, sometimes the enhancement of the tumor signal can make the delineation of the limit with the CSF more difficult, which makes it mandatory to systematically use both the noninjected and injected CISS. These high-resolution 3-D sequences allow good 3-D volume reconstruction, which is especially useful to visualize the complex 3-D relationship between the lesion and the nerves in the canal (fig. 2).

The third sequence is a 3-D T_1 axial sequence with gadolinium (MPRage, Siemens Magnetom 1.5 T; matrix 230 × 256, FOV 256 mm, TR 2,160 ms, TE 4.88 ms, angle 15°, 144 slices 1.5-mm thickness).

The advantages of this kind of sequence are: (1) good visualization of limits of the lesion with the bone and the CSF; (2) Good visualization of the extent of the lesion in the canal [6].

The disadvantages of this sequence are: (1) as a gradient echo sequence, this sequence is frequently more sensitive to magnetic field heterogeneity, distortions are frequently detected especially in the Z direction; (2) other structures than the VS can be enhanced (arachnoid hyperemia, surrounding vessels), which can lead to the inaccurate definition of the limits of the lesion; (3) global overestimation of the lesion volume due to the reconstruction algorithm, which underestimates the volume of the hypointense structures (schwannoma) in hyperintense environment (CSF) on T_2 sequences and overestimates the volume of the hyperintense lesion (schwannoma) in a hypointense environment (CSF) on T_1 sequences.

CT scan in bony window is systematically performed in our Institution for VS. Parameters of the acquisition are those used for high-resolution petrous bone investigations (with contrast).

The advantages of the CT scan are: (1) its low distortion (but not null) allows to use it as a reference to check the distortion of the MR sequences; the limits of the intracanalicular portion of the VS on MR sequences are compared with the limits of the bony canal itself as displayed on the CT scan (fig. 1); (2) the correct volume of the VS is better appreciated on the CT scan as a compromise between the overestimated volume of the 3DT1 gadolinium and 3DT2 MR sequences.

As demonstrated in table 1, none all these examinations have limits and are complementary, which means that they need to be associated in order to define accurately the real topology of the different portions of the lesion, its extent in the canal, relationship to the nerves and to the brainstem.

Dose Planning

Dose planning is certainly the most typical neurosurgical instant in the radiosurgical procedure for the treatment of VSs (fig. 3). Indeed, it is a key moment in which the therapeutic choices will have a major influence on the clinical results, in terms of efficacy and safety. The therapist has to inform the patient about the rationale of the treatment, its limitations, the expected results, and the specific risks. A serious knowledge of the radiosurgical technique, of the principles of dosimetry, and

Table 1. Four technically different periods

	Period			
	July 1992 to July 1997	July 1997 to May 2000	June 2000 to July 2006	After July 2006
CT and MRI	Yes	Yes	Yes	Yes
Dose, Gy	12–14	12–14	12–14	12–14
Dosimetry	Kula	GammaPlan	GammaPlan	New LGP
	Separated management of the images and dose planning	Simultaneous management of the images and dose planning coregistered in the same stereotactic space	Simultaneous management of the images and dose planning coregistered in the same stereotactic space	Simultaneous management of the images and dose planning coregistered in the same stereotactic space
LGK	Model B	Model B	Model C	PerfeXion model
APS	No	No	APS	Fully robotized
Fusion MRI/CT	No	Yes	Yes	Yes
Images	Manual definition on films	Direct transfer of digital images from the MR scan to the workstation	Direct transfer of digital images from the MR scan to the workstation	Direct transfer of digital images from the MR scan to the workstation

LGK = Leksell Gamma Knife; APS = Automatic Positioning System.

the therapist's personal experience, will allow an a posteriori analytic study of the influence of the dosimetry therapeutic choices on the patient's outcome. The correlation between the preoperative therapeutic choices and the postoperative clinico-radiological information is mandatory to optimize the therapeutic strategies. These therapeutic choices should be the result of a thinking integrating the clinical status of the patient, the understanding of the specific pathology of VS, the awareness of the other therapeutic choices, as well as the knowledge of the radiological and surgical anatomy.

The way a certain number of parameters will be defined during the dosimetry planning will have a major influence on the clinical results. This explains the great variability of clinical results from one operator to another, for the same radiological and radiosurgical tools. This reinforces the necessity of a specific and long-term training, associated with continuous education and a good knowledge of the latest literature.

Parallel to the technical improvement of modern imaging, both the Gamma Knife radiosurgery and dose planning techniques have been dramatically improved (table 2). The understanding of the relationship between dosimetric strategy and functional outcome has also improved with the increasing worldwide experience [7]. These technical and conceptual changes have been followed by a significant improvement of dose planning and clinical results, especially in terms of functional preservation [8, 9].

Dose Planning Procedure

Registration of the Stereotactic *Images in the Stereotactic Space.* The definition of the fiducial

Table 2. Contribution of each imaging modality

	MPR inj.	CISS	CISS inj.	FatSat	CT scan
Low distortion	–/+	++	++	–	++++
Partial volume effect	+	+++	+++	–	+++
Visualization of the nerves in the CSF	–	+++	++	–	–
Distinction vessels tumor	–	+	++	+	–
Distinction nerves tumor	–	+	+++	–	–
Distinction postop. fat and tumor	–	–	+	+++	+/–
Distinction brainstem tumor (Koos III–IV)	+++	–	++	+	+/–
Petrous bone structures (cochlea, vestibule, ...)	–	–	–	–	+++
Extent in the canal	++	+	++	–	–

MPR = Magnetisation Prepared Rapid Gradient Echo (contrast 3DT1 volumetric MRI); FatSat = Fat Saturated T1 MRI.

points from the indicator box (MR and CT scan) is made either manually or automatically. This is highly recommended at this stage as a grey scale is narrow enough to allow visualization of mainly the highest intensity part of these points. When slices at the beginning and end of the acquired volume display more distortion, manual fiducial registration excluding these slices can be recommended as long as a sufficient number of slices is kept to avoid tilt errors.

Delineation of the Contrast Enhancement on the 3DT1 Acquisition. This is very helpful in the accurate definition of the target and will allow calculation of conformity and selectivity indexes.

Elaboration of the First Draft Dose Planning on the 3DT1 Acquisition. Multisocentric strategy is, at least for Gamma Knife surgery dose planning, the best way to create extremely conformational and specific dose planning. Additionally, when well managed, this strategy allows a good control of the dose distribution in the target volume (homogeneity). The risk in insufficiently educated or experienced hands is to end up with an unnecessarily large number of isocenters with a severe deterioration of the dose gradient outside the target. The gradient index (for us the ratio PIV25%/PIV50%) should be less than 3.0. By the way, two dose plans with similar conformity and selectivity indexes can be of very different quality and differentiated by their gradient index.

Visualization of the Dose Planning on the Bony Window Images of the CT Scan. This stage allows to check the absence of distortion. When the limits of the intracanalicular part of the VS fit perfectly with the bony IAC, distortion of these two modalities is unlikely. Usually, this comparison shows that the 3DT1 is overestimating the real volume of the lesion.

Dose Planning Is Checked on the 3DT2 Sequence (CISS without Injection). If there is a discrepancy between CT and 3DT1 images, technical arguments must be found indicating which modality is distorted and the appropriate correction must be applied. Thus, comparison of the CISS with the two other sets of images is very helpful. Additionally, the CISS has a higher resolution than the 3DT1 and allows a more realistic evaluation of the limits and exact volume of the lesion. Fusion with CT bony window usually demonstrates this fact.

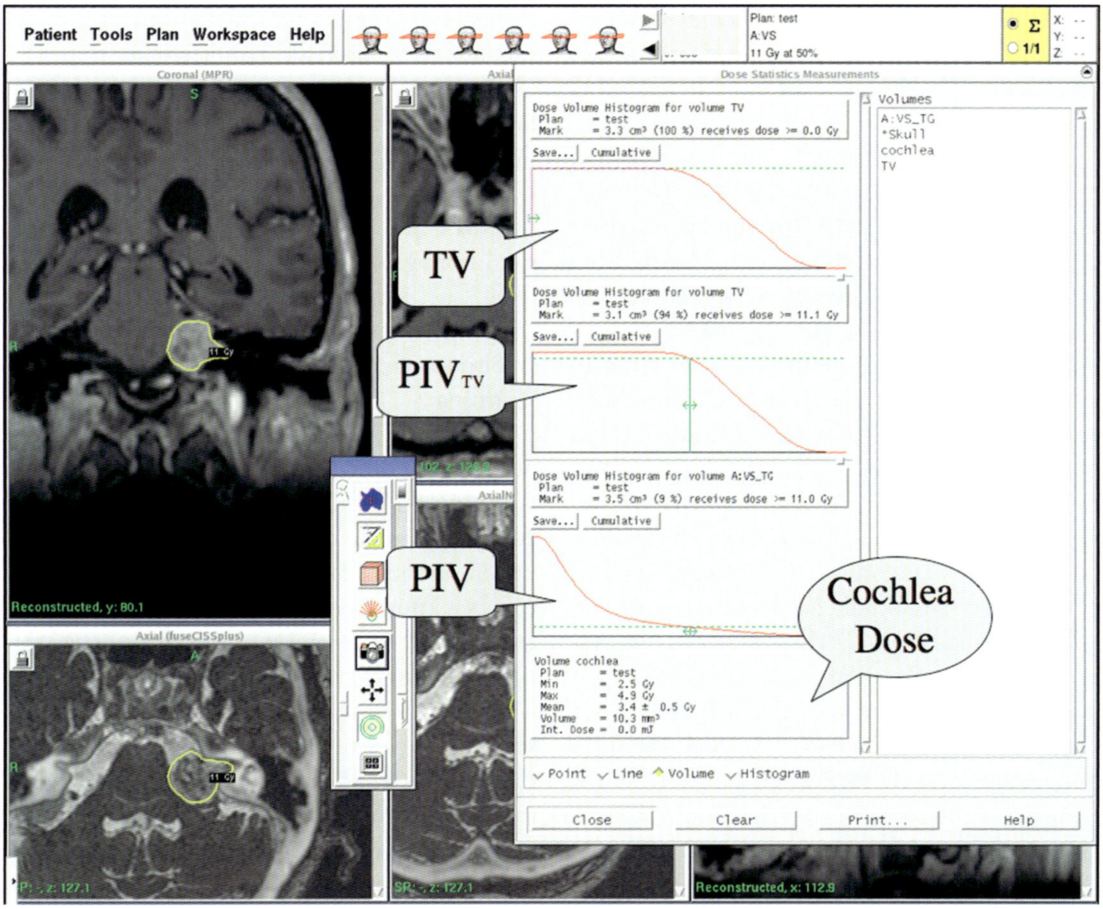

Fig. 3. Doseplanning for a KoosIII VS. Histogramms allow calculation of the Conformity, selectivity and gradient indexes by the measurement of the PIV (50% isodose volume), the TV (tumor volume), PIVTV (part of the TV covered by the PIV) and the volume of the 25% isodose volume.

Definition of the VIIth and VIIIth Nerves' Topography. In small (stage I and II) tumors, these nerves are always well visualized at their emergence or entry in the brainstem.

Local Corrections of the Dose Plan according to the 3DT2 Injected. The topology of the nerves at the contact of the lesion is ill defined in CISS sequences without contrast (both are black). Enhancement of the tumor by the injection allows the delineation of the nerves in their cisternal portion in spite of their contact with the tumor. The dose planning is then modified in order to minimize the dose delivery to these structures.

Management of the Dose Distribution inside the Target Volume. No healthy structures run through the tumor in unilateral VS. Thus, dose homogeneity is not a goal. On the contrary, we intend to create deliberate heterogeneity. We shape the dose distribution in the volume with the goal to displace the highest doses (high spot) in the extracanalicular part of the tumor far from the VIIth and VIIIth nerves. All the 'possible tips' are used to preserve the steepest falloff of dose at the interface of the tumor with these nerves and with the cochlea (in patients with serviceable hearing).

Conformity, Selectivity and Gradient Indexes. Conformity, selectivity and gradient indexes are calculated and eventually the dose planning corrected.

Dose Selection. Since 1992, our dose selection policy has not significantly changed. The marginal dose selected is 12 Gy. In patients with deafness and facial palsy who have previously been operated on microsurgically, we sometimes use higher doses [9, 10]. In patients with functional hearing (Gardner-Robertson 1–2) or large lesions, we frequently use 11 or 10 Gy. This dose regimen recommended by Georg Noren [11] has been demonstrated by Flickinger et al. [12] and Miller et al. [13] to be associated with a lower incidence of neuropathy. The stability of our dose policy allows us to evaluate the influence of other parameters, especially our learning curve and technical advances [14]. Thus, we have progressively observed the disappearance of facial palsy, which has now become extremely rare in our Center and in other centers with a high technical and human level of practice [15–21].

Quality Control

Gamma Knife radiosurgery treatment of VSs requires high accuracy for the prescribed dose definition and delivery. The main potential sources of error are [22]: (1) wrong patient identification; (2) wrong patient imaging; (3) frame loosely fixed; (4) wrong fiducial box fixation during imaging; (5) imaging distortion; (6) insufficient conformity selectivity of the dose planning; (7) unadapted dose selection; (8) wrong setting of the coordinates.

Imaging errors in stereotactic localization must be a permanent concern. The treatment is only as accurate as the least accurate process in the whole chain of events from patient scanning to patient treatment (accuracy of the Leksell frame, MR and Gamma Knife are 0.3, 0.7 and 0.3 mm, respectively). The main factors contributing to the error are the anatomical distortions of imaging modalities used for treatment planning.

Pixel position is coded with a unique magnetic field strength and any fluctuation from the theoretical value of the field creates geometrical distortion. Image distortion comes from: (1) magnetic field in homogeneity (static field or nonlinear gradients); (2) susceptibility artifacts (air/tissue, hemosiderin); (3) chemical shift; (4) eddy currents from the Leksell frame.

Shimming must be done systematically before scanning.

Theoretically, distortion measurement must be performed systematically both in phantom scanning with and without the frame and in patient scanning as long as there is individual patient-induced distortion. However, the phantom is a known object target but not the patient head. Thus, we cannot measure directly patient-induced distortion. What we can evaluate with a phantom is the inherent distortion from the scanner and frame. Consequently, we can reduce these distortions by modifying the scanning protocol. The optimal solution is to obtain a sequence giving a set of low distortion images that have isotropic voxels. QA is not optional. We use the most accurate radiosurgical device in the world. Unless we are serious about image distortion, we are wasting its accuracy. CT is considered as the reference for spatial accuracy after appropriate scanner quality control using the stereotactic fiducial system. MRI pulse sequence distortions are measured with a phantom designed for 3-D nonlinear local distortion evidence. A distortion correction transformation is computed from the phantom images and applied to the patient images. Results are verified using the stereotactic fiducial system.

Fiducial registration errors show spatial accuracy improvement, approaching CT quality, after distortion correction of magnetic resonance images.

The multimodal imaging approach for the dose planning of VS radiosurgery treatment is relevant. Quality control of spatial accuracy for imaging modalities is mandatory and realistic in clinical routine.

Conclusions

Thanks to the development of modern high-resolution MR, computers, visualization software, registration, fusion of anatomical images, radiosurgery in VSs can really be performed with a surgical mind. Neurosurgeons can really navigate in images which currently reach the high accuracy and precision at the scale of the high capacity of conformity and selectivity of the Gamma Knife surgery instrument, and thus operate still keeping permanently under control the location of the surrounding critical structures, in order to prevent their injury. However, this is possible only under the condition of a comprehensive approach where advantages, disadvantages and limits of each modality and sequence are understood and integrated in order to better adhere to the requirements related to the anatomical, physiopathological and clinical functional status context of the patient. Dose planning is the operating phase where the decisions taken have a real impact on the quality of the clinical result. That is a complex process requiring the integration of clinical, radiological, anatomical, radiobiological information deserving specially rigorous quality control.

It is mandatory to develop a local strategy for quality control of the stereotactic imaging and dose delivery in each center based on the critical analysis of the limits in terms of distortion and resolution of the local imaging equipments. Consequently, complication avoidance requires systematic use of quality control procedures adapted to the local context for identification, correction and compensation of all the sources of inaccuracy, imprecision or distortion.

References

1 Gussen R: Intramodiolar acoustic neurinoma. Laryngoscope 1971;81:1979–1984.
2 Khurana VG, Link MJ, Driscoll CL, Beatty CW: Evolution of a cochlear schwannoma on clinical and neuroimaging studies. Case report. J Neurosurg 2003;99:779–782.
3 Birzgalis AR, Ramsden RT, Curley JW: Intralabyrinthine schwannoma. J Laryngol Otol 1991;105:659–661.
4 Held P, Frund R, Seitz J, Nitz W, Haffke T, Hees H, Waldeck A: Comparison of a T2* w. 3D CISS and a T2 w. 3D turbo spin echo sequence for the anatomical study of facial and vestibulocochlear nerves. J Neuroradiol 2000;27:173–178.
5 Stuckey SL, Harris AJ, Mannolini SM: Detection of acoustic schwannoma: use of constructive interference in the steady state three-dimensional MR. AJNR Am J Neuroradiol 1996;17:1219–1225.
6 Kocaoglu M, Bulakbasi N, Ucoz T, Ustunsoz B, Pabuscu Y, Tayfun C, Somuncu I: Comparison of contrast-enhanced T1-weighted and 3D constructive interference in steady state images for predicting outcome after hearing-preservation surgery for vestibular schwannoma. Neuroradiology 2003;45:476–481.
7 Linskey ME, Lunsford LD, Flickinger JC: Radiosurgery for acoustic neurinomas: early experience. Neurosurgery 1990;26:736–745.
8 Flickinger JC, Kondziolka D, Pollock BE, Lunsford LD: Evolution in technique for Vestibular Schwannoma Radiosurgery and Effect on Outcome. Int J Radiation Oncology Biol Phys 1996;36:275–280.
9 Regis J, Delsanti C, Roche P, Soumare O, Dufour H, Porcheron D, Peragut JC, Thomassin JM, Pellet W: Preservation of hearing function in the radiosurgical treatment of unilateral vestibular schwannomas. Preliminary results. Neurochirurgie 2002;48:471–478.
10 Regis J, Roche PH, Delsenti C, Soumare O, Thomassin JM, Pellet W: Stereotactic Radiosurgery for Vestibular Schwannoma; in Pollock BE (ed): Contemporary Stereotactic Radiosurgery: Thechnique and Evaluation. Armonk, New York, Futura Publishing Company, 2002, pp 181–212.
11 Noren G: Long term results of Gamma knife treatment in acoustic neurinomas. Presented at Reunion Lilloise de Radiochirurgie Stereotaxique, Lille, March 26–27, 1993.

12 Flickinger JC, Kondziolka D, Lunsford LD: Dose and diameter relationships for facial, trigeminal and acoustic neuropathies following acoustic neuroma radiosurgery. Radiotherapy and Oncology 1996;41:215–219.
13 Miller R, Foote R, Coffey R, Sargent D, Gorman D, Schomberg P, Kline R: Decrease in cranial nerve complications after radiosurgery for acoustic neuromas: a prospective study of dose and volume. Int J Radiat Oncol Biol Phys 1999;43:305–311.
14 Regis J: New developments in the management of vestibular schwannomas in the modern era of radiosurgery. Neurochirurgie 2004;50:156–158.
15 Delbrouck C, Hassid S, Massager N, Choufani G, David P, Devriendt D, Levivier M: Preservation of hearing in vestibular schwannomas treated by radiosurgery using Leksell Gamma Knife: preliminary report of a prospective Belgian clinical study. Acta Otorhinolaryngol Belg 2003;57:197–204.
16 Kondziolka D, Lunsford L, Flickinger J: Gamma knife radiosurgery for vestibular schwannomas. Neurosurg Clin N Am 2000;11:651–658.
17 Kondziolka D, Lunsford LD, Flickinger JC: Gamma knife radiosurgery for vestibular schwannomas. Neurosurg Clin N Am 2000;11:651–658.
18 Noren G: Long-term complications following gamma knife radiosurgery of vestibular schwannomas. Stereotact Funct Neurosurg 1998;70(suppl 1): 65–73.
19 Prasad D, Steiner M, Steiner L: Gamma surgery for vestibular schwannoma. J Neurosurg 2000;92:745–759.
20 Regis J, Delsanti C, Roche PH, Thomassin JM, Pellet W: Functional outcomes of radiosurgical treatment of vestibular schwannomas: 1,000 successive cases and review of the literature. Neurochirurgie 2004;50:301–311.
21 Regis J, Pellet W, Delsanti C, Dufour H, Roche PH, Thomassin JM, Zanaret M, Peragut JC: Functional outcome after gamma knife surgery or microsurgery for vestibular schwannomas. J Neurosurg 2002;97:1091–1100.
22 Wikler D, Metens T, David P, Levivier M: Imaging for stereotaxic treatment of vestibular schwannomas. Error factors and corrections. Neurochirurgie 2004;50:282–288.

Prof. Jean Régis
Service de Neurochirurgie Fonctionnelle et Stéréotaxique
Hôpital d'Adulte de la Timone
264 bvd Saint Pierre
FR–13385 Marseille Cedex 05 (France)
Tel. +33 4 91 38 65 62, Fax +33 4 91 38 70 56, E-Mail jregis@ap-hm.fr

Régis J, Roche P-H (eds): Modern Management of Acoustic Neuroma.
Prog Neurol Surg. Basel, Karger, 2008, vol 21, pp 65–72

Extended Middle Cranial Fossa Approach for Vestibular Schwannoma: Technical Note and Surgical Results of 896 Operations

R. Shiobara[a] · T. Ohira[a] · Y. Inoue[b] · J. Kanzaki[b] · T. Kawase[a]

Departments of [a]Neurosurgery and [b]Otorhinolaryngology, School of Medicine, Keio University, Tokyo, Japan

Abstract

From 1976 to 2006, 896 vestibular schwannomas were operated on using an extended middle cranial fossa approach. With this approach, the operative field can be extended according to tumor size and the facial and cochlear nerves can be preserved more easily with cooperation between the neurosurgeon and ENT surgeon. The mortality rate among 896 vestibular schwannoma patients was 0.3%. In the 760 initially operated vestibular schwannomas with total removal of the tumor, facial nerves were anatomically preserved in 715 or 94.1% of the cases. In 61.0% of 270 cases in which hearing preservation was attempted, hearing was preserved, and in 46.7% of those 270 cases useful hearing was preserved postoperatively. However, in the last 10 years the useful hearing preservation rate of the 140 attempted cases was 53.6%. Most of the complications of this approach were cerebrospinal fluid leakage; by using fat tissue, fibrin glue and spinal drainage from 1992 to 2005, cerebrospinal fluid leakage occurred in 59 or 10.6% of 569 cases, with 13 or 2.3% being repaired surgically. Moreover, in the last 10 years, the surgical results have improved along with improved surgical experience, improved instruments and better monitoring methods.

Prior to 1975, we used various operative routes for vestibular schwannomas, and thereafter employed an extended middle cranial fossa approach [1], combining the translabyrinthine-transtentorial approach of Morrison and King [2] and the Bochenek and Kukwa's extended approach through the middle cranial fossa [3]. This procedure, performed in cooperation with neurosurgeons and ENT surgeons, lowered the rate of postoperative mortality, increased the preservation rate of the facial and cochlear nerves, and avoided selection of the approach according to the size of the tumor. This approach to vestibular schwannoma and other cerebellopontine angle tumors is the most flexible one. In the present paper, the operative procedures and the surgical results are presented.

Material and Methods

In the 30 years from 1976 to 2006, 896 vestibular schwannomas underwent operations using an extended middle cranial fossa approach. The age of the patients with vestibular schwannomas ranged from 8 to 80 years, with a mean age of 47.5 years. Of the 896 operations, 442 were performed on males and 454 on females; 441 operations were performed on the right side, 455 on the left side, and 2 were performed bilaterally. There were 300 large tumors more than 3 cm in diameter, 559 small and medium-sized tumors and 37 intracanalicular tumors.

Preoperative Procedure
In the 15 years from 1976–1990, no particular preoperative procedures were associated with the extended middle cranial fossa approach. However, in the last 15

years, spinal drainage has been applied both pre- and postoperatively to minimize the risk of brain compression due to intraoperative intracranial hypertension and to protect against postoperative cerebrospinal fluid (CSF) leakage.

Anesthetic Considerations

Anesthesia is performed as is usual for a craniotomy, with an intravenous drip infusion of 500 ml of mannitol (20%) started at the beginning of the procedure.

Patient Position

The patient is placed in the supine position, with the head slightly elevated and rotated so as to place the affected side in the superior (upward) position with the ipsilateral auricle on top. The key to obtaining the correct position depends upon the surgeon's ability to correctly and accurately study the angle and position of the external auditory meatus, which further forms the basis for envisioning the anatomy of the tympanic cavity, the vestibule, the cochlea, the labyrinth, the internal auditory canal and so on.

Monitoring Electrode Setup

Electrodes for monitoring intraoperative facial nerve response are positioned on the orbicularis occuli and orbicularis oris muscles, with other nonsensory electrodes set up as necessary on the stylomastoid and elsewhere. In those operative procedures where hearing preservation is a priority, an earphone and electrode are set up to monitor auditory brain stem response. For patients requiring a cochleogram to be recorded, a needle electrode is inserted from the edge of the craniotomy directly into the tympanic cavity, or through the tympanic membrane. Prior to draping, the auricle is folded forward temporarily and held with two or three sutures, thus covering the earphone and external auditory meatus.

Skin Incision: Craniotomy

In the surgical procedure for vestibular schwannomas or cerebellopontine angle meningiomas by way of the extended middle cranial fossa approach' the skin incision is the same regardless of the size of the tumor or the concern for hearing preservation. A rough semicircular incision is carried out and is centered on the auricle and external auditory meatus; this incision starts anteriorly from the centre of the mid-cranial skull base and extends posteriorly to the rear of the mastoid, thus ensuring adequate exposure of the mid-cranial skull base (fig. 1) [4]. Following flapping of the skin aside, a slightly smaller incision is made in the temporal fascia, temporal muscle and periosteum, thereby separating them from the temporal bone all the way up to the external auditory meatus, where they are folded over with the skin flap.

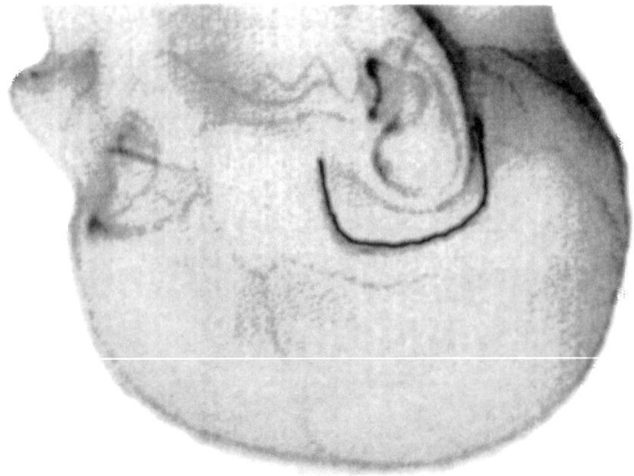

Fig. 1. Drawing showing skin incision. Reprinted with permission from Shiobara [4].

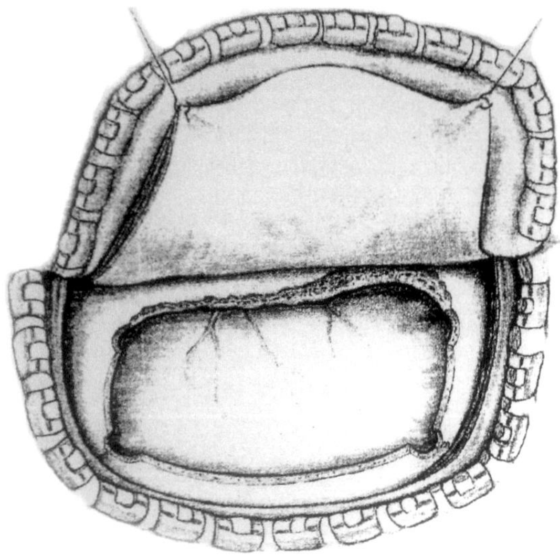

Fig. 2. Drawing showing craniotomy. Reprinted with permission from Shiobara [4].

In the next stage, a free bone flap is constructed, extending the bone window all the way down to the bottom of the middle cranial base using a rongeur and a drill. At the posterior portion of the bone window, the mastoid air cells are gradually removed until a portion of the sigmoid sinus is exposed (fig. 2) [4].

Epidural Approach to the Pyramidal Ridge

After the craniotomy, the dura mater of the middle cranial fossa is separated from the mid-cranial base and raised on the inner side to the pyramidal ridge or sulcus of the

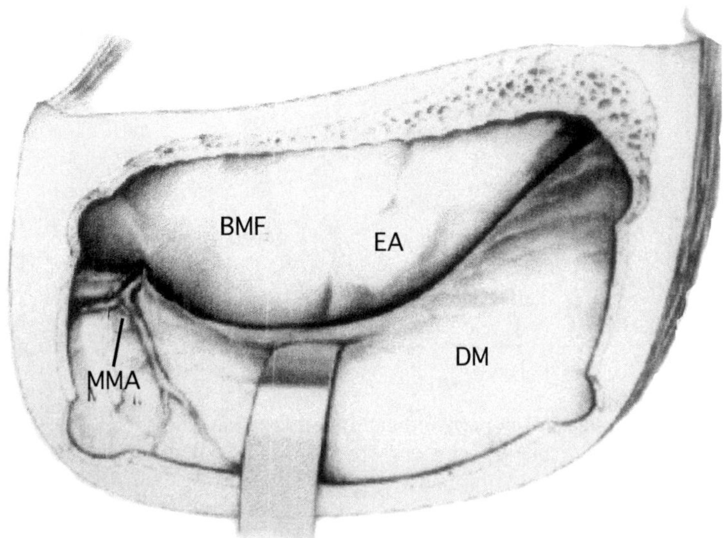

Fig. 3. Drawing showing epidural approach to the pyramidal ridge. BMF = Base of middle cranial fossa; DM = dura mater of middle cranial fossa; EA = eminentia arcuata; MMA = middle meningeal artery. Modified with permission from Shiobara [4].

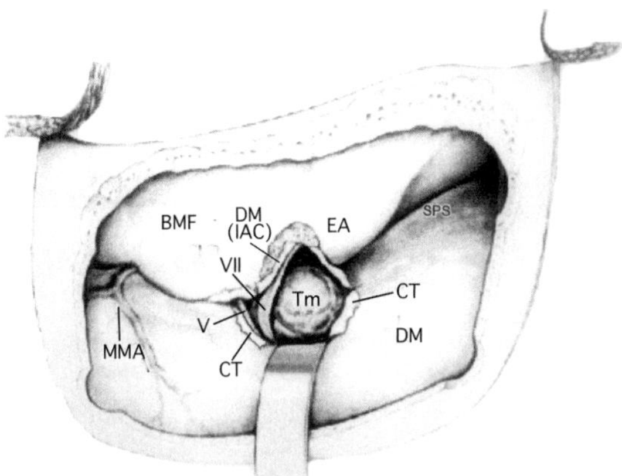

Fig. 4. Drawing showing opening of the internal auditory canal and exposure of a medium-sized tumor. CT = Cerebellar tentorium; DM(IAC) = dura mater of internal auditory canal; Tm = tumor; V = trigeminal nerve; VII = facial nerve. Modified with permission from Shiobara [4].

petrosal sinus, while the anterior side is raised up to the foramen spinosum (fig. 3) [4].

Operative Procedure with Attempted Hearing Preservation
Once the upper portion of the pyramidal ridge is exposed extradurally, only the upper wall of the internal auditory canal is opened. After recognizing the relative anatomy of the external auditory meatus, eminentia arcuata, major petrosal nerve and its sulcus, the upper part of the internal auditory canal is opened by drilling along the base of the eminentia arcuata. Once the internal auditory canal is reached and successfully opened, the dura mater is incised and the tumorectomy is carefully begun. Care is taken to preserve the facial and cochlear nerves (fig. 4) [4]. While performing tumorectomies inside the internal auditory canal, internal tumor decompression is applied from the upper posterior part of the canal, while identification and monitoring of the facial nerve occurs (which is compressed by the anterior upper wall of the canal). Simultaneously from time to time the cochlear nerve is identified (which is compressed by the anterior lower canal wall). When the middle cranial fossa approach or extended middle cranial fossa approach are employed, the favorable operative site in the internal auditory canal very often allows for easy identification of the four nerves of interest, namely the facial, cochlear, superior and inferior vestibular nerves.

Operative Procedure without Attempted Hearing Preservation
In those patients with medium- or large-sized tumors, where effective hearing has been lost preoperatively, the tumorectomy is carried out following suitable enlargement of the operative site. In other words, the procedure for release of the internal auditory canal is followed by a labyrinthectomy and partial mastoidectomy. Connecting the area for drilling, the internal auditory canal is opened anteriorly, while the posterior pyramidal portion of the temporal lobe is adequately removed from the canal. The dura mater of the posterior surface or posterior fossa surface of the pyramidal portion is exposed externally,

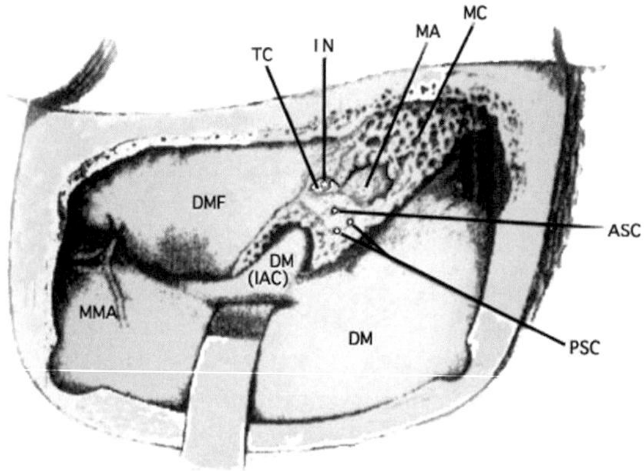

Fig. 5. Drawing showing labyrinthectomy and exposure of the intracanalicular dura mater by partial mastoidectomy. ASC = Anterior semicircular canal; IN = incus; MA = mastoid antrum; MC = mastoid cells; PSC = posterior semicircular canal; TC = tympanic cavity. Modified with permission from Shiobara [4].

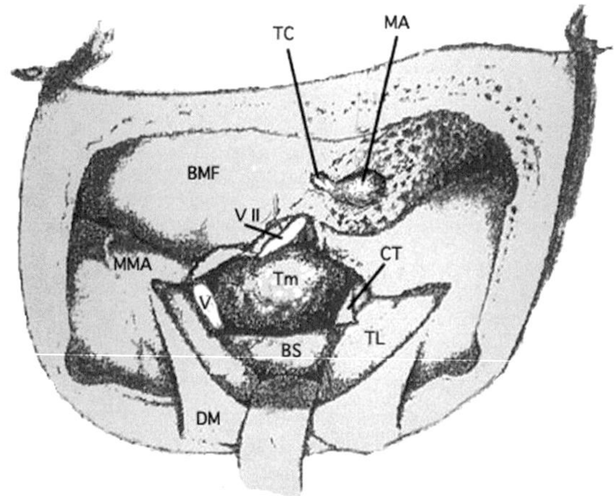

Fig. 6. Drawing showing exposure of a large tumor. BS = Brain stem; TL = temporal lobe. Modified with permission from Shiobara [4].

which also exposes part of the superior petrosal and sigmoid sinuses (fig. 5) [4]. An almost complete extirpation of the semicircular canal is carried out. The middle cranial and posterior dura mater are widely excised, while in the central region the operative site is extended to involve the free edge of the cerebellar tentorium, following which the superior sinus is excised, thus completely removing the cerebellar tentorium (fig. 6) [4]. The operative site is further enlarged by extending the incisions posteriorly. By rolling back the incised cerebellar tentorium, dura mater and superior petrosal sinus, the bulk of the tumor can then be excised. As already described, extirpation of the tumor will be performed while preserving and monitoring the facial nerve (fig. 7) [4].

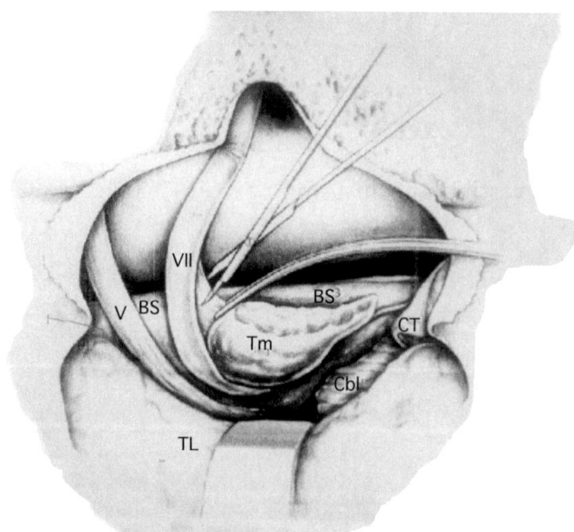

Fig. 7. Drawing showing removal of the tumor and preservation of the facial nerve. Cbl = Cerebellum. Modified with permission from Shiobara [4].

Preservation of Cerebrospinal Fluid Leakage, Skull Base Repair, and Closing Up

In procedures based on the extended middle cranial fossa approach in which hearing preservation has been a priority, areas of the internal auditory canal or the mastoid portion of the temporal bone are sealed using materials such as fat flaps (usually harvested from the abdominal area) or temporal muscle flaps and temporal fascia flaps, followed by fixation with fibrin glue. In the removal of larger tumor where hearing preservation has not been attempted, it is quite possible that creation of the operative site has involved drilling into the tympanic cavity itself. In such cases, after removing the incus from the middle ear, the tympanic cavity is completely packed with a fat flap and fibrin glue. Removal of the incus makes complete packing of the cavity much easier. Following this, fibrin glue is spread over the drilled bone surface and that is sealed with a fat flap. Any areas of chipping damage caused by the drilling are covered with a larger fascia flap, and all of the repair work is, in turn, sealed over with fat flaps and thoroughly fixed with fibrin glue. Finally, the dura mater is sutured back together, repairing any damaged areas with artificial dura mater and fibrin glue. The skull bone is returned to its original position and superficial tissues are folded down and sutured back in place.

Table 1. Mortality rate in 896 cases of vestibular schwannoma

	1976–1995	1996–2005	1976–2005
Initially operated	0.5%	0.2%	0.4%
	2/377	1/437	3/814
Reoperated	0	0	0
	0/48	0/34	0/82
Total	0.5%	0.2%	0.3%
	2/425	1/471	3/896

Results

There were only 3 postoperative deaths of vestibular schwannoma patients among 1,056 patients with cerebellopontine angle tumor, yielding a cerebellopontine angle tumor mortality rate of 0.3%. The overall mortality rate in 896 vestibular schwannomas was 0.3%; in 760 initially operated vestibular schwannomas with total removal of tumor, the mortality rate was 0.1% (table 1). In the 814 initially operated vestibular schwannomas, the tumors were totally removed in 760 or 93.4%, and in 724 or 94.1% of the 760 cases facial nerves were anatomically preserved. In 35.5% of 760 cases in which hearing preservation was attempted, hearing was preserved in 164 or 61.0% postoperatively, and useful hearing (hearing loss ≤50 dB, speech discrimination score ≥50%) preservation was achieved in 126 or 46.7% of the attempted cases (table 2). Most complications of this approach were CSF leakage, and there were 15 such cases from 1976 to 1991, representing 7.5% of 201 cases. From 1976 to 1991, there were 38 CSF leakage cases, representing 18.9% of 201 cases, and 15 or 7.5% of 201 were repaired surgically. Meanwhile, by using fat tissue, fibrin glue and spinal drainage from 1992 to 2005, there were 59 CSF leakage cases, representing 10.6% of 559 cases, and 13 or 2.3% of 559 were repaired surgically (table 3).

However, for the past 10 years, the surgical results have improved because of improved microsurgical techniques and increased surgical experience, as well as improved instruments and better monitoring methods. Therefore, in 410 initially operated vestibular schwannomas with total removal during the last 10 years, the rate of the anatomically preserved facial nerves was 97.8%, the rate of the usefully preserved hearing was 53.6% of 140 cases in which hearing preservation was attempted (table 2), and the rate of the surgically repaired CSF leakage was 2.3% of 559 cases (table 3).

Discussion

After Balance [5] reported a successful suboccipital craniotomy operation in 1894, many early neurosurgeons developed a variety of approaches such as the subtemporal transtentorial or the translabyrinthine approach [6–9]. In the 1970s, King [2, 10] and King and Morrison [11] developed a translabyrinthine-transtentorial approach, which retains the advantages of the translabyrinthine route, and allows for a high rate of total removal and a low incidence of operative mortality. Bochenek and Kukwa [3] then obtained favorable results with a modification of that approach. In order to distinguish the approach described in

Table 2. Facial and hearing preservation of 760 cases with initial operation and total removal of tumor

		1976–1995	1996–2005	1976–2005
Anatomical preservation of facial nerve		89.7%	97.8%	94.1%
		314/350	401/410	715/760
Preserved facial nerve	H-B I, II	76.0%	89.5%	83.3%
		266/350	367/410	633/760
	H-B III, IV	10.0%	6.8%	8.3%
		35/350	28/410	63/760
	H-B V, VI	3.0%	1.5%	2.5%
		13/350	6/410	19/760
Hearing preservation attempted		37.1%	34.1%	35.5%
		130/350	140/410	270/760
Hearing preservation of attempted cases		50.8%	70.0%	61.0%
		66/130	98/140	164/270
Useful hearing[1] preservation of attempted cases		39.2%	53.6%	46.7%
		51/130	75/140	126/270

H-B = House and Brackmann grading.
[1]Hearing loss ≤50 dB, speech discrimination score ≥50%.

this report from both of the previous approaches (those of King and Morrison and Bochenek and Kukwa), we have designated it an 'extended middle cranial fossa approach' [1, 12, 13] and have used it for the 30 years since 1976.

Anatomically, the route to the cerebellopontine angle and the anterior inferior lateral site of the tumor is shortest via this approach, whereas the distance to these areas is longest via the suboccipital approach [14]. The extended middle cranial fossa approach has the advantage of causing less (and only slight) compression of the temporal lobe; the decompression that occurs in the posterior cranial fossa is equal to or more than occurs with the suboccipital approach owing to the wide drilling of the temporal bone and the incision of the cerebellar tentorium. As the extended middle cranial fossa approach allows for extension according to tumor size, even a large tumor can be removed in one stage by this approach.

The identification of the nerve by various devices has been attempted [15–17]. The intraoperative monitoring of facial nerve evoked potentials and, recently, antidromic facial nerve action potentials were found to be useful in cerebellopontine angle operations, including vestibular schwannomas in this series. In our experience, the function of the anatomically preserved nerve paralleled the antidromic facial nerve action potential tracings which were monitored intraoperatively just after the removal of the tumor and preservation of the nerve. We believe that these potentials are more useful in intraoperative monitoring of the nerve than facial nerve evoked potentials and can

Table 3. Results of the initial 768 operative cases with total tumor removal

	1976–1991	1992–2005[1]	1976–2005
CSF leakage	18.9%	10.6%	12.8%
	38/201	59/559	96/760
CSF leakage repaired surgically	7.5%	2.3%	3.7%
	15/201	13/559	28/760

[1]From 1992, fat tissue, fibrin glue and spinal drainage were used to protect CSF leakage pre-, intra- and postoperatively.

predict postoperative function and suggest the timing of anastomosis of the preserved nerve.

We believe that monitoring of the acoustic nerve compound action potentials is the best means of intraoperative monitoring for hearing preservation. By this method, the surgeons obtain instantaneous feedback, and can decide whether to stop or continue the operative procedure based on the real-time changes in the amplitudes and the latencies of these potentials. The auditory brain stem response requires a few minutes for averaging additions, display, and printing, and the electrocochleograms do not indicate the whole electrical function of the cochlear nerve. Postoperative improvement on the preoperative level of hearing is very difficult to achieve. Not all patients who have preoperative hearing are good candidates for an attempt to preserve hearing. Wade and House [18], in a report on 20 patients, stated that 'the ideal candidate for attempt at hearing preservation by any approach is a patient whose tumor size is less than 1.5 cm and whose hearing is no worse than a 30 dB pure tone loss with 70% speech discrimination'. Jannetta et al. [19], Samii and Ohlemutz [20], and Sterkers et al. [21] stated that an attempt should be made to save the hearing of all patients who have preserved hearing before surgery, regardless of the size of the tumor. In the present study, patients with a pure tone loss average of 50 dB or less and a speech discrimination score of 50% or more were selected for preservation of hearing. In this report, postoperative hearing was preserved in 70.0% of 140 cases, and useful hearing (≤50 dB, ≥50%) was preserved in 53.6% of 140 cases.

Conclusions

We have compiled extensive data regarding the outcomes of patients operated on using the extended middle cranial fossa approach. Based on these results, we conclude that this approach is one of the most flexible and advantageous approaches available for surgically treating cerebellopontine angle tumors (especially for vestibular schwannomas).

References

1 Shiobara R: A modified extended middle cranial fossa approach for acoustic tumors. Neurol Med Chir (Jpn) 1980;20:173–182.

2 King TT: Combined translabyrinthine-transtentorial approach to acoustic nerve tumours. Proc R Soc Med 1970;63:780–782.

3 Bochenek Z, Kukwa A: An extended approach through the middle cranial fossa to the internal auditory meatus and the cerebello-pontine angle. Acta Otolaryngol 1975;80:410–414.

4 Shiobara R: 1. Acoustic neurinoma, meningioma, epidermoid; in Yamaura A (ed): Operative atlas of neurosurgery. Tokyo: Igaku-Shoin, 2004, Vol 1, pp 328–334 (Jpn).
5 Balance CA: Some Points in the Surgery of Brain and Its Membranes. London: Macmillan, 1907, p 276.
6 Cushing H: Tumors of the Nervus Acusticus and the Syndrome of the Cerebellopontine Angle. Philadelphia: WB Saunders, 1917.
7 Dandy WE: Results of removal of acoustic tumors by the unilateral approach. Arch Surg 1941;42:1062–1033.
8 House WF: Surgical exposure of the internal auditory canal and its contents through the middle cranial fossa. Laryngoscope 1961;71:1363–1385.
9 Rand RW, Kurze T: Micro-neurosurgical resection of acoustic tumors by a transmeatal posterior fossa approach. Bull Los Angeles Neurol Soc 1965;30:17–20.
10 King TT: Results and complications of translabyrinthine and transtentorial approaches to 60 acoustic nerve tumors. J Neurol Neurosurg Psychiatry 1975;38:411 (Abstract).
11 King TT, Morrison AW: Translabyrinthine and transtentorial removal of acoustic nerve tumors. J Neurosurg 1980;52:210–216.
12 Kanzaki J, Shiobara R, Toya S: Acoustic neuroma surgery. Translabyrinthine-transtentorial approach via the middle cranial fossa. Arch Otorhinolaryngol 1980;229:261–269.
13 Shiobara R, Ohira T, Kanzaki, Toya S: A modified extended middle cranial fossa approach for acoustic nerve tumors. Results of 125 operations. J Neurosurg 1988;68:358–365.
14 Ogata M: On the anatomical measurements of the posterior fossa using dry skulls – from neurosurgical standpoint. No Shinkei Geka 1984;12:717–723 (Jpn).
15 Olgado TE, Buchheit WA, Rosenholtz HR: Intraoperative monitoring of facial muscle evoked responses obtained by intracranial stimulation of the facial nerve: more accurate technique for facial nerve dissection. Neurosurg 1979;4:418–421.
16 Moller AR, Jannetta PJ: Preservation of facial function during removal of acoustic neuromas. Use of monopolar constant-voltage stimulation and EMG. J Neurosurg 1984;61:757–760.
17 Ohira T, Shiobara R, Toya S, et al: Intraoperative monitoring of facial muscle responses for preservation of the facial nerved in cerebellopontine angle tumors. Facial Nerv Res Jpn 1984;4:143–148.
18 Wade PJ, House W: Hearing preservation in patients with acoustic neuromas via the middle cranial fossa approach. Otolaryngol Head Neck Surg 1984;92:184–193.
19 Jannetta PJ, Moller AR, Moller MB: Technique of hearing preservation in small acoustic neuromas. Ann Surg 1984;200:513–523.
20 Samii M, Ohlemutz A: Preservation of eight cranial nerve in cerebellopontine angle tumors; in Samii M, Jannetta PJ (eds): The facial Nerve. Berlin: Springer-Verlag 1981, pp 116–120.
21 Sterkers JM, Sterkers O, Maudelonde C, et al: Preservation of hearing by the retrosigmoid approach in acoustic neuroma surgery. Adv Otorhinolaryngol 1984;34:187–192.

R. Shiobara
Department of Neurosurgery, School of Medicine, Keio University
35 Shinanomachi, Shinjuku-Ku
Tokyo 160-8582 (Japan)
Tel. +81 3 3353 1211, ext. 62329, Fax +81 3 3354 8053, E-Mail shiobara@1961.jukuin.keio.ac.jp

Régis J, Roche P-H (eds): Modern Management of Acoustic Neuroma.
Prog Neurol Surg. Basel, Karger, 2008, vol 21, pp 73–78

Translabyrinthine Approach for Vestibular Schwannomas: Operative Technique

Pierre-Hugues Roche[a] · William Pellet[a] · Takuzo Moriyama[c] · Jean-Marc Thomassin[b]

[a]Service de Neurochirurgie, Hôpital Sainte-Marguerite, [b]Fédération d'Oto-Rhino-Laryngologie, Hôpital la Timone, Assistance Publique-Hôpitaux de Marseille, Marseille, France; [c]Department of Neurosurgery, Miyazaki Medical College, Miyazaki, Japan

Abstract

For large vestibular schwannomas (VSs) for which removal is the primary therapy, the goals are complete tumor resection and maintenance of normal neurological function. The authors analyzed their results about facial nerve preservation, extent of resection and complications following resection of large VSs via a widened translabyrinthine approach. Between 1991 and 2001, 110 patients with a unilateral large VS (Koos stage IV) were operated on using the same technique in the same institution. The main steps of the operative technique were detailed and the clinical outcomes analyzed and compared with the results that were extracted from matched series in the literature. The main postoperative complications were cerebrospinal fluid leakage through the scalp wound in 4%, cerebrospinal fluid rhinorrhea in 4% requiring surgical revision in 3%. One percent of meningitis, 1% of posterior fossa hematoma and 4% of transient lower cranial nerve palsies were observed. There was no death related to the surgery. Total tumor removal was achieved in 85% of cases, near-total in 11% and subtotal in 4% of cases. Sixty-two percent of patients obtained normal to near-normal facial function (House-Brackmann grades 1 and 2). The authors suggest that the translabyrinthine approach is a suitable route for the safe removal of large VSs.

Management of small- to middle-sized vestibular schwannomas (VSs) has gradually moved toward nonsurgical treatments. However, microsurgical resection remains the gold standard treatment of large VS. Among several techniques, the translabyrinthine approach (TLA) is routinely used by many experienced teams in order to achieve a radical resection with facial nerve preservation. The main goal of this chapter is to describe the technical steps of this approach and provide helpful information concerning usual difficulties during this surgery. We will also comment the results and indications of this surgery.

Material and Method

The different steps of the approach are detailed following the data obtained from temporal bone dissections and dissections of cadaveric heads injected with colored fluid. Between 1991 and 2001, the authors operated on 110 large unilateral stage IV (Koos [1]) VSs. Sixty percent of patients were female and 40% were male. Mean age at the time of surgery was 50.1 years ranging from 16 to 82 years. Main symptoms at the time of diagnosis were unilateral hypoacousia (65%), dizziness or vertigo (19%), tinnitus (15%), hydrocephalus (1%). Patient's characteristics have been described in a previous study [2].

The results are extracted from our own operative experience and from the main series in the literature. In the Medline search we made, we have selected exclusively the translabyrinthine series dedicated to large tumors.

Operative Technique

The technique has been described in several main papers [3–7], but we detail here our individual concept.

Positioning
Patient is positioned supine, the head is turned to the opposite side, the neck and the shoulders are free in order to avoid jugular vein compression. Rigid fixation of the head with a Mayfield system is not necessary. A multichannel intraoperative facial nerve monitoring (4 electrodes) is necessary and recording is started at the time of mastoidectomy.

Superficial Step
A curved postauricular skin incision is performed after making local anesthesia using xylocaine-adrenaline solution. The incision is started at the level of the mastoid tip and proceeds upward and forward at the level of the temporal squama, 4 cm above the root of zygoma. The scalp is elevated sharply. The temporal muscle above and sternocleidomastoid muscle below are dislocated. This step allows the identification of the following bony landmarks: Henle spike, asterion, posterior margin of root of zygoma, mastoid tip. The retrolabyrinthine and labyrinthine segment of the petrous bone can now be removed (fig. 1a).

Mastoidectomy and Retrolabyrinthine Exposure
This step (fig. 1b) is first conducted using a large cutting burr or a pineapple-shaped drill. The cortical bone is removed within the boundaries delineated by the outer triangle delineated by the asterion, the root of zygoma and the mastoid tip. The drilling is done gradually toward the depth, while maintaining a uniform horizontal working surface. During this step, the compact bone over the sigmoid sinus will be exposed and skeletonized with a diamond drill. Identification of the sinodural angle is then an important step and provides a good landmark to expose the presigmoid dura and the floor of the middle fossa. Then, the surgeon opens the mastoid cells and identifies the mastoid antrum. Exposure of this space is a key landmark to locate the compact bone of the lateral semicircular canal (SCC). At the same depth, drilling the mastoid air cells below this loop will give access to the jugular bulb and to the inner surface of the digastric groove. Proceeding just anteriorly and medially gives the projection of the stylomastoid foramen and the vertical course of the fallopian canal. It is important to remove the bone behind the sigmoid sinus and above the superior petrosal sinus, in order to widen the approach.

Translabyrinthine Drilling
The SCCs are then drilled (fig. 1c, d). The lateral and posterior SCCs are first opened. The anterior end of the lateral SSC should be drilled cautiously because of its close relationship to the tympanic portion of the facial nerve. Drilling in front of the common crus allows the identification of the vestibular aqueduct and vestibule. The medial wall of the vestibule corresponds to the posterior border of the internal auditory canal (IAC). Exposure of the posterior rim of the IAC can now be achieved using a small diamond drill under the microscope. At the most lateral part of the IAC, the dura becomes thinner and a bony crest named the transverse crest dividing horizontally the fundus is exposed. Under the porus of the IAC, the petrous bone should be drilled as far as the pyramidal fossa (lower margin of the cochlear acqueduct) is exposed. This is the landmark of the cerebellomedullary cistern and lower cranial nerves. Usually the final step of the drilling is conducted with a small diamond drill and leaves small fragments of bone over the dura. Before opening, the fragments have to be detached from the dura with a sharp small dissector.

Opening of the Presigmoid Dura
The dura opening is an important step because it should be optimized and fitted to the bony approach. An 'M'-shaped incision is performed, starting horizontally just under and parallel to the superior petrosal sinus (fig. 1d). Then it goes next to the porus, leaving the dura of the IAC unopened and then returns at the level of the vertical portion of the sigmoid sinus, under the endolymphatic sac. In case of a huge extension of the tumor cranially, coagulation and division of the superior petrosal sinus is required to cut the tentorium toward the free edge, improving the working corridor. In order to facilitate the dura opening, extradural retractors can be positioned over the temporal dura and the sigmoid sinus; in this way, the sinodural angle is increased and improves the presigmoid dura exposure.

Tumor Resection
Once the dura has been opened, the cerebellum is protected by cottonoids. It is important to locate and preserve the arachnoid sheath that overlays the tumor capsule, and separate it away from the parenchyma in order to stay in the appropriate plane. The posterior pole of the tumor is now clearly identified, and it is advised to put the stimulator over the tumor capsule in order to rule out a posterior course of the facial nerve [6]. It is useful to go downward early in order to cut the arachnoid under the inferior pole of the tumor and then release the cerebrospinal fluid from the cerebellomedullary cistern. It gives significant cerebellar relaxation and avoids application of retractors. The surgeon can now debulk the tumor mass staying inside the capsule and using ring curettes or ultrasonic aspiration, depending on the tumor consistency. For young surgeons, this step is usually insufficient because care is taken not to go through the capsule and damage the

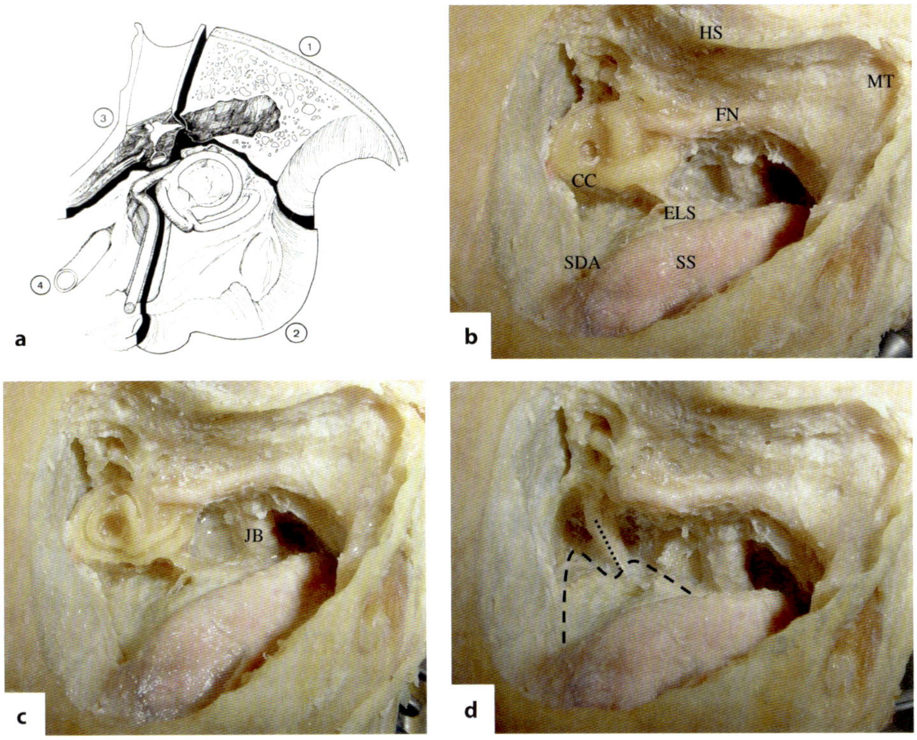

Fig. 1. Key steps of the widened TLA. **a** Petrous bone segmentation following Pellet et al. [7]. During the petrous bone resection, segment 1 (retrolabyrinthine segment) and segment 2 (labyrinthine segment) are consecutively resected while segment 3 (tympanic) and 4 (carotid) are not exposed. **b** Retrolabyrinthine drilling is achieved and the following structures are exposed: common crus (CC), endolymphatic sac (ELS), Henle spike (HS), facial nerve (FN, third portion), mastoid tip (MT), sinodural angle (SDA), sigmoid sinus (SS). **c** The translabyrinthine step is started by drilling the SCCs. JB = Jugular bulb. **d** The TLA is achieved. The M-shaped dashed line indicates the shape of the presigmoid dura opening, while the straight dotted line shows the opening of the IAC.

facial nerve. A better understanding of the tumor volume in the surgical field comes with experience and facilitates gradually the achievement of this step and thus saves time. The tumor capsule is then gradually elevated and the brain protected by the application of soft cottonoids. The facial nerve needs to be identified while it emerges from the pontomedullary fissure. Several landmarks may be used. Location of the foramen of Lushka and choroids plexus just above the IXth nerve is important because the facial nerve is usually lying just above it. The nerve is also located around 2–3 mm in front of the cochleovestibular bundle, and appears as a white avascular tract running upward and frontward. Sometimes, when the anatomy is dramatically shifted by tumor mass, stimulation of the nerve precedes its visual identification. Inside the cerebellopontine angle (CPA), the facial nerve is dissected from the tumor capsule in the medial to lateral direction. The continuous use of the stimulator helps to determine the trajectory of the nerve over the tumor periphery, considering its variability [6]. If the plane of dissection between the nerve and the tumor cannot be kept anymore in the case of facial nerve infiltration or extreme adhesion, we recommend to leave a small fragment of tumor in order to preserve the facial nerve function.

In a second step, the lateral tumor portion is managed in the IAC. The dura has been incised horizontally under high magnification. The two vestibular nerves are identified and cut at the fundus. The facial nerve is stimulated (0.05 mA) in front of the superior vestibular nerve. In between them, the bill's barr is also located. Dissection of the tumor from the facial nerve is conducted from lateral to medial. A Fisch microinstrument or another kind of sharp spatula is used to separate the tumor from the nerve. This maneuver is usually easily done inside the IAC because there is no true adhesion, but more difficulties arise at the level of the porus because of adhesion to the dura and numerous microvascular feeders. Coagulation and traction should be avoided at this point, but the facial nerve is definitely put at risk during this step.

At the end of the procedure, the facial nerve integrity is checked as well as the electric activity. If responses are obtained while the delivered stimulation intensity is maintained at 0.05 mA at the level of the exit zone of the VIIth nerve, a good facial motor function may be expected [8]. The cottonoids are then removed under warmed saline irrigation. Coagulation should be avoided on the pontine surface and of course on the facial nerve. Hemostasis is usually obtained by application of oxidized cellulose on the bleeding points.

Closure Step

The communication with the middle ear is closed with bone dust and fibrin glue. The temporal bone cavity and the dural defect are closed by multiple pieces of fat that have been harvested in the abdominal area. A meticulous closure is essential to minimize the probability of cerebrospinal fluid (CSF) leakage. The procedure is achieved by a tight closure of the musculofascial flap over the fat graft and the stitching of the skin in two layers. A pressure dressing is applied for 2 days.

Postoperative Management

The patient is kept in bed at an intensive care unit during 24 h in order to diagnose early a potentially life-threatening posterior fossa hematoma or early general complication.

Variations during Surgery

Several modifications from the patient or the tumor may influence the conduction of the procedure. Concerning the patient, the level of pneumatization may facilitate or complicate the completeness of the drilling. A far advanced sigmoid sinus reduces the sinodural angle and hampers the presigmoid drilling. In this case, an enlarged subtemporal and presigmoid drilling is required. When the position of the jugular bulb is high, it is necessary to lower the bulb using technical refinements described elsewhere [7, 11].

In case of extra-large tumors, it is advised to optimize the internal debulking and sometimes to cut the dura of the tentorium. Tumor vascularization and hardness are rarely compromising. Arterial feeders come from the anteroinferior cerebellar artery, rarely from the PICA and from the dura at the level of the porus. Dissection of veins at the brain stem may be difficult to achieve but usually the transverse pontine vein is not involved. Great care should be taken to preserve veins, particularly large ones because of the risk of infarction. It is advised to put a small piece of Surgicel and a microcottonoid on the bleeding point and work at another place during at least 5 min and check the hemostasis after removal of the cottonoid.

Results

Completeness of Tumor Removal

Using the TLA, total tumor removal is usually possible even for extra-large tumors, ranging from 91 to 96% of cases [2, 4, 9–13]. There is no place that cannot be reached. The inferior extension toward the lower cranial nerves or the upper pole involvement toward the tentorium can be easily controlled if the translabyrinthine exposure is properly done. In the present series, total tumor removal was achieved in 85% of cases, near-total in 11% and subtotal in 4% of cases. In most cases, incomplete resection was an intentional decision due to the adhesion of the facial nerve with the tumor at the porus or in the CPA.

Complications

Resection of large VSs is still challenging but no postoperative death was observed in the present series. Posterior fossa hematoma occurred in 1% of our operated cases and required emergency surgery without any additional consequences. In addition to the risk to the VIIth cranial nerve, lower cranial nerve deficit occurred in 4% of our cases and did not require any feeding tube or tracheostomy. All of them recovered in the months that followed surgery. We observed CSF leakage through the scalp wound in 4%. This complication was treated by administration of acetazolamide tablets during a few days, iterative lumbar punctures (once a day during 3 consecutive days) and compressive dressing. CSF rhinorrhea was reported in 4% requiring surgical revision in 3%. One case of postoperative meningitis (1%) justified intravenous antibiotics. This rate of complications is similar to what has been described using the same approach for large VSs [4, 6, 9, 10, 13].

Facial Nerve Preservation

In our series, the facial nerve preservation was 60% (House and Brackmann grade 1 or 2 [14]) for large VSs, which is comparable to the other series from the literature. We learned from our own experience of the translabyrinthine removal of large VSs that special portions of the facial nerve could be particularly threatened. Usually the nerve runs cranially at its exit zone from the brain stem and its identification and dissection can be achieved safely at this place. While its trajectory changes abruptly and becomes transversal and ventral in the CPA, we usually observe a phenomenon of folding of the fibers over the tumor capsule and this area is difficult to dissect. The other critical area is the anterior margin of the porus acousticus where another radical change of trajectory is observed. Moreover, the tumor capsule receives many arterial feeders at this point, which provide more adhesion and additional risk of heat injury in case of bipolar coagulations. We routinely use the stimulation probe as a microdissector of the nerve, keeping the intensity of stimulation very low (0.05 mA). At the end of the procedure we can always expect a good postoperative facial motion (grade 1 or 2) if such stimulation (0.05 mA) of the nerve's origin provides good responses. We are now very confident with this technique and do not hesitate to give this information to the patient's family immediately after the surgery.

Discussion

From a historical perspective, the TLA to the CPA was first proposed by Panse in 1904 [15] but was developed and routinely used in the 1960s by William House [16], a famous neuro-otologist. This approach is justified by several arguments: Whatever the size of the tumor, the facial nerve is early identified via reliable bony landmarks at the fundus of the IAC; distal infiltration of the fundus can be removed; the cerebellum is never retracted; the brain stem is safely approached laterally in the second part of the procedure, allowing a good control of vessels. In rare cases of unexpected facial nerve interruption during the procedure, it is possible to perform an end-to-end anastomosis. The exposure and mobilization of the intrapetrous part of the facial nerve avoid any tension in the anastomosis. However, the use of the TLA necessitates the coordination of a neuro-otologist and a neurosurgeon. The duration of the approach by itself is longer than the retrosigmoid approach, and complete hearing loss is unavoidable. Mastoidectomy is sometimes responsible for a skull deformity that is felt by the patient. The tissue graft used for the closure is harvested from the abdomen and needs another skin incision.

There is no doubt that the appropriate treatment of large VSs is optimal resection, but there is also no question that facial nerve palsy is unacceptable for the patients. Moreover, it is predictable that in the near future this double mission (facial nerve preservation and radical removal) may be more difficult to achieve. Considering that most cases of small- to middle-sized VS will be treated electively by radiosurgery may lengthen the learning curve of young neurosurgeons who will be involved in the microsurgical treatment of large VSs. An option that still needs to be validated would be to recommend a two-stage combined strategy described as follows. A primary resection is undertaken as far as the facial nerve can be safely preserved. At the point where the nerve may be damaged, tumor capsule is left and this observation is detailed on the operative chart and clearly announced to the patient. Then, the residual tumor is treated adjunctively with radiosurgery after it has been clearly identified on a postoperative MR evaluation. We started to propose this therapeutic combination at our institution for 4 years and are observing promising results of facial nerve preservation.

Conclusions

In our current experience, we give high priority to the translabyrinthine route in the attempt to remove large VS even though many experienced teams prefer the retrosigmoid approach for the same type of tumor. Both techniques are able to provide radical cure with the same level of facial nerve preservation, and the criterion for choosing the approach mainly depends on the individual practice and confidence of the team in the one or the other approach.

There is still a need to reduce the rate of postoperative facial deficit, and in this way, a two-stage microsurgical and radiosurgical management may be an acceptable alternative that needs to be validated.

References

1 Koos WT, Day JD, Matula C, Levy DI: Neurotopographic considerations in the microsurgical treatment of small acoustic neurinomas. J Neurosurg 1998;88:506–512.
2 Deveze A, Roche PH, Facon F, Gabert K, Pellet W, Thomassin JMT: Résultats de l'exérèse par voie translabyrinthique élargie des schwannomes vestibulaires. Neurochirurgie 2004;50:244–252.
3 Day JD, Chen DA, Arriaga M: Translabyrinthine approach for acoustic neuroma. Neurosurgery 2004;54:391–396.
4 Lanman TH, Brackmann DE, Hitselberger WE, Subin B: Report of 190 consecutive cases of large acoustic tumors (vestibular schwannoma) removed via the translabyrinthine approach. J Neurosurg 199;90:617–623.
5 Mc Elveen JT: The translabyrinthine approach to the cerebellopontine angle tumors; in Wilkins RH, Rengachary SS (eds): Neurosurgery, McGraw-Hill, 1996, vol 1, pp 1107–1113.
6 Tos M, Thomsen J, Harmsen A: Results of translabyrinthine removal of 300 acoustic neuromas related to tumour size. Acta Otolaryngol (Suppl) 1988;452:38–51.
7 Pellet W, Cannoni M, Pech A: Otoneurosurgery 1990, Springer-Verlag.
8 Roche PH, Lari N, Régis J, Thomassin JM: Letter to the editor. J Neurosurg 2006;104(1):175–176.
9 Anderson DE, Leonetti J, Wind JJ, Cribari D, Fahey K: Resection of large vestibular schwannomas. Facial nerve preservation in the context of surgical approach and patient-assessed outcome. J Neurosurg 2005;102:643–649.
10 Briggs RJS, Luxford WM, Atkins JS, Hitselberger WE: Translabyrinthine removal of large acoustic neuromas. Neurosurgery 1994;34:785–792.
11 Roche PH, Moriyama T, Thomassin JM, Pellet W: High Jugular Bulb in the translabyrinthine approach to the cerebellopontine angle: anatomical considerations and surgical management. Acta Neurochir 2006, in press.
12 Sampath P, Rini D, Long DM: Microanatomical variations in the cerebellopontine angle associated with vestibular schwannomas (acoustic neuromas): a retrospective study of 1006 consecutive cases. J Neurosurg 2000;92:70–78.
13 Sluyter S, Graamans K, Tulleken CAF, Van Veelen WM: Analysis of the results obtained in 120 patients with large acoustic neuromas surgically treated via the translabyrinthine-transtentorial approach. J Neurosurg 2001;94:61–66.
14 House JW, Brackmann DE: Facial nerve grading system. Bull Am Acad Otolaryngol Head Neck Surg 1985;4:4.
15 Panse R: Ein Gliom des Akustikus. Arch Ohrenheilk 1904;61:251–255.
16 Mc Elveen JT: The translabyrinthine approach to the cerebellopontine angle tumors; in Wilkins RH, Rengachary SS (eds): Neurosurgery, McGraw-Hill, 1996, vol 1, pp 1107–1113.
17 House WF: Evolution of transtemporal bone removal of acoustic tumors. Arch Otolaryngol 1964;80:731–742.

Prof. Pierre-Hugues Roche
Service de Neurochirurgie de l'Hôpital Nord
Assistance Publique-Hôpitaux de Marseille
Chemin des Bourrelly
FR–13915 Marseille Cedex 20 (France)
Tel. +33 4 91 96 86 20, Fax +33 4 91 96 89 15, E-Mail proche@mail.ap-hm.fr

Régis J, Roche P-H (eds): Modern Management of Acoustic Neuroma.
Prog Neurol Surg. Basel, Karger, 2008, vol 21, pp 79–82

Management of Large Vestibular Schwannomas by Combined Surgical Resection and Gamma Knife Radiosurgery

Stéphane Fuentes · Yasser Arkha · Grégoire Pech-Gourg · François Grisoli · Henry Dufour · Jean Régis

Service de Neurochirurgie Fonctionnelle et Stéréotaxique, Hôpital d'Adulte de la Timone, Marseille, France

Abstract

In this report, we evaluated the treatment results of a combination of surgery and radiosurgery for large vestibular schwannomas. The series of 8 patients included in this study underwent surgery followed by radiosurgical treatment between January 2000 and January 2006. The patients included 5 males and 3 females aged 24–78 years (mean age: 53 years). The average maximum diameter of the tumor was 40 (35–45) mm. At the time of radiosurgery, the treatment size became 18 (9–20) mm. The mean peripheral dose administered was 11.8 (range 11–13) Gy, and the mean dose administered in the centre of the tumor was 23.75 (22–26) Gy. The mean follow-up period was 46 months after radiosurgery. Excellent facial nerve function (House-Brackmann grade 1 or 2) was preserved in 7/8 patients (87.5%). In the case of large vestibular schwannomas, the combined management is one option for maintaining cranial nerve function and tumor growth control.

Surgery is still the main option available for treating large vestibular schwannomas. The latest surgical, electrophysiological and anesthetic reanimation methods have greatly reduced the postoperative morbidity and mortality rates associated with this approach [1, 2].

However, the functional preservation of the facial nerve still remains a challenge. Postoperative facial nerve damage has been reported to occur in about 48% of the patients in some series [1, 3–6].

Even when the facial nerve is left anatomically intact, surgical interventions of this kind can have severe esthetic and functional consequences, which greatly reduce patients' quality of life [1, 7].

Some authors have therefore suggested performing subtotal endocapsular resection on large vestibular schwannomas, followed by Gamma Knife radiosurgical treatment of the residual tumor [7].

Here, we report on our own experience with this combined therapeutic strategy, in which partial resection is performed on large vestibular schwannomas taking a retrosigmoid approach, and the residual fragment is subsequently treated using Gamma Knife radiosurgery.

Material and Methods

The series of 8 patients included in this study underwent surgery followed by radiosurgical treatment between January 2000 and January 2006. In all these cases, it was deliberately intended at the outset to use this combined approach.

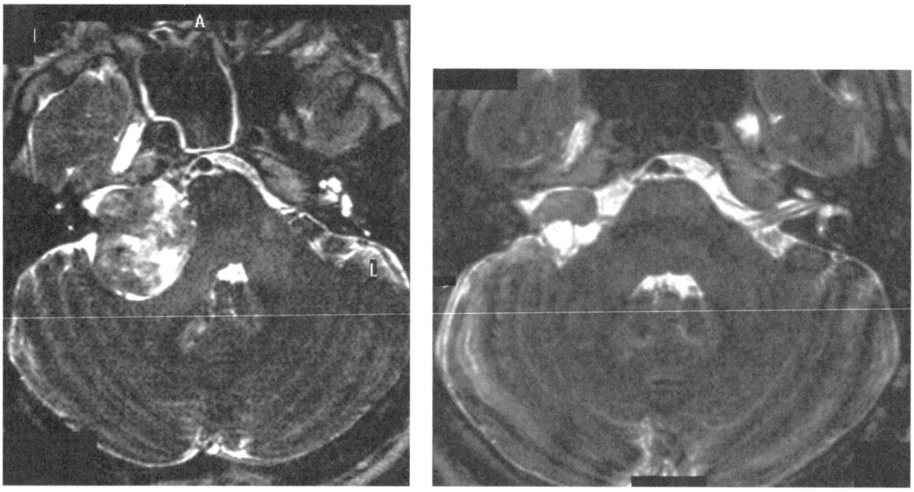

Fig. 1. **a** Preoperative T_2-weighted MRI showing the right vestibular schwannoma. **b** T_2-weighted MRI demonstrating residual tumoral fragment with a mainly intrameatal location prior to Gamma Knife radiosurgery.

The patients included 5 males and 3 females aged 24–78 years (mean age: 53 years). All the patients had hearing deficits: one patient had a grade 2 useful hearing score on the Gardner-Robertson classification scale, 3 patients were rated grade 4, and 4 were rated grade 5 on this scale. Two patients complained of facial neuralgia, and 5 had cerebellar symptoms.

The extrameatal diameter of the tumors was found to be 35 mm in 2 patients, 40 mm in 5 patients and 45 mm in one patient.

Surgical resection was performed on all the patients, taking a retrosigmoid approach.

During the operation, patients under 70 years of age (n = 5) were placed in the sitting position, and the older patients (n = 3) were placed in the ventrolateral decubitus (park bench) position.

The facial nerve was monitored in all the patients. The internal auditory canal was systematically opened in order to locate and stimulate the facial nerve. The tumoral fragment was left in situ along the whole trajectory and when it came into contact with the facial nerve (fig. 1 and 2).

The time elapsing between surgery and Gamma Knife radiosurgical treatment was 6–12 months (mean interval: 9 months). The mean size of the residual tumoral fragment treated with Gamma Knife radiosurgery was 18 mm (range 9–20 mm). The mean volume of the residual tumor was 1.16 (range: 0.31–2.20) cm^3. The mean peripheral dose administered was 11.8 (range: 11–13) Gy, and the mean dose administered in the centre of the tumor was 23.75 (22–26) Gy.

Results

No cases of cerebrospinal fluid leakage or meningitis occurred in this series. No mortalities occurred.

On the House-Brackmann classification scale, our patients were rated as follows postoperatively, prior to radiosurgical treatment: 6 grade 1 patients, 1 grade 2 patient, and 1 grade 3 patient. All the patients showed signs of brain stem and cerebellar compression, which improved postoperatively. The operation lasted for 5 h on average (range: 4–8 h). The patients' mean length of stay at the neurosurgical ward was 7 (range: 5–10) days. Their mean stay at the neurosurgical ward for the Gamma Knife treatment was 48 h. The mean follow-up time after the radiosurgical intervention was 46 (range: 12–73) months. No complications were observed after the radiosurgical treatment. The patients were given MRI follow-up after 6 months, 1 year, and then every year. No increase was observed in the volume of the treated tumoral residues, and no facial nerve dysfunction occurred as the result of the radiosurgical treatment.

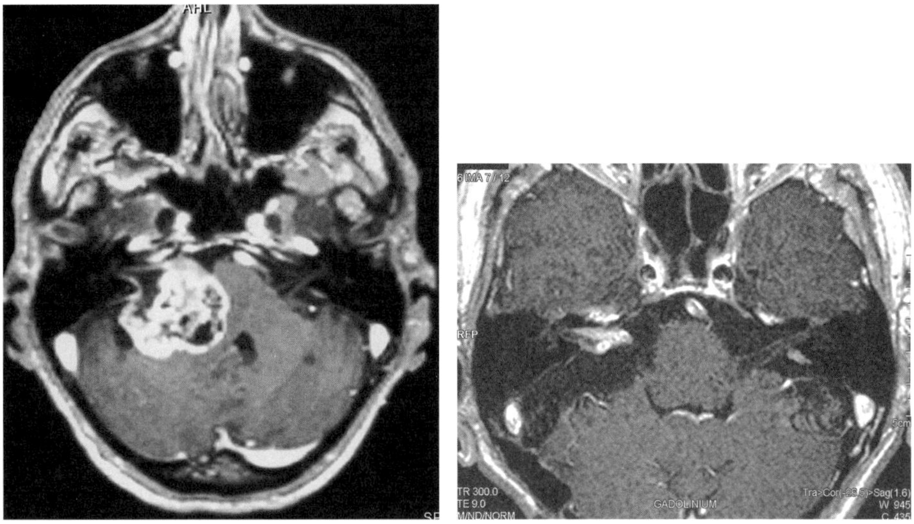

a b

Fig. 2. **a** Preoperative T_1-weighted MRI with gadolinium contrast showing the right vestibular schwannoma. **b** T_1-weighted MRI with gadolinium contrast (prior to Gamma Knife radiosurgery) showing the tumoral fragment in contact with the facial nerve.

Patients with grade 1 or 2 functional scores accounted for 87.5% of the series.

Discussion

Thanks to the great progress made in the surgical treatment of pontocerebellar tumors, the risk of mortality associated with these interventions has been practically abolished. The only risk which remains to be overcome is therefore that of facial nerve or other cranial nerve dysfunction [1, 3–6].

The rates of preserved facial function after surgical treatment of large vestibular schwannomas have varied from one series to another in the literature. They depend mainly on the type of approach taken, but also on the quality of the tumor resection. However, facial function seems to have been preserved in 52.6–68% of patients with large tumors [1, 3–6, 8].

The enlarged translabyrinthine approach seems to give the best resection quality, but it is associated with longer operating times, higher rates of postoperative facial paralysis, and in particular, with a risk of cerebrospinal fluid leakage (6.2–20%) [1, 3, 4, 6]. The risk of cerebrospinal fluid leakage has led to a further surgical intervention in 3.1–13.6% of patients [1, 3, 4, 6].

Vestibular schwannomas can relapse 10–15 years postoperatively (10% of patients), even when surgeons have the impression that they have been completely removed [9, 10]. Residual tumoral fragments can increase with time, and it has been estimated that an increase in tumor volume will occur in 44–53% of patients undergoing intracapsular resection [7, 8, 11].

Radiosurgery has proved its worth as a means of treating small vestibular schwannomas: a tumoral control rate of 91–97.7% has been achieved, and in particular, the risk of facial paralysis has been reduced to 1.3% [12, 13].

Iwai et al. [7] previously reported on a series of patients with large vestibular schwannomas who were treated using a combined surgical and radiosurgical approach. The results obtained in the latter series were encouraging, since the rate of facial nerve preservation was 85.7%, and an excellent rate of tumoral control was achieved.

Similar results were obtained in the present series, where the mean rates of facial function (87.5% of patients were rated grade 1 or 2 on the House-Brackmann scale) and tumoral control rates recorded 46 months after Gamma Knife radiosurgery were most encouraging.

Conclusion

Large vestibular schwannomas can be effectively treated by deliberately adopting the strategy consisting in combining the surgical retrosigmoid approach, which is a relatively noninvasive approach, with Gamma Knife radiosurgery. This twofold therapeutic method seems to give an excellent functional outcome and high rates of tumoral control. Further studies are now required, however, in which larger numbers of patients are followed for longer periods of time, in order to confirm the validity of this method.

References

1 Deveze A, Roche PH, Facon F, Gabert K, Pellet W, Thomassin JM: Résultats de l'exérèse par voie translabyrinthique élargie des schwannomes vestibulaires. Neurochirurgie 2004;50:244–252.

2 Samii M, Matthies C: Management of 1,000 vestibular schwannomas (acoustic neuromas) : surgical management and results with an emphasis on complications and how to avoid them. Neurosurgery 1997;40:11–20.

3 Sluyter S, Graamans K, Tulleken CA, Van Veelen CW: Analysis of the results obtained in 120 patients with large acoustic neuromas surgically treated via the translabyrinthine-trantentorial approach. J Neurosurg 2001;94:61–66.

4 Tos M, Thomsen J, Harmsen A: Results of translabyrinthine removal of 300 acoustic neuromas related to tumour size. Acta Otolaryngol Suppl 1988;452:38–51.

5 Tos M, Youssef M, Thomsen J, Turgut S: Causes of facial nerve paresis after translabyrinthine surgery for acoustic neuroma. Ann Otol Rhinol Laryngol 1992;101:821–826.

6 Wu H, Sterkers J: Translabyrinthine removal of large acoustic neuromas in young adults. Auris Nasus Larynx 2000;27: 201–205.

7 Iwai Y, Yamanaka K, Ishiguro T: Surgery combined with radiosurgery of large acoustic neuromas. Surg Neurol 2003;59: 283–291.

8 Lownie SP, Drake CG: Radical intracapsular removal of acoustic neuromas. Long-term follow-up review of 11 patients. J Neurosurg 1991;74:422–425.

9 Sterkers JM, Viala P, Benghalem A: Récidives des neurinomes de l'acoustique. Rev Laryngol Otol Rhinol 1988;109:71–73.

10 Thomassin JM, Pellet W, Epron J, Braccini F, Roche PH: Les récidives des neurinomes de l'acoustique après exérèse chirurgicale. Ann Otolaryngol Chir Cervicofac 2001;118:3–10.

11 Mazzoni A, Calabrese V, Moschini L: Residual and recurrent acoustic neuroma in hearing preservation procedures: neuroradiologic and surgical findings. Skull Base Surgery 1996;6:105–112.

12 Konzioka D, Lunsford LD, McLaughlin MR, Flickinger JC: Long-term outcomes after radiosurgery for acoustic neuromas. N Engl J Med 1998;339:1426–1433.

13 Regis J, Delsanti C, Roche PH, Thomassin JM, Pellet W: Résultats fonctionnels de la radiochirurgie des schwannomes vestibulaires. A propos de 1000 cas successifs et revue de la littérature. Neurochirurgie 2004;50:301–311.

Dr. Stéphane Fuentes
Service de Neurochirurgie Fonctionnelle et Stéréotaxique
Hôpital d'Adulte de la Timone, 264 bvd Saint Pierre
FR–13385 Marseille Cedex 05 (France)
Tel. +33 491 385 543, Fax +33 491 385 511, E-Mail sfuentes@ap-hm.fr

Régis J, Roche P-H (eds): Modern Management of Acoustic Neuroma.
Prog Neurol Surg. Basel, Karger, 2008, vol 21, pp 83–88

The Wait and See Strategy for Intracanalicular Vestibular Schwannomas

Pierre-Hugues Roche[a] · Outouma Soumare[a] · Jean-Marc Thomassin[b] · Jean Régis[c]

[a]Service de Neurochirurgie, Hôpital Sainte-Marguerite, [b]Fédération d'Oto-Rhino-Laryngologie, [c]Service de Neurochirurgie Stéréotaxique et Fonctionnelle, Hôpital la Timone, Assistance Publique-Hôpitaux de Marseille, Marseille, France

Abstract

To refine our therapeutic policy for intracanalicular tumors, we reviewed our series of patients who where initially treated conservatively. Forty-seven patients (22 men and 25 women) harboring an intracanalicular vestibular schwannoma were followed prospectively. Mean age at the time of inclusion was 54.4 (20–71) years. The mean follow-up period was 43.8 months (±40 months) ranging from 9 to 222 months. Failure was defined as significant tumor growth and/or hearing deterioration that required a microsurgical or radiosurgical treatment. Failure was observed in 35 cases while a conservative treatment is still ongoing in 12 patients. Ten patients kept an unchanged tumor size (21.3%), while 36 patients experienced a tumor growth (76.6%), and 1 patient experienced a mild decreased tumor size (2.1%). Among the 40 patients who where available for hearing level study, 24 patients (60%) did not change their Gardner and Robertson hearing class. Fifteen patients (37.5%) experienced a >10-dB hearing loss and 2 of them became deaf. One patient (2.5%) improved her hearing level from 56.3 to 43.8 dB over a 39.5-month follow-up period. These data suggest that the wait and see policy exposes the patient to degradation of hearing and tumor growth. Both events may occur in an independent way in the middle-term period. This information has to be given to the patient, and a careful sequential follow-up may be adopted when the wait and see strategy is chosen.

During the past 3 decades, there have been dramatic advances in the diagnosis and treatment of vestibular schwannomas (VSs). However, there are still patients in whom a conservative management approach might represent a suitable alternative. The natural history of untreated VS remains a matter of concern, particularly for the subgroup of intracanalicular tumors. The aim of this study was to analyze our own experience of conservatively treated intracanalicular VS with special emphasis on tumor volume behavior and hearing maintenance.

Method

From 1981 to 1999, a conservative attitude has been systematically proposed for 60 consecutive intracanalicular tumors. Thirteen patients did not agree to come back for follow-up investigation and data were obtained in 47 patients who accepted this protocol. For the purpose of this paper, the referring physician or directly the patient was asked to provide missing data (hearing level data and MRI films). Comparison of means was made using Student's test, Mann-Whitney U test and Kruskal-Wallis test. The χ^2 test and Fisher test were used to compare the repartition. Actuarial survival curves were calculated by the Kaplan-Meier method.

Method for the Study of the Volume and Kinetics

For the patients in whom diagnosis was made from March 1990, MRI was routinely used for the sequential follow-up. Study of tumor growth was based on the following parameters:

– Tumor growth rate was measured in millimeters per year (difference between the final and the initial diameter) divided by the length of follow-up (years).
– Tumor growth rate used the volume and the same formula, given in cubic millimeters per year. Tumor volume was given using y • x • x/2 where y was the transverse diameter and x the anteroposterior diameter of the tumor, assuming that anteroposterior and cranicaudal extensions were very similar.
– Tumor doubling time (TDT) used the following formula [1]:

TDT = log2 • T/(log last measured volume – log initial volume).

Change of tumor size was also described following the Koos staging system [2].

Parameters used for the search of statistical correlation with tumor growth were: age, sex, initial auditory brain stem response (ABR), hearing level (pure tone average – PTA, speech discrimination score – SDS), homogeneous versus heterogeneous contrast loss, internal auditory canal (IAC) deformation.

Method for the Analysis of the Hearing Level and Kinetics

PTA was calculated by averaging the hearing loss at the 500-, 1,000-, 2,000-, 4,000-Hz thresholds. SDS was also systematically recorded and a Gardner and Robertson grading could thereby be given. Patients in whom a deaf status was recorded at the time of diagnosis and those with missing data were excluded from the interpretation of the kinetics. The level of hearing was defined as unchanged when the difference between the initial and the final PTA did not exceed 10 dB.

Population

Forty-seven patients underwent a conservative management of their VSs. There were 22 male and 25 female patients. Mean age at the time of inclusion was 54.4 years, ranging from 20 to 71 years. Mean follow-up was 43.8 months (±40 months) ranging from 9 to 222 months, and median time was 34.7 months.

The first manifestation was hypoacousia in 37 cases (78.7%). Sudden hearing loss was noted in 16 cases (34%; permanent in 1 patient, partial recovery in 10 patients, complete recovery in 5 patients). Progressive hearing loss was observed in 21 cases (44.7%). In the other cases, the first manifestation was distributed as follows: Sudden vertigo and progressive hearing loss in 1 patient, dizziness in 3 patients followed by progressive hearing loss in 2 of them, dizziness and imbalance in 2 patients. Dizziness, imbalance and tinnitus altogether were noticed in 2 patients, and tinnitus in 1, while incidental discovery was observed in 1 patient with a single hearing ear.

At the time of diagnosis, hypoacousia was observed in 46 patients and included deafness in 4 patients, tinnitus in 26 patients (55.32%), dizziness in 16 patients (34.04%), imbalance in 21 patients (44.68%), and full ear feeling in 3 patients (6.38%).

Radiological Findings at the Initial CT or MRI Scan

Homogenous contrast enhancement of the tumor was observed in 45 cases, while heterogeneous in 2 cases. In 22 cases, the tumor extended to the fundus of the IAC. On bone window CT scan, the IAC displayed a normal shape in 34 cases, widening of the porus in 10 cases and osteolysis in 3 cases.

Results

Failure of conservative management was defined by the necessity of radiosurgery or microsurgical treatment (fig. 1). This failure was observed in 35 cases, while a conservative treatment is still ongoing in 12 patients. Mean follow-up of failed cases was 41.3 (±37.08) months with a median of 34.7 (10.6–222) months. Mean follow-up of the 12 remaining cases was 49.95 (±46.49) months with a median of 33.94 (9.2–167) months. One of these patients required a translabyrinthine removal because of progression to a Koos stage IV after 46 months. Thirty patients underwent Gamma Knife radiosurgery (GKR; 1 stage III, 24 stage II, 5 stage I), and 4 patients are scheduled for GKR (3 stage I and 1 stage II).

Analysis of Tumor Behavior

During the follow-up period, 10 patients displayed an unchanged size (21.3%), 36 patients experienced tumor growth (76.6%), and 1 patient had a moderately decreased tumor size (2.1%). For the 36 patients who experienced tumor growth, mean follow-up was 39.7 (±37.1) months and median was 33.4 months. Mean tumor growth (MTG) was 2.8 mm/year (±1.9; median 2.4).

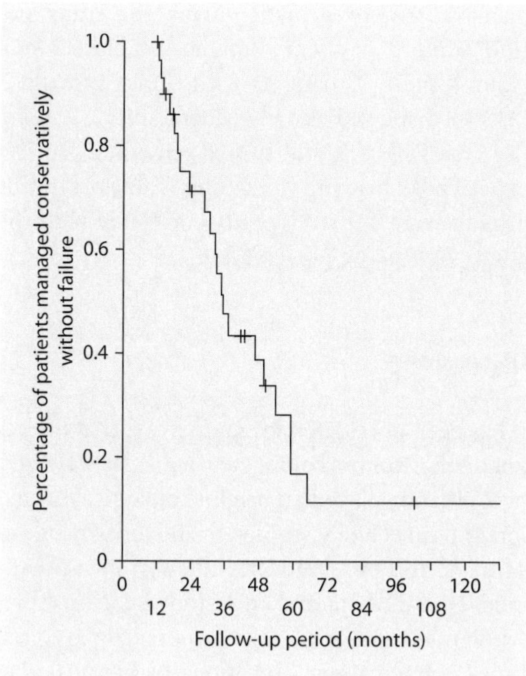

Fig. 1. Graph showing the actuarial survival curve without failure for the 47 patients. Failure of conservative management was defined by the necessity of radiosurgery or microsurgical treatment in patients displaying tumor growth and/or hearing deterioration.

When the whole population was included, mean initial transverse diameter was 8.1 (±2.5) mm and mean final transverse diameter was 13.1 (±4.6) mm ($p < 0.001$). Mean initial volume was 84.5 (±48.9) mm^3 and mean final volume was 409.5 (±841.7) mm^3 ($p < 0.001$). MTG was 2.1 (±2) mm/year. For 45 patients, MTG was 122 (±244) mm^3/year. For the 10 tumors that remained stable, mean and median follow-ups were 60.4 (±46.4) months and 45.2 months, respectively. TDT was obtained in 35 growing cases and ranged from 4.8 to 164.7 months with a mean of 27.8 (±32.6) months during a median period of 16.2 months. TDT was less than 1 year in 11 patients (31.4%), between 1 to 3 years in 18 patients (51.4%) and more than 3 years in 6 (17.4%). No statistical correlation could be found between the tumor growth or TDT and the following parameters: age, gender, initial PTA, initial SDS, ABR, postcontrast enhancement and IAC deformation findings.

Analysis of Hearing

Among the 47 patients, 40 were available for study of the hearing level (4 where already deaf at the time of inclusion and 3 were lacking audiometric data). The hearing class (PTA) of 24 patients (60%) remained unchanged. Fifteen patients (37.5%) presented a >10-dB hearing loss and 2 of them became deaf. One patient (2.5%) improved her hearing level from 56.3 to 43.8 dB (PTA) over a 39.5-month period. Mean and median follow-up periods of the unchanged hearing group were 35.1 (±42.5) and 22.3 months, respectively. Mean and median follow-up periods of the worsened hearing group were 57.8 months (±24.2) and 55.3 months, respectively. No statistical difference was found between the 2 groups regarding tumor growth rate, TDT, and also the following initial parameters: SDS, ABR, first symptom, gender, age, radiological findings. There was no evidence of any predictive parameter of hearing loss at the time of initial management.

Study of the Useful Hearing

Among the 47 patients, 31 (66%) presented with a useful hearing at the time of diagnosis (PTA ≤50 dB and SDS ≥50%). During the follow-up period, 21 patients (67.7%) kept a useful hearing and 10 patients (32.3%) lost it (fig. 2). Another patient improved from a nonuseful (56.25 dB of initial PTA) to a useful hearing (43.75 dB PTA at 39.5 months). Mean follow-up of the 31 patients was 40 (±39.4) months and median follow-up 32.2 months. Mean follow-up of the 21 patients who preserved their hearing level was 40.8 (±45) months (median: 32.2 months). Mean follow-up of the 10 patients with hearing worsening was 38.21 (±26) months (median: 33 months). Among the 31 patients with

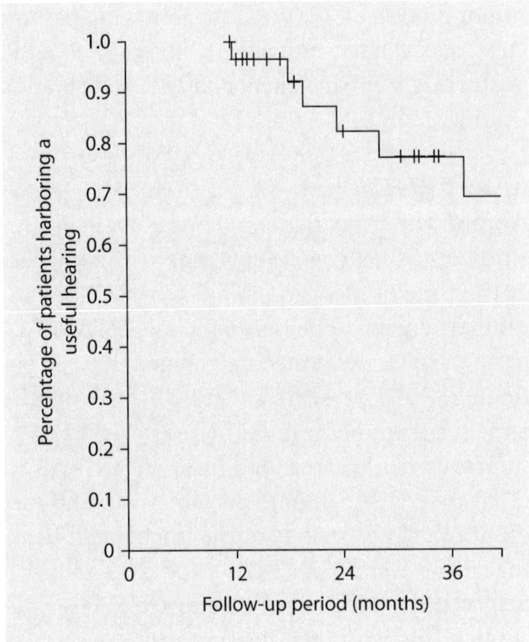

Fig. 2. Actuarial survival curve without hearing decrease to a non-useful level (31 patients with useful hearing at the time of enrolment).

a useful hearing at the time of enrolment, 25 patients (80.6%) experienced tumor growth, 5 patients (16%) presented a stable tumor and 1 patient (3%) presented a decreased tumor size. In the group of patients who experienced tumor growth, 8 patients (32%) lost their useful hearing, and among the patients with stable tumors, 1 patient (20%) lost his useful hearing. Tumor growth was not correlated with the risk of hearing loss (table 1).

Study of Patients with a Near-Normal Hearing Level

Among the 47 patients, 16 presented with a near-normal hearing at the time of their inclusion (PTA ≤30 dB and SDS ≥70%). During the follow-up (mean: 34.2 (±23.7) months, median: 26.3 months), 11 of the 16 patients (68.8%) kept the same hearing level, while 5 of them deteriorated (fig. 3). Among the 16 patients, 13 (81.2%) displayed tumor growth during the study period while 3 of them remained stable (18.8%). Among these 13 patients with tumor growth, 3 (23.1%) displayed hearing degradation. Among the 3 patients without tumor growth, 2 (66.7%) experienced hearing worsening. Values of tumor growth were not statistically correlated with the ability of hearing preservation.

Discussion

It has been postulated for many years that intracanalicular tumors belonged to a distinct category of VS that displayed an original biological behavior. Martin et al. [3] studied the histopathology of 144 VSs and observed that 100% of intracanalicular tumors displayed an Antoni A architecture, while the majority of large tumors displayed a B type (76.8%) pattern. Additionally, Kasantikul et al. [4] underlined the predilection of male patients for intracanalicular tumors and a female predilection for large VS. Taken collectively, these data suggested that intracanalicular VSs were less aggressive and that most of these tumors were able to maintain stability in the long-term. We shared this opinion when GKR was introduced in our institution and thus decided to adopt a wait and see policy in this group of patients (table 2). At the same time, we recommended a sequential follow-up of this population with special attention paid to volume modification and hearing status.

In the management of VS, the wait and see policy may be adopted for several reasons that can be listed as follows: patients with asymptomatic VS, patients in whom the only hearing ear is involved, elderly patients with mild symptoms, patient refusal of any treatment. In the series from Deen et al. [5], the proportion of each cause was 4, 4, 55, and 21%, respectively. For an individual tumor case, conservative attitude may also depend on the experience of the surgical team when the issue of hearing preservation is at stake. Another important issue is to know if microsurgery after

Table 1. Correlation between hearing degradation and growth

	Mean initial PTA	Mean final PTA	p
Patients with stable tumor	41.09	51.25	0.049
Patients with growing tumor	30.56	43.56	0.001
p	0.179	0.269	

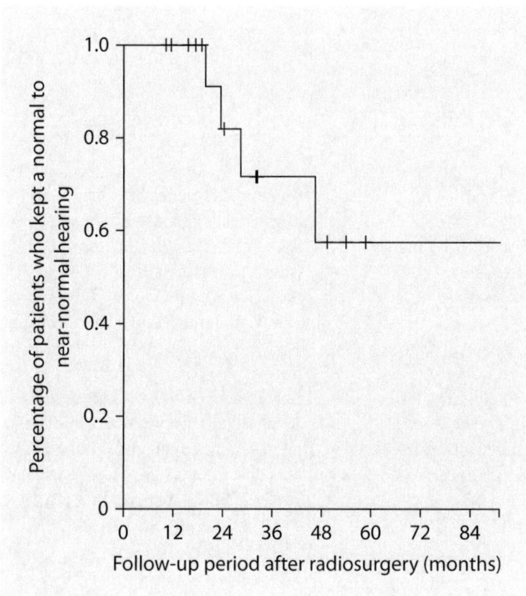

Fig. 3. Actuarial survival curve without hearing decrease in the subgroup of near-normal hearing patients (Gardner-Robertson class I).

failed conservative policy (observation of tumor growth) gives less chance for the patient when compared with early proactive treatment. Raut et al. [6] analyzed both groups and, except hearing results, found similar functional outcome and comparable tumor cure rate in matched cases.

When analyzing the literature about the wait and see policy in small VSs, many methodological pitfalls [7] weaken the value of conclusions that are drawn (table 2) [5, 6, 8]. Studies were mainly retrospective and lacking sequential MRI scanning. Numerous patients were lost to follow-up and were not consecutively enrolled but highly selected for this strategy. Moreover, the studies did not select exclusively intracanalicular VS. We attempted to avoid such drawbacks in our own protocol but our study also suffered from an insufficient follow-up and a limited number of enrolled patients.

Regarding the issue of hearing preservation, results from the literature are in line with our own observations. First, hearing decline occurs in a significant percentage of patients, and second, hearing deterioration is independent of tumor volume changes.

Conclusions

Results from this study indicate that conservative management of small VS exposes the patient to a significant risk of tumor growth or hearing loss in the years that follow this decision. Thus, such option should be proposed in highly selected cases and its risks should be explained to the patient. If adopted, conservative management requires a sequential follow-up with interval scanning. These conclusions led us to change our policy in the management of intracanalicular VS and to propose an early proactive radiosurgical treatment when hearing was still useful at the time of diagnosis.

Table 2. Summary of the main recent series of conservatively managed patients

Author/year	Patients	Study design	Mean follow-up	Stable tumor volume %	Growth %	Hearing decrease %	Additional microsurgery or radiosurgery
Deen, 1996	68	retrospective TDM-MRI	3.4 years	71	29		15%
Raut, 2004	72	prospective serial MR	80 months (52–242)	41.7	32		32%
Bozorg, 2005	111	retrospective	33 months	47	47	56	15%
Present series	47	prospective	44 months	22	76	37.5	35/47

References

1 Ogawa K, Kanzaki J, Ogawa S, Tsuchihashi N, Ikeda S: Progression of hearing loss in acoustic neuromas. Acta Otolaryngol Suppl 1991;487:133–137.

2 Koos WT, Day JD, Matula C, Levy DI: Neurotopographic considerations in the microsurgical treatment of small acoustic neurinomas. J Neurosurg 1998;88:506–512.

3 Martin C, Prades JM, Mayaud R, Chelik L: Facteurs d'évolutivité des neurinomes de l'acoustique. JFORL 1992;41:18–22.

4 Kasantikul V, Netsky MG, Glasscock MEd, Hayes JW: Intracanalicular neurilemmomas: clinicopathologic study. Ann Otol Rhinol Laryngol 1980;89:29–32.

5 Deen HG, Ebersold MJ, Harner SG, Beatty CW, Marion MS, Wharen RE, Green JD, Quast L: Conservative management of acoustic neuroma: an outcome study. Neurosurgery 1996;39:260–264.

6 Raut VV, Walsh RM, Bath AP, Bance ML, Guha A, Tator CH, Rutka JA: Conservative management of vestibular schwannomas – second review of a prospective longitudinal study. Clin Otolaryngol Allied Sci 2004;29:505–514.

7 Sackett DL, Haynes RB, Guyat GH, Tugwell P: Macking a prognosis; in Sackett DL, Haynes RB, Tugwell P, Guyatt GH: Clinical Epidemiology: A Basic Science for Clinical Medicine, ed 2. Boston, Little, Brown and Company, 1991, ed 2, pp 173–185.

8 Bozorg Grayeli A, Kalamarides M, Ferrary E, Bouccara D, ElGharem H, Rey A, Sterkers O: Conservative management versus surgery for small vestibular schwannomas. Acta Otolaryngol 2005;125:1063–1068.

Prof. Pierre-Hugues Roche
Service de Neurochirurgie de l'Hôpital Nord
Assistance Publique-Hôpitaux de Marseille
Chemin des Bourrelly
FR–13915 Marseille Cedex 20 (France)
Tel. +33 4 91 96 86 20, Fax +33 4 91 96 89 15, E-Mail proche@mail.ap-hm.fr

Régis J, Roche P-H (eds): Modern Management of Acoustic Neuroma.
Prog Neurol Surg. Basel, Karger, 2008, vol 21, pp 89–92

Recurrence of Vestibular Schwannomas after Surgery

Pierre-Hugues Roche[a] · Telmo Ribeiro[a] · Muhamad Khalil[a] · Outouma Soumare[a] · Jean-Marc Thomassin[b] · William Pellet[a]

[a]Service de Neurochirurgie, Hôpital Sainte-Marguerite, and [b]Fédération d'Oto-Rhino-Laryngologie, Hôpital La Timone, Assistance Publique-Hôpitaux de Marseille, Marseille, France

Abstract

The issue of recurrence of vestibular schwannomas is poorly studied by the surgical literature and is probably underestimated. Our own long-term retrospective analysis after translabyrinthine approach has indicated a 9.2% recurrence rate. This long-term event is mainly due to regrowth of microfragments that have been left in the operative field along the course of the facial nerve or at the surface of the pons. Management of recurrence depends on the tumor size and patient's condition. Our current policy is to propose a Gamma Knife radiosurgical treatment in eligible cases. Prospective long-term follow-up studies using serial MR imaging after radical removal should bring reliable data about the incidence of vestibular schwannoma recurrence.

Recurrence of vestibular schwannomas (VSs) is defined by radiological evidence of a new tumor that appears in the operative field during follow-up while the initial surgery has been considered as total and confirmed by normal postoperative images. This restrictive definition excludes the case of tumor regrowth after incomplete surgery and also occurrence of a new tumor on the same nerve, which may sometimes happen in neurofibromatosis type 2 (NF2) patients. The aim of this chapter is to review the data about incidence of recurrence after microsurgery, and also the way to diagnose and to manage this situation.

Incidence of Recurrence

Assuming that VS is a benign tumor, it was not recommended to propose sequential clinical or radiological follow-up for patients who where managed with radical total removal. Moreover, before the area of MRI, radiological evaluation was inefficient to identify small remnant tumors. Thus, surgeons usually waited for clinical symptoms to confirm recurrence. Nowadays, we are still missing a prospective long-term follow-up MR study to evaluate the incidence of recurrence.

In an attempt to evaluate the true incidence of VS after microsurgery, we conducted a retrospective study about the follow-up of patients who where treated using an enlarged translabyrinthine approach in our institution [1]. Two hundred and four patients were asked to check their clinical and posterior fossa MR status at 8–16 years after microsurgery. 97 of them (47.5%) accepted to be enrolled. Radiological evidence of recurrence following strict criterions was 9.2% (9% after total removal and 11% after radical subtotal removal). Obviously, this study suffered from many weaknesses: retrospective design, small proportion of enrolled patients, radical subtotal instead of total removal in several cases. However, this high rate of recurrence has been observed in several other studies, with two authors reporting a 10% rate [2, 3]. Conversely, other studies report very low rates. For instance, the House Ear Institute experience indicates a 0.3% recurrence rate in 1,668 patients, but no data are provided about the methodology of follow-up [4]. This team underlined the fact that the average time of recurrence was 10 years after first surgery. The recent study from Schmerber et al. [5] reported no radiological recurrence after the translabyrinthine removal of unilateral VS. The mean follow-up period for MRI was 11 years (range, 5–21 years). However, among the 148 patients who were included in this study, only 91 provided enough data. Moreover, the repartition of size was very heterogeneous (7 stage I, 48 stage II, 22 stage III, 14 stage IV). The small number of large tumors that have been operated on in this cohort is insufficient to stress a definitive conclusion regarding the actual rate of recurrence.

Influencing Parameters

It may be assumed that the attempt of hearing preservation may increase the risk of nonradical surgery and recurrence. In this situation, the surgeon may not wish to take the risk of direct manipulation of the last piece of tumor along the course of the cochlear nerve or compromise its vascularization. When perioperative auditory brain stem response indicates some degradation of the recorded waves, surgery may be deliberately interrupted, leaving some remnant tumor against the cochlear nerve. Samii and Matthies [6] reported a 1.4% recurrence rate when an attempt of hearing preservation was made versus 0.48 when this attempt was not made. Atlas et al. [2] observed a 10% rate in the 3–5 years that followed microsurgery with the attempt of hearing preservation.

Selection of the approach could theoretically interfere with the potential of recurrence. The retrosigmoid route leaves blind the 2 last millimeters at the end of the internal auditory canal (IAC), while the translabyrinthine technique explores the fundus and usually does not leave any blind area. However, no difference has been demonstrated in terms of recurrence between both approaches. Moreover, it is now routinely possible to check what has been left in the fundus of the IAC using an endoscope.

Tumor size at the time of management can also be discussed; removal of extra-large tumors may lead to some tumor microfragments being left against the brain stem, trigeminal root, lower cranial nerves or elsewhere in the CPA. However, this issue has never been specifically studied.

Biological parameters may be incriminated. Despite the same histological features that are shared by sporadic and NF2 schwannomas, we know that NF2 patients may have multifocal schwannomas on the same nerve; these tumors display a multilocular shape, are more adherent to the surrounding structures, particularly to the cochlear nerve. Thus, the potential of recurrence in these cases may be more important. Hwang et al. [7] analyzed the pathological findings of 15 VSs with rapid regrowth or recurrence after surgery between 1978 and 2000. They observed a statistically more elevated rate of cellularity, pleomorphism and proliferative index in this group in comparison with a control group.

Diagnosis of Recurrence

Nowadays, diagnosis of recurrence is mainly based on postoperative image checking, but in rare occasions clinical manifestations are at the origin of the diagnosis. Several presentations may occur. Apart from ataxia or axial signs in cases of large recurrences, worsening or onset of new cranial nerve deficits is the most common finding, including trigeminal symptoms, hearing decrease after initial preservation, and facial nerve symptoms (hemifacial spasm, facial motion worsening). Neuroimaging techniques, particularly MR imaging using special sequences

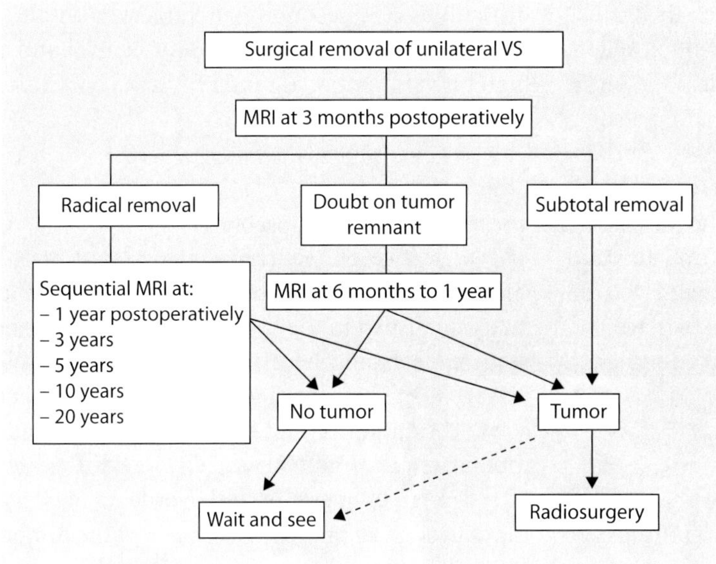

Fig. 1. Radiological follow-up scheme after removal of unilateral VS. The dotted arrow indicates an option that can be proposed in case of a small and stable residual tumor in elderly patients.

(fat suppression, post-gadolinium T_1 sequences) are the most valuable methods for detection of tumor recurrence. Several locations of recurrent schwannomas have been described, but most of them occur along the course of the facial nerve. These places are: the fundus of the IAC, the porus of the IAC, the pons at the entry zone of the dorsal root of the trigeminal nerve. In some circumstances, it may be difficult to make the difference between a scar tissue and true recurrence. Linear thin images located on the dura, particularly in the IAC may belong to the former while globular mass close to the brainstem may belong to the latter category. If any doubt remains, sequential MR scanning will bring the solution if a growing feature appears.

Follow-Up Scheme after Microsurgery

Immediate postoperative MRI study is not useful owing to the difficulties to clearly identify a remnant tumor in a modified postoperative area. Indeed, there is a risk of misinterpretation with scar tissue, edematous response of cranial nerves or artifacts. Additionally, evidence of tumor remnant does not justify early treatment. Thus, we recommend the first MRI at 3 months following surgery (fig. 1). The radiologist should have enough information about the approach that has been done in order to give the appropriate sequences. The use of a translabyrinthine route requires fat sat sequence to differentiate the fat that fills the bony defect from potential remnant tumor inside the lateral part of the IAC.

When subtotal removal has been performed with evidence of typical residual tumor on the postoperative MRI, an adjunctive treatment may be considered. The timing of this treatment depends on several parameters: size of the residual tumor, postoperative functional status, opinions from the surgeon and patient. If additional treatment is not planned, yearly MRI seems justified. The precise behavior of untreated remnant tumor is not clearly assessed, but data from the literature indicate a 20–40% regrowth rate.

When total removal has been achieved (based upon the operative chart and confirmed by a tumor-free postoperative MRI), we recommend another MRI of the posterior fossa at 1 year after surgery, and additional MRI each 3 years until 20 years after microsurgery. Additional ultralong-term follow-up remains questionable. One of the major difficulties to collect long-term information is to keep the patient focused on this issue, particularly if he/she could go back to his/her previous status without any permanent complication. However, we recently observed the case of an ultra-late recurrence of a benign unilateral VS in a patient who underwent a radical tumor removal 20 years ago.

Management of Recurrence

This issue is discussed in individual chapters but briefly, three alternatives have to be discussed: conservative treatment, radiosurgery, microsurgery. Conservative treatment may be proposed in elderly patients with small and moderately growing tumors. Microsurgery is proposed for large recurrent tumors but it carries additional difficulties due to previous surgery. If tumor size is compatible, radiosurgery is our preferred option as it is not invasive. Radiosurgery avoids the difficulties of a second open surgery with altogether a satisfactory rate of tumor control and a high rate of functional preservation.

Conclusion

The incidence of recurrence is underestimated since there is no long-term follow-up imaging study published in the literature. Management of recurrence should be discussed by a multidisciplinary team and depends on tumor size, patient age and symptoms. However, assuming that additional microsurgery may bring more difficulties after a previous operation and in order to preserve the neurological microenvironment of the tumor, our policy is to recommend radiosurgical treatment if possible. In our experience, functional results with this approach are comparable to those obtained after first intention radiosurgery.

To avoid ultra-late large recurrences, it is advised to propose a sequential clinical and MR follow-up protocol in the long-term, even in cases of estimated radical surgery.

References

1 Thomassin JM, Pellet W, Epron J, Braccini F, Roche PH: Les récidives des neurinomes de l'acoustique après exérèse chirurgicale. Ann Otolaryngol Chir Cervicofac 2001;118:3–10.

2 Atlas MD, Harvey C, Fagan PA: Hearing preservation in acoustic neuroma surgery: a continuing study. Laryngoscope 1992;102:779–783.

3 Cerullo LJ, Grutsch JF, Heiferman K, Osterdock R: The preservation of hearing and facial nerve function in a consecutive series of unilateral vestibular nerve schwannoma surgical patients. Surg Neurol 1993;39:485–493.

4 Shelton C: Unilateral acoustic tumors: how often do they recur after translabyrinthine removal? Laryngoscope 1995;105:958–966.

5 Schmerber S, Palombi O, Boubagra K, Charachon R, Chirossel JP, Gay E: Long-term control of vestibular schwannoma after a translabyrinthine complete removal. Neurosurgery 2005;57:693–698.

6 Samii M, Matthies C: Management of 1,000 vestibular schwannomas: surgical management and results with an emphasis on complications and how to avoid them. Neurosurgery 1997;40:11–23.

7 Hwang SK, Kim DG, Paek SH, Kim CY, Kim MK, Chi JG, Jung HW: Aggressive vestibular schwannomas with postoperative rapid growth: clinicopathological analysis of 15 cases. Neurosurgery 2002;51:1381–1391.

Prof. Pierre-Hugues Roche
Service de Neurochirurgie de l'Hôpital Nord
Assistance Publique-Hôpitaux de Marseille
Chemin des Bourrelly
FR–13915 Marseille Cedex 20 (France)
Tel. +33 4 91 96 86 20, Fax +33 4 91 96 89 15, E-Mail proche@mail.ap-hm.fr

Régis J, Roche P-H (eds): Modern Management of Acoustic Neuroma.
Prog Neurol Surg. Basel, Karger, 2008, vol 21, pp 93–97

Morphological Changes of Vestibular Schwannomas after Radiosurgical Treatment: Pitfalls and Diagnosis of Failure

Christine Delsanti[c] · Pierre-Hughes Roche[a] ·
Jean-Marc Thomassin[b] · Jean Régis[c]

[a]Service de Neurochirurgie, Hôpital Sainte-Marguerite, [b]Fédération d'Oto-Rhino-Laryngologie, et [c]Service de Neurochirurgie Stéréotaxique et Fonctionnelle, Hôpital la Timone, Assistance Publique-Hôpitaux de Marseille, Marseille, France

Abstract

Rationale: Evaluate the morphological changes following radiosurgery in order to better define failure parameters. **Methods:** 332 non-neurofibromatosis type 2 vestibular schwannomas not previously treated surgically or radiosurgically were subjected to Gamma Knife radiosurgery between 1992 and 2004 at the Gamma Knife Center in Marseille with at least three sequential MRI scans after radiosurgery. Five length measurements were systematically obtained. **Results:** Mean follow-up was 4.6 years. Transient loss of contrast enhancement appeared in 213 patients (68%). Significant increase was present at 6 months in 178 patients. In 74 patients, the volume at 3 years was still higher than on the day of radiosurgery but remained stable. Failure occurred in 16 patients. Most showed progressive growth at all MRI controls after radiosurgery but late failure after initial response was possible. **Conclusions:** Sequential MRI scans after radiosurgery are necessary. A progressive and continuous growth at 3 years is essential to make diagnosis of failure.

Morphological changes of vestibular schwannomas (VSs) after radiosurgery are sometimes misinterpreted. As almost all the new onset neuropathies are temporary and will resolve without treatment, clinical changes are a poor indicator of failure. A correct interpretation of follow-up imaging and the knowledge of the different patterns of evolution are therefore the only way to prevent unnecessary and inappropriate surgery.

In this report, we will try to give guidelines for a correct interpretation of morphological changes based on the analysis of the series of VSs treated by radiosurgery in Marseille.

Materials and Methods

This study focused on non-neurofibromatosis type 2 VSs not previously treated surgically or radiosurgically. They were part of the 1,000 first VSs that were treated at our Gamma Knife Center in Marseille between July 1992 and January 2004.

Most of the VS patients are followed by the referent institution and we do not possess sequential MRI scans for them. For 332 patients, we possess at least 3 sequential MRI scans after radiosurgical treatment, 1 during the 1st year after treatment and a least 2 after the 1st year. The two groups of patients are comparable in terms of age, gender, mean volume on the day of treatment and Koos distribution.

For each patient, we do 5 measurements on MRI and calculate the corresponding volume according to

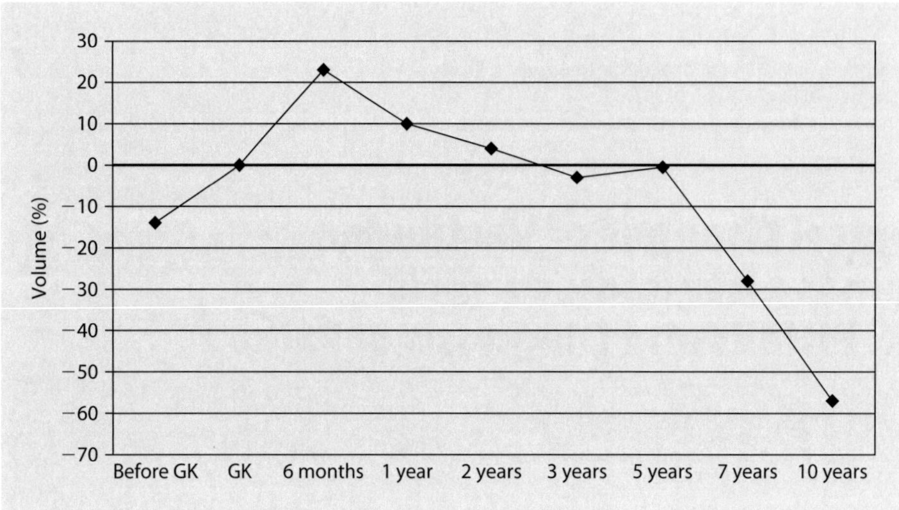

Fig. 1. Overall evolution of volume of treated VSs.

Linskey et al. [1]. Each volume is compared with the volume on the day of treatment and the difference is expressed in terms of percentage of the volume on the day of treatment.

Modification of contrast enhancement is also reported for each MRI.

Results

For these 332 patients, the mean follow-up was 4.6 years (minimum 1.6 years, maximum 13 years, median 4 years).

Loss of Contrast Enhancement

Loss of contrast enhancement is the most frequent modification after radiosurgery. We studied it on 312 patients with noncystic VS.

We observed transient loss of contrast enhancement for 213 (68%) patients. This loss of contrast enhancement was present for 55% (173 patients) at 6 months, 36% (111 patients) at 1 year and only 5% (17 patients) at 3 years. This loss of contrast enhancement was almost always transient. Only 3 patients still had loss of contrast enhancement at the last follow-up.

Modifications in Volume

Figure 1 demonstrates overall evolution of the volume of the treated VSs. At 6 months, a swelling was present in 178 patients. For 91 patients, the swelling was more than 30% in volume and may have reached up to 200%. For axial measurement, the VS may increase more than 5 mm in one axis.

Figure 2 shows comparison of different subgroups of patients. As described by Pollock [2], some VSs are larger at 3 years than on the day of treatment, but these patients are not considered as failure because they are stable despite the initial growing. We have 74 patients belonging to this subgroup. A long follow-up for this subgroup, can demonstrate that it is probably a delayed response to radiosurgery.

If we compare this subgroup with patients considered as failure (16 patients), the mean initial growth at 6 months is almost the same (53% for failure vs. 50% for increased without failure) but the VSs of the failure subgroup grow more rapidly (at 1 year, mean growth 75 vs. 52%, at 2 years mean growth 207 vs. 58%).

Figure 3 shows all the available measurements for failure patients.

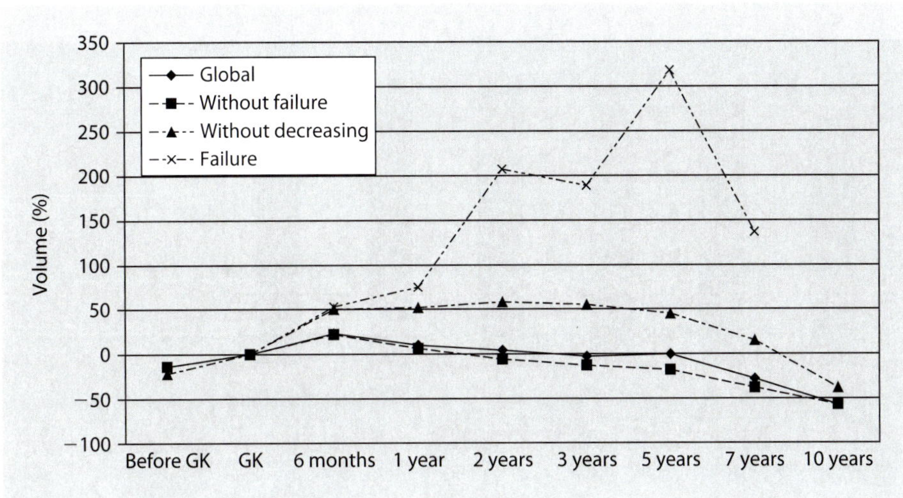

Fig. 2. Comparison of different subgroups of patients.

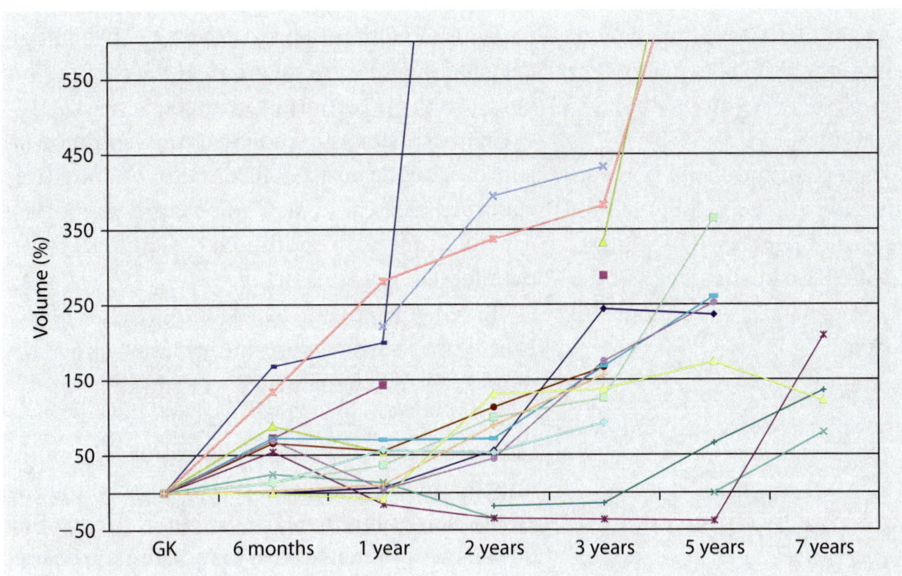

Fig. 3. Available measurements for failure patients.

No statistical analysis is possible for this subgroup of patients, but we can see three groups of patients. In the first group, the growth of the tumor is significant at the first control and continues up to surgery. In the second group, the initial growth is followed by stabilization at 1 year or sometimes 2 years, and then it continues up to surgery. The third group is the group of late failure. We have only 2 patients in this group, which was previously not described [3]. After an initial phase of tumor control, they showed a dramatic increase at 5 years for the first and 7 years for the second.

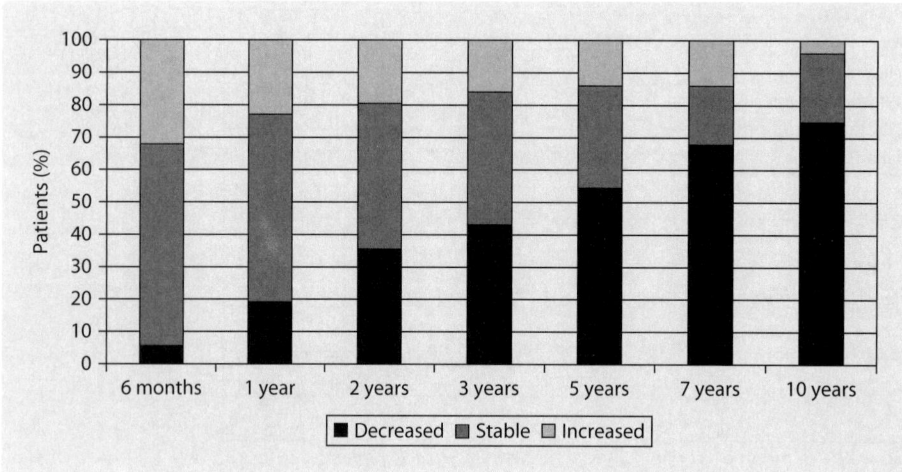

Fig. 4. Evolution of the percentage of stable patients and patients without failure whose tumors increased or decreased in volume.

The second patient had cranial nerve impairment concomitant to tumor growth. She underwent surgery without problem. Anatomopathologic analysis revealed no atypias.

Figure 4 shows the evolution of the percentage of stable patients and patients without failure whose tumors increased or decreased in volume. More than 50% of patients had shrinkage of the lesion at 5 years. At 10 years, only one patient still had an increased lesion.

Discussion

Unexpected Course of VS after Gamma Knife Radiosurgery

The course of VS after Gamma Knife radiosurgery (GKR) is not uniform and continuous refinements of radiology allow us to describe several patterns of volumetric and morphological changes of VS after GKR. The proper way to describe these changes is to obtain a sequential iterative MRI scan for each patient after treatment. This strategy [4] has been used in this and also in recent studies from which it is possible to extract interesting data [2, 5]. Pollock [2] described several patterns of volume change following chronological criteria while Hasegawa et al. [5] focused his study on the postcontrast changes.

In the historical studies, it was common to summarize the post-GKR course of VS into three subtypes: decreased size, unchanged size or escapement requiring additional treatment. Other details were not considered.

Taken collectively, our data together with recent studies bring more information about the patterns of VS changes.

It is very frequent to observe tumor growth after GKR. This growth take places in the 3–12 months after treatment and is mainly transient without any additional symptoms (Pollock type 1). Depending on the method that is used to measure the changes (2-mm diameter rule, 10% increased computerized volume) the incidence of such growth varies from 10 to 50% of patients. Such growth is usually correlated with morphological changes, particularly loss of central contrast enhancement, named type C by Hasegawa et al. [5]. The exact meaning of such loss of contrast is poorly understood (necrosis, apoptosis, subacute inflammatory period).

Another pattern is the growth after GKS followed by stabilization at an increased volume.

Such population, if followed for long enough, indicates no additional modification in the long-term and does not require any other treatment (Pollock type 2).

In another group of patients, continuous growth after GK may be observed.

Careful long-term control is still needed because each series mentions several cases of ultra-late failure while tumor remained stable during the first 5 years.

Factors Affecting Tumor Expansion

Although it is difficult to predict tumor expansion at the time of GKR, several factors have been suspected. Tumor size exceeding 15 cm^3 and cystic component are the most strongly suspected but other factors have been advocated: low doses, female gender ($p < 0.05$ in the multivariate analysis from Hasegawa).

How to Manage These Unexpected Tumor Changes

First point is to tell the patient and referring physician that these changes may happen and that the patient has to maintain close contact with the neurosurgeon who made the procedure.

Enough follow-up time should be allowed after this observation and perhaps more sequential follow-up MR protocol recommended (each 6 months may be necessary).

The kinetics of growth and the intratumorous changes should be carefully analyzed. Special attention may be given to cystic modifications because the cysts usually do not stop growing.

The patient should be checked for clinical symptoms (trigeminal symptoms, gait ataxia, severe imbalance are the main signs of clinical failure). In the case of Pollock type 1 or type 2 modifications with no cystic features, nothing more is needed. In the case of progressive enlargement on serial imaging, whether solid or cystic, additional treatment may be required, particularly in the case of clinical worsening. Cystic changes necessitate surgical procedure while solid tumor can justify an attempt of additional second GKR, if the volume is still compatible.

Conclusion

Diagnosis of failure in the radiosurgical treatment of VSs is still controversial. Sequential imaging during the first 3 years after treatment is essential to detect failure and avoid unnecessary surgery. Continuous increase in volume at 3 years (VS larger than on the day of treatment and the previous control) must be considered as failure. Follow-up after 3 years is necessary do detect late failure. We propose MRI at 5, 7 and 10 years after treatment.

References

1 Linskey ME, Lunsford LD, Flickinger JC, Kondziolka D: Stereotactic radiosurgery for acoustic tumors. Neurosurg Clin North Am 1992;3:191–205.

2 Pollock BE: Management of vestibular schwannomas that enlarge after stereotactic radiosurgery: treatment recommendations based on a 15 year experience. Neurosurgery 2006;58:241–248.

3 Noren G: Gamma Knife radiosurgery for acoustic neurinomas; in Gildenberg PL, Tasker RR (eds): Textbook of Stereotactic and Functional Neurosurgery. New York, Mc Graw-Hill, 1996, vol 1, pp 835–844.

4 Régis J, Pellet W, Delsanti C, Dufour H, Roche PH, Thomassin JM, Zanaret M, Peragut JC: Functional outcome after gamma knife surgery or microsurgery for vestibular schwannomas. J Neurosurg 2002;97:1091–1100.

5 Hasegawa T, Kida Yoshihisa, Yoshimoto M, Koike J, Goto K: Evaluation of tumor expansion after stereotactic radiosurgery in patients harboring vestibular schwannomas. Neurosurgery 2006;58:1119–1128.

Dr. Christine Delsanti
Service de Neurochirurgie Stéréotaxique et Fonctionnelle, Hôpital de la Timone, AP-HM
FR–13385 Marseille (France)
Tel. +33 4 91 38 65 62, Fax +33 4 91 38 70 56, E-Mail cdelsanti@free.fr

Régis J, Roche P-H (eds): Modern Management of Acoustic Neuroma.
Prog Neurol Surg. Basel, Karger, 2008, vol 21, pp 98–102

Tissue Changes after Radiosurgery for Vestibular Schwannomas

Marc Levivier

Centre Universitaire Romand de Neurochirurgie, Lausanne – Geneva, and Department of Neurosurgery, CHUV, Lausanne, Switzerland

Abstract

The specific effects of radiosurgery on brain tumor tissue are not well understood. We review several approaches that have been used to address this issue. Correlating the radiobiology of radiosurgery with the radioclinical outcome may help to understand these tissue changes. In vivo imaging investigations are usually performed with MRI, but the use of functional and metabolic imaging, such MR spectroscopy, positron emission tomography or single-photon emission computed tomography may provide additional information on the effects of radiosurgery. Finally, histological observations represent an invaluable source of information, when systematically analyzed in their clinical context.

The specific effects of radiosurgery on brain tumor tissue still needs better understanding. The concept of radiosurgery developed by Leksell aimed at the precise destruction of a chosen target by ionizing beams delivered in a single session, without significant destruction of the adjacent tissues. In the original conception of radiosurgery, the desired goal was a total destructive effect within the selected target volume. Originally, Leksell developed Gamma Knife as an alternative method to electrode-based lesioning of deep-seated tracts or nuclei for functional neurosurgery. As such, the doses delivered were very high, with the aim of inducing a necrotic lesion at the target point. Since then, several animal studies and clinical observations have validated this effect [1]. However, as stated by Norén [2] in his historical perspective of Gamma Knife radiosurgery for vestibular schwannomas (VSs), 'there is no doubt that Lars Leksell had acoustic neurinomas in mind when he presented the concept of radiosurgery in 1951'. Indeed, in his first paper, Leksell suggested the use of the technique also for the treatment of deep-seated circumscribed tumors. Accordingly, the first patients with VS were also treated with very high doses when compared to current protocols, leading to a high rate of VIIth and Vth cranial nerve neuropathies. In parallel to the advancements in image-based targeting and in the dosimetry techniques, the clinical results also improved thanks to the progressive changes in dose prescription [3]. Indeed, accumulated experience has shown that in tumoral radiosurgery, the use of high doses, aiming at a total tumoral necrotic destruction, are associated with high complication rate. In benign tumors especially, the use of lower doses has shown to provide a high rate of tumoral cell inactivation, yielding high tumoral control. However, this evolution was empirical and there is little objective knowledge and rationale on the relationship between the dose used and the tissue changes induced in VS treated with radiosurgery. In benign lesions in patients with a high survival expectancy, understanding the tissue changes after radiosurgery can be addressed in several ways, as reviewed below.

Radiobiology of Radiosurgery and Radioclinical Correlates

Ionizing radiation produces of a physical break in one or both of the helical strands of DNA. A single-strand break has a high likelihood of repair while two or more breaks on the same DNA strand are more likely to cause permanent damage to the cell, without the possibility of repair. Double-strand breaks lead to the physical disruption of the DNA structure. Consequently, the damage to that cell will be permanent leading to the desired therapeutic effect.

Radiosurgery increases the chance of ionizing radiation to induce permanent DNA damage as it allows the delivery of a much higher dose to the irradiated cells (i.e. it increases the number of delivered photons, increasing the statistical likelihood of a collision). Moreover, compared to fractionated radiotherapy which uses lower doses that require DNA to be maximally condensed to have a high likelihood of achieving a double-strand DNA break (i.e. indicated in tumors with a high proliferative index and that are considered to be radiosensitive), radiosurgery can act in benign tumors with a low proliferative index, such as VS, that are considered radioresistant.

As reviewed by Linskey [4] when comparing radiosurgery and radiotherapy for patients with VS, there are four potential outcomes for VS cells in which a double-strand DNA break occurs. Firstly, although theoretically possible, there is only an infinitesimal chance that the break spontaneously reanneals in the correct orientation. However, if this occurs in enough cells within the tumor, the radiosurgical treatment would be ineffective. The second possibility would be that the DNA damage leads to the activation of the endogenous cellular genomic surveillance system, which in turn would lead to the activation of immediate programmed cell death or apoptosis. The clinical corollary of this phenomenon would be early tumor shrinkage resulting from cell loss. The third possibility would occur if the radiation-induced DNA damage only triggered activation of the endogenous cellular genomic surveillance system when the cell entered the active cell cycle. This would result in delayed apoptosis with the clinical corollary of delayed tumor shrinkage over time. Because schwannoma cells generally have long cell cycle times and a low proliferative index, we would expect to see continued tumor shrinkage over many years after radiosurgery. This phenomenon is well described in the clinical GKS setting of VS. Fourthly, DNA damage might lead to a state of irreversible cellular growth arrest. In this state, schwannoma cells will remain intact and alive but will be unable to enter the active cell cycle and divide. The clinical corollary would be permanent stability in tumor size with loss of previously documented linear growth potential, despite intact tumor cellular architecture on histopathological examination. This phenomenon is also well described in the radiosurgery clinical setting of VS.

Moreover the direct radiation effects on schwannoma cells are not the only factors potentially leading to tumor control and/or shrinkage. Indeed, the tumor vasculature is also susceptible to radiation effects. Potential pathological results include tumor cell ischemia and hypoxemic cell death with subsequent cell loss. The clinical corollary is loss of central tumor contrast enhancement and delayed tumor shrinkage once ischemic cell loss predominates over ischemic cell swelling.

Image-Based in vivo Investigations

Serial follow-up with MR imaging has become the standard technique for the evaluation of the response of VS to radiosurgery [5–7]. Serial MR studies of unilateral VS treated with Gamma Knife radiosurgery show temporary enlargement of the tumor (41% of cases in the study of Nakamura et al. [5]) which occurs mostly within the first 2 years after radiosurgery. Subsequent regression of the tumor volume is usually observed during and after the 2nd year following radiosurgery. Because of such enlargement followed by regression, close follow-up with neuroimaging is desirable after radiosurgery for VS. Transient loss of contrast enhancement on MR is also often recognized in most cases, but this sign is not necessarily a useful prognostic sign of the response to radiosurgery. In most cases, serial MR studies may show that the tumor is stable after the 3rd year following radiosurgery. However, diagnosis of failure in the radiosurgical treatment of VS is still controversial, as discussed by Delsanti et al. [this vol., pp. 93–97]. Thus, this confirms that serial imaging during the first 3 years after treatment is essential to detect failure and avoid unnecessary surgery. The authors conclude that continuous increasing at 3 years (VS larger than the day of treatment and the previous control) must be considered as a failure, and also that follow-up after 3 years is necessary (e.g. 5, 7 and 10 years after treatment) to detect late failure.

Although serial MR is very important in the follow-up, the morphological changes visible with this technique may not reflect the tissue changes induced by radiosurgery in VS. Some signs, like the persistence of a peripheral hypersignal area, associated with contrast enhancement, together with central hypointensity, might correlate well with the corresponding histology. This has been observed in a case report of an NF2 type VS that was partially resected several months following Gamma Knife radiosurgery, because of tumor volume growth and clinical deterioration [8]. However, this is in contrast with most cases where histology was reported after surgery, because in those cases, surgery was performed after failed radiosurgery. These patients usually present with growing tumor and new contrast enhancement on MR, and histology is rather characteristic of typical VS with few or no residual signs of radiosurgery [9].

A promising approach to better understand the in vivo tissue changes following radiosurgery might be the use of functional and metabolic images. Although some data already exist with the use of MR spectroscopy, positron emission tomography or single-photon emission computed tomography, these studies have been performed in primary SCN tumors or in metastases of systemic cancers, and their primary goal was to evaluate the contribution of these imaging techniques in differentiating between radiation necrosis and tumor recurrence or progression. In that respect, functional and metabolic images appear to be very useful [10–12], but no study has specifically evaluated the in vivo serial changes of functional and metabolic images as a potential prognostic factor of the therapeutic response to radiosurgery, and only anecdotic information exists concerning their use in VS, as in our case report [13].

Histological Observations

Few systematic reports exist on the histological observations of tissue changes in VS after radiosurgery. Moreover, most of the reported observations focus on the surgical impact of the tissue changes induced by radiosurgery (such as fibrosis and adherences) and their consequences of the microsurgical removal of those tumors [14–16]. Recently, Szeifert et al. [17] have reviewed a series of 22 patients that underwent craniotomy for VS removal after failed radiosurgery, as part of a larger series of 1,350 patients with VS that were treated with radiosurgery in the Gamma

Knife center of Marseille, France. The originality of this report is that it focuses specifically on the histopathological analysis of these tumors. Thus, this study, which is summarized below, provides a specific description of some of the tissue changes that may be induced by radiosurgery in VS. Indeed, since this series has to be considered as a series of failure after radiosurgery, the histopathological observations may lack some of the changes observed in the majority of those patients that have benefited from radiosurgery with a long-term tumor control.

Szeifert et al. [17] reported that histopathological changes affected both the parenchyma and the stroma of the radiosurgically treated VS. The basic histopathological lesion was a necrotic core surrounded by a middle transitional zone covered by an outer capsule. The inner core of tumors consisted of necrotic debris containing scattered shrunken apoptotic neoplastic cells, with narrow cytoplasmic rim and dark pycnotic basophilic nuclei without recognizable nucleoli. This histological picture was characteristic of coagulation necrosis or ischemic infarction. This area was sharply demarcated from the surrounding tissues. The outer capsule or mantle zone of VS usually presented densely packed Schwann cell nests with storiform pattern or nuclear palisade arrangement. Scar tissue formation among and around tumor cell nests was a common finding with thick collagen bundles, hyaline degeneration, proliferating fibroblasts and fibrocytes. As the time interval increases from radiosurgery, this zone becomes more hypocellular and is replaced by bulky connective tissue. Interestingly, living tumor tissue remnants were demonstrated in all treated VS cases, even 92 months following radiosurgery. Further immunohistochemical studies showed that *Ki67* proliferative activity was decreased 6 months after radiosurgery, and it was only occasional at 16 months after radiosurgery, although moderate but still existing proliferative capacity was still visible even 48 months after radiosurgery. Thus, from the morphological point of view the biological effect of high-dose irradiation on VS tumor tissues evokes that the tumor parenchyma is the primary target of the radiation-induced cell death either via coagulation necrosis or inducing apoptosis, although some VS may retain a proliferative potential for a very long period of time. However, complementary immunohistochemical investigations (FVIII, CD31, CD34) also reveal that another target of radiosurgery is the stroma of the tumor, where it induces endothelial destruction and wall damage of the vessels with granulation tissue proliferation. Results of these immunohistochemical reactions suggest that the endothelial cell layer of vessels is very sensitive and reacts early to high-dose irradiation in tumor tissue changes.

References

1 Szeifert GT, Kondziolka D, Lunsford LD, Nyary I, Hanzely Z, Salmon I, Levivier M: The contribution of pathology to radiosurgery. Prog Neurol Surg 2007;20:1–15.

2 Norén G: Gamma knife radiosurgery of acoustic neurinomas. A historic perspective. Neurochirurgie 2004;50:253–256.

3 Regis J, Levivier M, Wikler D, Porcheron D: Dosimetric planning for radiosurgical treatment of vestibular schwannomas. Neurochirurgie 2004;50:289–300.

4 Linskey ME: Stereotactic radiosurgery versus stereotactic radiotherapy for patients with vestibular schwannoma: a Leksell Gamma Knife Society 2000 debate. J Neurosurg 2000;93(suppl 3):90–95.

5 Nakamura H, Jokura H, Takahashi K, Boku N, Akabane A, Yoshimoto T: Serial follow-up MR imaging after gamma knife radiosurgery for vestibular schwannoma. AJNR Am J Neuroradiol 2000;21:1540–1546.

6 Prasad D, Steiner M, Steiner L: Gamma surgery for vestibular schwannoma. J Neurosurg 2000;92:745–759.

7 Regis J, Pellet W, Delsanti C, Dufour H, Roche PH, Thomassin JM, Zanaret M, Peragut JC: Functional outcome after gamma knife surgery or microsurgery for vestibular schwannomas. J Neurosurg 2002;97:1091–1100.

8 Szeifert GT, Massager N, DeVriendt D, David P, De Smedt F, Rorive S, Salmon I, Brotchi J, Levivier M: Observations of intracranial neoplasms treated with gamma knife radiosurgery. J Neurosurg 2002;97(suppl 5): 623–626.
9 Kwon Y, Khang SK, Kim CJ, Lee DJ, Lee JK, Kwun BD: Radiologic and histopathologic changes after Gamma Knife radiosurgery for acoustic schwannoma. Stereotact Funct Neurosurg 1999;72(suppl 1):2–10.
10 Chernov M, Hayashi M, Izawa M, Ochiai T, Usukura M, Abe K, Ono Y, Muragaki Y, Kubo O, Hori T, Takakura K: Differentiation of the radiation-induced necrosis and tumor recurrence after gamma knife radiosurgery for brain metastases: importance of multi-voxel proton MRS. Minim Invasive Neurosurg 2005;48:228–234.
11 Kimura T, Sako K, Tanaka K, Gotoh T, Yoshida H, Aburano T, Tanaka T, Arai H, Nakada T: Evaluation of the response of metastatic brain tumors to stereotactic radiosurgery by proton magnetic resonance spectroscopy, 201TlCl single-photon emission computerized tomography, and gadolinium-enhanced magnetic resonance imaging. J Neurosurg 2004;100:835–841.
12 Tsuyuguchi N, Takami T, Sunada I, Iwai Y, Yamanaka K, Tanaka K, Nishikawa M, Ohata K, Torii K, Morino M, Nishio A, Hara M: Methionine positron emission tomography for differentiation of recurrent brain tumor and radiation necrosis after stereotactic radiosurgery in malignant glioma. Ann Nucl Med 2004;18:291–296.
13 Levivier M, Massager N, David P: In vivo evaluation of tumor response to radiosurgery: application to vestibular schwannomas. Neurochirurgie 2004;50:320–326.
14 Beatty CW, Ebersold MJ, Harner SG: Residual and recurrent acoustic neuromas. Laryngoscope 1987;97: 1168–1171.
15 Pollock BE, Lunsford LD, Kondziolka D, Sekula R, Subach BR, Foote RL, Flickinger JC: Vestibular schwannoma management. Part II. Failed radiosurgery and the role of delayed microsurgery. J Neurosurg 1998;89:949–955.
16 Slaterry WR, Brackmann D: Results of surgery following stereotactic irradiation for acoustic neuromas. Am J Otol 1995;16:315–321.
17 Szeifert GT, Figarella-Branger D, Roche PH, Regis J: Histopathological observations on vestibular schwannomas after Gamma Knife radiosurgery: the Marseille experience. Neurochirurgie 2004;50:327–337.

Marc Levivier, MD, PhD
Rue du Bugnon, 46
BH-10163 – CHUV
CH–1011 Lausanne (Switzerland)
Tel. +41 21 314 26 02, Fax +41 21 314 26 05, E-Mail Marc.Levivier@chuv.ch

Régis J, Roche P-H (eds): Modern Management of Acoustic Neuroma.
Prog Neurol Surg. Basel, Karger, 2008, vol 21, pp 103–107

Facial Nerve Outcome after Microsurgical Resection of Vestibular Schwannoma

Rafik Marouf · Rémi Noudel · Pierre-Hugues Roche

Service de Neurochirurgie, Hôpital Nord, Assistance Publique-Hôpitaux de Marseille, Marseille, France

Abstract

The risk of facial nerve palsy after microsurgical removal of vestibular schwannoma cannot be totally eradicated. Beyond the functional problem, patients have to overcome the consequences of cosmetic disturbances, particularly the psychosocial difficulties and the decrease in quality of life due to this palsy. Taken together, the data from our personal experience and analysis of the literature indicate that the major predictor of postoperative facial deficit is tumor size. This information must be given to the patient when counseling for treatment option. When confronted with large tumors, we personally changed our surgical goals and considered that facial nerve conservation and tumor control are interconnected priorities instead of radical removal.

Despite gradual refinements of the microsurgical techniques, the occurrence of facial nerve palsy remains a common event after the surgical treatment of vestibular schwannomas (VSs). Based on our personal experience and on the review of the recent international literature, we report the incidence of this event in relation to tumor size and approach, and analyze the main predictive parameters of this complication.

Results

In table 1, we have analyzed the results obtained by several skull base teams whom expertise in the field of VS surgery is well known [1–13]. We have separated the table in two parts. In the first one, results are given independently of tumor size; a majority of these series included patients harboring small- to middle-sized tumors. Good facial motion at the last follow-up examination (House-Brackmann, H-B, grade 1 or 2) was found in 61–97% of patients. In the second part of the table, we selected the publications which gave enough data on large tumors. A uniform definition of 'large tumors' is not widely accepted, but our selection criteria for the purpose of this study were: main tumor diameter exceeding 3 cm or Koos stage IV [14]. In this subgroup, good facial motion was found in 38–84% of cases.

Discussion

How to Evaluate

The H-B classification is nowadays uniformly validated, although the accuracy of the grading

Table 1. Some relevant studies of operated VS that have been published in the last 15 years (especially tumor size and postoperative facial nerve results were considered)

First author	Tumor diameter in CPA	Number of cases	Surgical approach	Total resection, %	Facial nerve preservation[1] at last follow-up, %
Ebersold, 1992 [1]	all size	255	RS	97	61.7
Fischer, 1992 [2]	all size	270	RS	92	65.6
Sterkers, 1994 [3]	all size	576	RS	91	97
Wigand, 1996 [4]	all size	485	middle fossa	98	79
Samii, 1997 [5]	all size	1000	RS	98	64
Isaacson, 2005 [6]	all size	221	MF and TL		87
Results for large tumors					
Gormley, 1997 [7]	>4 cm	28	all approaches	99	38
Lanmann, 1999 [8]	>3 cm	190	TL	96	52
Sluyter, 2001 [9]	>2 cm	120	TL	92	56
Devèze, 2004 [10]	Koos IV	110	TL	82	60
Yamakami, 2004 [11]	>3 cm	50	RS	86	84
Zhang, 2005 [12]	>4 cm	105	RS	86.7	56.7
Anderson, 2005 [13]	>3 cm	71	all approaches	95.8	80

RS = Retrosigmoid; TL = translabyrinthine; CPA = cerebellopontine angle.
[1]H-B grades 1 and 2.

system is perfectible. When analyzing grade 3, there is a great heterogeneity in the severity of the deficit while patients are classified in the same grade. Moreover, this classification needed to evaluate the intermedius nerve component, which has been done at the Tokyo conference.

Self-assessment by patients is also an important way to evaluate. In this perspective, the Acoustic Neuroma Association mailed a detailed questionnaire to 2,372 members to identify preoperative and postoperative problems. 82.2% of them reported their experiences with facial nerve dysfunction: 11% experienced some degree of preoperative facial weakness or eye problems. 45.5% experienced worsened facial weakness caused by surgery, and of these, 72% reported that it was permanent. Twenty-eight percent of responders felt significantly affected by facial weakness [15].

Predictive Parameters of Facial Nerve Outcome

Tumor size is uniformly considered as the main predictor of the quality of facial nerve motion in the postoperative course (table 1). All neurosurgeons know the difficulties to identify, dissect and preserve the integrity of the facial nerve without damage in cases of large tumor.

Neurofibromatosis type 2 (NF2) is a situation where tumor shape is multilobulated and where the nerve is more frequently infiltrated by the tumor capsule. Preservation of facial nerve is usually more difficult in NF2 patients when compared with unilateral VS.

Preoperative facial deficit is hopefully an unusual presentation even in cases of very large tumors. However, its evidence may indicate early damage of the nerve fibers and additional difficulties of dissection during surgery.

Previous microsurgery of the same tumor is usually associated with postoperative degradation of facial motion. Freeman et al. [16] recently reported a series of 35 patients that were reoperated. Nine of them presented with a poor preoperative status of their facial nerve, and a further 10 deteriorated by at least 3 grades by 1 year postoperatively.

Peri-operative neuromonitoring gives reliable information for the postoperative course: Grayeli et al. [17] used of a four-channel monitoring system and reported that a proximal threshold between 0.01 and 0.04 mA had a positive predictive value of 94% for good facial function (H-B grade 1 or 2). In the study from Neff et al. [18], a response amplitude of 240 μV or greater predicted an H-B grade 1 or 2 outcome with 98% probability.

Concerning cystic organization of the schwannoma, Fundova et al. [19] compared the surgical results of 44 cystic VSs with 151 solid VSs, and found that cystic subtypes were associated with a greater risk of permanent facial palsy and generally less favorable surgical outcome, which is in keeping with many other reports.

For other parameters, there is more controversy. Patient age has been evaluated in several studies. Mirzayan et al. [20] did not observe any difference in results between patients under 21 years of age and a matched series of adult patients. In a paper published by Oghalai et al. [21], a cohort of 150 older patients (>60 years) were compared with 55 younger patients (<40 years). It was shown that older patient age lowers the chance of hearing preservation but does not affect facial outcomes. Selection of the approach has been a matter of debate. The translabyrinthine route was considered as the safest approach since it allowed early identification of the facial nerve at the fundus of the internal auditory canal. The middle fossa approach was associated with an increased risk because the facial nerve is pushed upward in the internal auditory canal and potentially damageable during tumor manipulation. Several studies have shown that in matched cases, there is no influence of the approach on the quality of facial nerve results [6].

Consequences of Facial Palsy

Beyond functional and cosmetic problems that are encountered in cases of facial nerve deficit, psychosocial difficulties and degradation of quality of life (QOL) are often described by patients while the surgeon's eye considers the result as acceptable. In a recent study about how patients and surgeons perceived QOL after surgery for large VS [22], it was shown that psychological problems were the preponderant symptoms, and their presence was the most powerful predictive variable for global and daily QOL. Physicians should bear in mind the impact of facial dysfunction on QOL when counseling patients regarding optimal management of VS.

How to Minimize the Risk of Postoperative Facial Palsy

– Be able to predict the nerve course before surgery. Despite high level of definition, our current 1.5-tesla MRI does not provide anatomical images of the nerve course in cases of large tumors. Preoperative visualization using diffusion tensor tractography [23] is not fully satisfactory. We are still referring to our individual experience and to statistical data about neurotopographic considerations [14] to better identify the nerve during surgery.

– Select carefully the indications for microsurgery.

– Master the surgical technique. The ideal system is to learn the surgical steps in small- to medium-sized tumors before managing large tumors. For young neurosurgeons, this scheme will become less available since more and more small tumors are frequently managed with radiosurgery. This means that this surgery will not remain in the field of general neurosurgery and will be reserved to skull base teams, which is already the current organization in many countries.

– Adopt an alternative strategy to radical surgery. The facial nerve is at risk in any place in the cerebellopontine angle, but it may be more damaged while penetrating at the level of the porus acousticus and in the 5–10 mm medial to the porus. In our opinion, it makes sense to leave some fragments of the tumor along the facial nerve at these specific places instead of achieving a radical resection with potential nerve damage. We have recently adopted this strategy for large VS and improved significantly our results in terms of facial motion preservation. There is a debate about the potential of regrowth of the remnant tumors and additional radiosurgery can be proposed as a second step. One can expect that such combined strategy will be widely adopted in the future.

References

1 Ebersold MJ, Harner SG, Beatty CW, Harper CM, Quast LM: Current results of retrosigmoid approach to acoustic neuroma. J Neurosurg 1992;76:901–909.

2 Fischer G, Fischer C, Remond J: Hearing preservation in acoustic neuroma surgery. J Neurosurg 1992;76:910–917.

3 Sterkers JM, Morrison GA, Sterkers O, El-Dine MM: Preservation of facial, cochlear, and other nerve functions in acoustic neuroma treatment. Otolaryngol Head Neck Surg 1994;110:146–155.

4 Wigand ME, Hait CT, Berg M, Wolf SR: Indications and technique for an advantages of the enlarged middle fossa approach; in Sterkers JM, Sterkers O (eds): Acoustic Neuroma and Skull Base Surgery. Proceedings of the 2nd International Conference on Acoustic Neuroma Surgery and 2nd European Skull base Society Congress, Paris, 22–26 Avril 1995. Amsterdam, Kugler Publish, 1996, pp 231–234.

5 Samii M, Matthies C: Management of 1,000 vestibular schwannomas (acoustic neuromas): Surgical management and results with an emphasis on complications and how to avoid them. Neurosurgery 1997;40:11–23.

6 Isaacson B, Telian SA, El-Kashlan HK: Facial nerve outcomes in middle cranial fossa vs translabyrinthine approaches. Otolaryngol Head Neck Surg 2005;133:906–910.

7 Gormley WB, Sekhar LN, Wright DC, Kamerer D, Schessel D: Acoustic neuromas: Results of current surgical management. Neurosurgery 1997;41:50–60.

8 Lanmann TH, Brackmann, DE, Hitselberger WE, Subin B: Report of 190 consecutive cases of large acoustic tumors (vestibular schwannoma) removed via the translabyrinthine approach. J Neurosurg 1999;90: 617–623.

9 Sluyter S, Graamans K, Tulleken CAF, Van Veelen WM: Analysis of the results obtained in 120 patients with large acoustic neuromas surgically treated via the translabyrinthine-transtentorial approach. J Neurosurg 2001;94:61–66.

10 Devèze A, Roche PH, Facon F, Gabert K, Pellet W, Thomassin JMT: Résultats de l'exérèse par voie translabyrinthique élargie des schwannomes vestibulaires. Neurochirurgie 2004; 50:244–252.

11 Yamakami I, Uchino Y, Kobayashi E, Yamaura A, Oka N: Removal of large acoustic neurinomas (vestibular schwannomas) by the retrosigmoid approach with no mortality and minimal morbidity. J Neurol Neurosurg Psychiatry 2004;75:453–458.

12 Zhang X, Fei Z, Chen YJ, Fu LA, Zhang JN, Liu WP, He XS, Jiang XF: Facial nerve function after excision of large acoustic neuromas via the suboccipital retrosigmoid approach. J Clin Neurosci 2005;12:405–408.

13 Anderson DE, Leonetti J, Wind JJ, Cribari D, Fahey K: Resection of large vestibular schwannomas: facial nerve preservation in the context of surgical approach and parient-assessed outcome. J Neurosurg 2005;102:643–649.

14 Koos WT, Day JD, Matula C, Levy DI: Neurotopographic considerations in the microsurgical treatment of small acoustic neurinomas. J Neurosurg 1998;88:506–512.

15 Ryzenman JM, Pensak ML, Tew JM: Facial paralysis and surgical rehabilitation: a quality of life analysis in a cohort of 1,595 patients after acoustic neuroma surgery. Otol Neurotol 2005;26:516–521.

16 Freeman SR, Ramsden RT, Saeed SR, Alzoubi FQ, Simo R, Rutherford SA, King AT: Revision Surgery for residual or recurrent vestibular schwannomas. Otol Neurotol 2007;28:1076–1082.

17 Grayeli AB, Guindi S, Kalamarides M, El Garem H, Smail M, Rey A, Sterkers O: Four-Channel electromyography of the facial nerve in vestibular schwannoma surgery: sensitivity and prognostic value for short-term facial function outcome. Otol Neurotol 2005;26:114–120.

18 Neff BA, Ting J, Dickinson SL, Welling DB: Facial nerve monitoring parameters as a predictor of postoperative facial nerve outcomes after vestibular schwannoma resection. Otol Neurotol 2005;26:728–732.

19 Fundova P, Charabi S, Tos M, Thomsen J: Cystic vestibular schwannoma: surgical outcome. J Laryngol Otol 2000;114:935–939.
20 Mirzayan MJ, Gerganov VM, Lüdemann W, Oi S, Samii M, Samii A: Management of vestibular schwannomas in young patients-comparison of clinical features and outcome with adult patients. Childs Nerv Syst 2007;23:891–895.
21 Oghalai JS, Buxbaum JL, Pitts LH, Jackler RK: The effect of age on acoustic neuroma surgery outcomes. Otol Neurotol 2003;24:473–477.
22 Nicoucar K, Momjian S, Vader JP, De Tribolet N: Surgery for large vestibular schwannomas: How patients and surgeons perceive quality of life. J Neurosurg 2006;105:205–212.
23 Taoka T, Hirabayashi H, Nagakawa H, Sakamoto M, Myochinr K, Hirohashi S, Iwasaki S, Sakaki T, Kichikawa K: Displacement of the facial nerve course by vestibular schwannoma: preoperative visualization using diffusion tensor tractography. J Magn Reson Imaging 2006;24:1005–1010.

Prof. Pierre-Hugues Roche
Service de Neurochirurgie de l'Hôpital Nord
Assistance Publique-Hôpitaux de Marseille
Chemin des Bourrelly
FR–13915 Marseille Cedex 20 (France)
Tel. +33 4 91 96 86 20, Fax +33 4 91 96 89 15, E-Mail proche@mail.ap-hm.fr

Régis J, Roche P-H (eds): Modern Management of Acoustic Neuroma.
Prog Neurol Surg. Basel, Karger, 2008, vol 21, pp 108–118

Facial Nerve Function Insufficiency after Radiosurgery versus Microsurgery

Manabu Tamura[a] · Noriko Murata[b] · Motohiro Hayashi[b] · Pierre-Hugues Roche[a] · Jean Régis[a]

[a]Stereotactic and Functional Neurosurgery, Timone University Hospital, Marseille, France;
[b]Department of Neurosurgery, Tokyo Women's Medical University, Tokyo, Japan

Abstract

Background: Due to the synergic role of the facial nerve and the nervus intermedius in the mechanical protection of the eye and taste, vestibular schwannomas and/or their treatment may prove to be dangerous for the visual function and taste. Our goal was to evaluate and compare the impact of the tumor itself and the impact of microsurgery (MS) or Gamma Knife radiosurgery (GKS). **Materials and Methods:** A functional questionnaire evaluating, among other items, patient complaints related to the eye and taste has been given out to a series of 200 patients 3 years after the GKS of a unilateral vestibular schwannoma not previously resected. Their answers were compared with those of a group of 200 patients operated on microsurgically. A Schirmer test was additionally performed before radiosurgery (RS) and more than 2 years after RS in 66 patients. **Results:** The risk of dry eye and burning eye is much higher in patients operated by MS compared to patients operated by GKS due to the high incidence of facial palsy (FP) in the former (57/99) and its absence in the later (0/80). In the population operated on microsurgically, the presence of a permanent FP (57 patients among 99 responding to the questionnaire) was, of course, associated with a high rate of complaint, with burning eye in 27 and crying eye in 39. In patients from the two arms with no FP, a dry eye was reported in 8/64 after GKS and 7/42 after MS (not significant) and a burning eye in 9/64 after GKS and 9/42 after MS (not significant). Thus, 14% of patients with no clinical signs of impairment of the VIIth motor nerve presented signs indicating the injury of the intermedius nerve, with the same probability whatever the kind of surgery. When no permanent FP was observed, a crocodile tear syndrome was more frequently observed after MS (4/42 versus 1/64; p = 0.07). This suggests an early lesion of the VIIth motor nerve and nervus intermedius and a subsequent abnormal regrowth. The only patient reporting a crocodile tear syndrome after GKS turned out to have a transiently presented mild deficit of the orbicular muscle signing a transient partial facial nerve injury. In the absence of FP, a 'crying eye' was reported more frequently after MS (16/42 vs. 9/64; p = 0.01) leading us to suspect a frequent subclinical injury of the VIIth nerve in those patients operated on using MS with no obvious FP. Patients tested with the Schirmer test before and more than 2 years later were improved in 27.3%, stable in 56.1% and worse in 16.7% of cases. The answers about taste showed that 8.1% of patients after GKS and 45.5% of patients after MS complained of taste. **Conclusions:** This study is the first demonstrating that RS can induce nervus intermedius injury in a small percentage of cases (14%). These patients have been treated 11 years ago with what we can consider as 'archeo-GKS technology' compared to today's radiosurgical instruments. Influence of modern GKS on the nervus intermedius is currently under evaluation in our group. However, symptoms related to the eye and taste either due to the injury of the nervus intermedius or the VIIth motor nerve or both are much more frequent after MS than after RS.

Very little attention has been paid in the literature to the nonmotor functions of the VIIth nerve and their impairment after surgery [1]. Fortunately, the surgical treatment of vestibular schwannomas (VSs) has dramatically improved during the last 2 decades. Thanks to very significant advances like modern anesthesiology, operative microscope, perioperative monitoring and radiosurgery (RS) the operative mortality has decreased (or even disappeared with RS) and the functional preservation improved very significantly. If nowadays, in skillful hands, the rate of the facial motor function preservation for Koos Stages I–II tumors is reaching 89% and 75% for Koos Stage III tumors [2–9], this rate tends to reach 100% with Gamma Knife surgery (GKS) with high-accuracy devices and skilled medical professionals . Relying on the use of a questionnaire that was completed by patients more than 3 years after microsurgery (MS) or RS and evaluating their functional outcome, we have been able to demonstrate a very significant improvement of the functional outcome in patients operated on using GKS instead of MS [10]. Preservation of the facial motor function is one of the most obvious advances in RS or MS [10, 11]. This represents a real revolution for the patients. However, this exceptional level of functional preservation with GKS leads us to question the preservation of the 'lower' functions of the VIIth nerve: lacrimal, gustatory and sensory functions.

Materials and Methods

GKS operation was performed according to our usual procedure [12].

A functional questionnaire evaluating, among other items, patient complaints related to the eye has been given out to a series of 68 patients 3 years after the GKS of a unilateral VS not previously resected. Their answers were compared to those of a group of 99 patients operated on microsurgically. Otherwise, for the taste evaluation a series of 135 patients after GKS was compared with that of 66 patients after MS.

In order to address the issue of the potential injury of the lacrimal component of the nervus intermedius, we have prospectively performed a Schirmer test before and more than 2 years after RS in 66 patients. The test was done for the duration of 1 min. The length of the tear progression on the test paper was cautiously recorded on both sides. The other side served as a reference. Patients with neurofibromatosis type 2 were excluded from the studied group. The follow-up was longer than 2 years in all the patients (range 2–11.4, median 4.0, and mean 4.8 years). The marginal dose was usually 12 Gy (median 12.0, mean 12.5, range 8–16). The median volume of the lesion was 718.7 mm^3 (mean 1,201.0, range 32–4,856). According to the Koos classification [13], 2 VS were in stage I, 42 in stage II, 20 in stage III, 2 in stage IV. The median age of the patients was 59 years (mean 55.4; range 17–78). At clinical examination before RS, 8 patients presented with slight facial palsy (FP; House grade 2), the other 58 patients had no FP; none of these patients had undergone MS before [14].

Results

We have analyzed answers to our questionnaire about eye complaints in 200 patients after MS and 200 patients after GKS. Ninety-nine patients who underwent MS and 68 patients who underwent GKS answered the questionnaire completely (fig. 1). Although 57 (58%) MS patients experienced facial motor dysfunction, none of those treated with Gamma Knife reported any complaint related to facial motor dysfunction. Four patients experienced facial motor deficit before GKS. We also separately analyzed (fig. 2) those who did not experience facial motor deficit before MS (42 cases) and GKS (64 cases). We analyzed answers to the questionnaire about taste complaints in the 66 MS patients and 135 GKS patients who answered all questions. Thirty (45.5%) patients complained of taste disturbance after MS, while 11 (8.1%) patients complained after GKS.

We performed and compared the Schirmer test before and after GKS in 66 patients. We divided the results of the test into three groups: worse, stable and better. Results were worse in

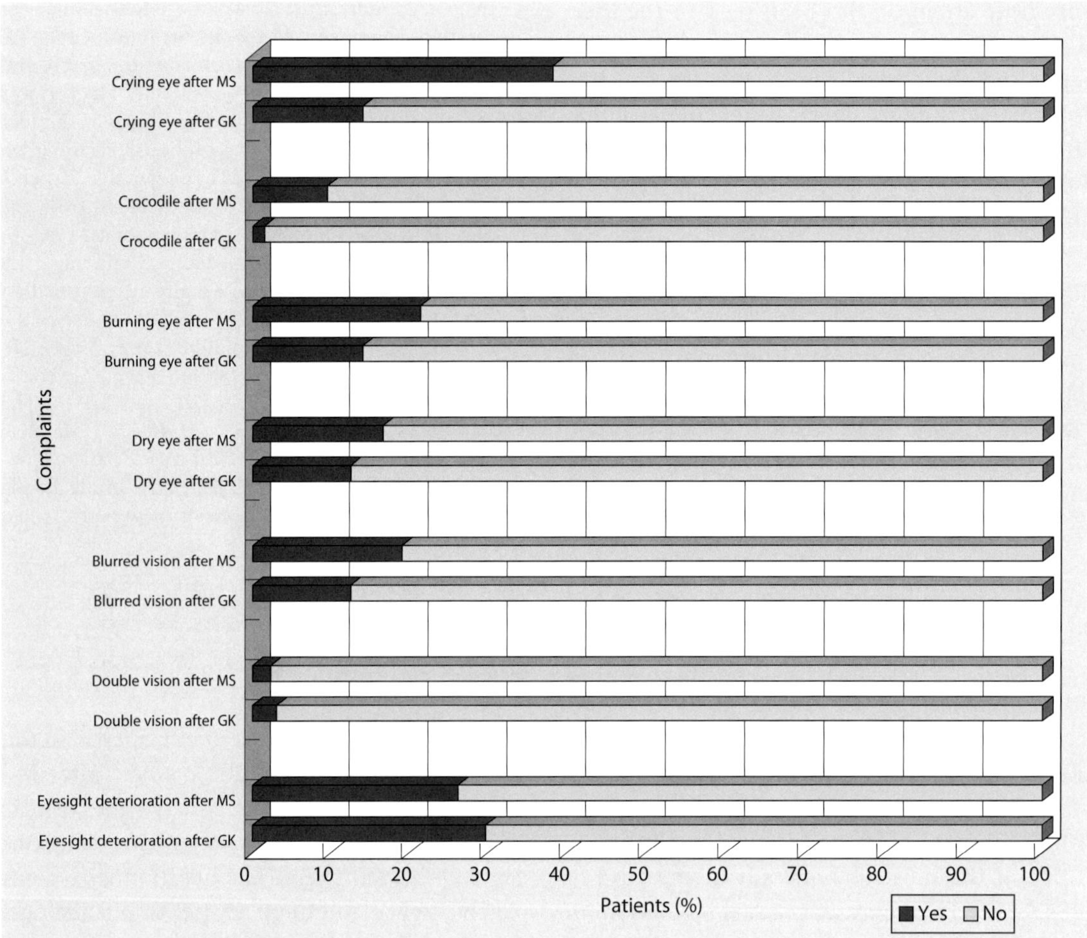

Fig. 1. Patient self-assessed functional outcome for items related to the eyes after MS and GKS (cases with or without facial motor nerve dysfunction).

11 patients, stable in 37 patients, and better in 18. The result was quoted 'worse' when the secretion in the Schirmer test after GKS was significantly decreased as compared to before, 'stable' when the secretion was the same and 'better' when the test was more symmetrical than before GKS. We were also interested in the normalization of initial abnormal lacrimation. The Schirmer test has shown a clear initial deficit of lacrimation in 27 of 66 patients (41%). In 17 of these 27 patients (63%), lacrimation was normalized at the time of the postoperative control and improved from 52.6% to 25.6% deficit (51.4% improvement). In this population with injury of the intermedius nerve before GKS, 6 developed a worsening of this preexisting deficit (22%). Among the 39 patients with no lacrimal deficit before GKS, 5 patients (12.8%) had deteriorated lacrimation after GKS and 34 cases (87.2%) kept their normal lacrimation after GKS (table 1).

The overall percentage of patients with abnormal lacrimation (which means the secretion was not symmetrical) after GKS was significantly

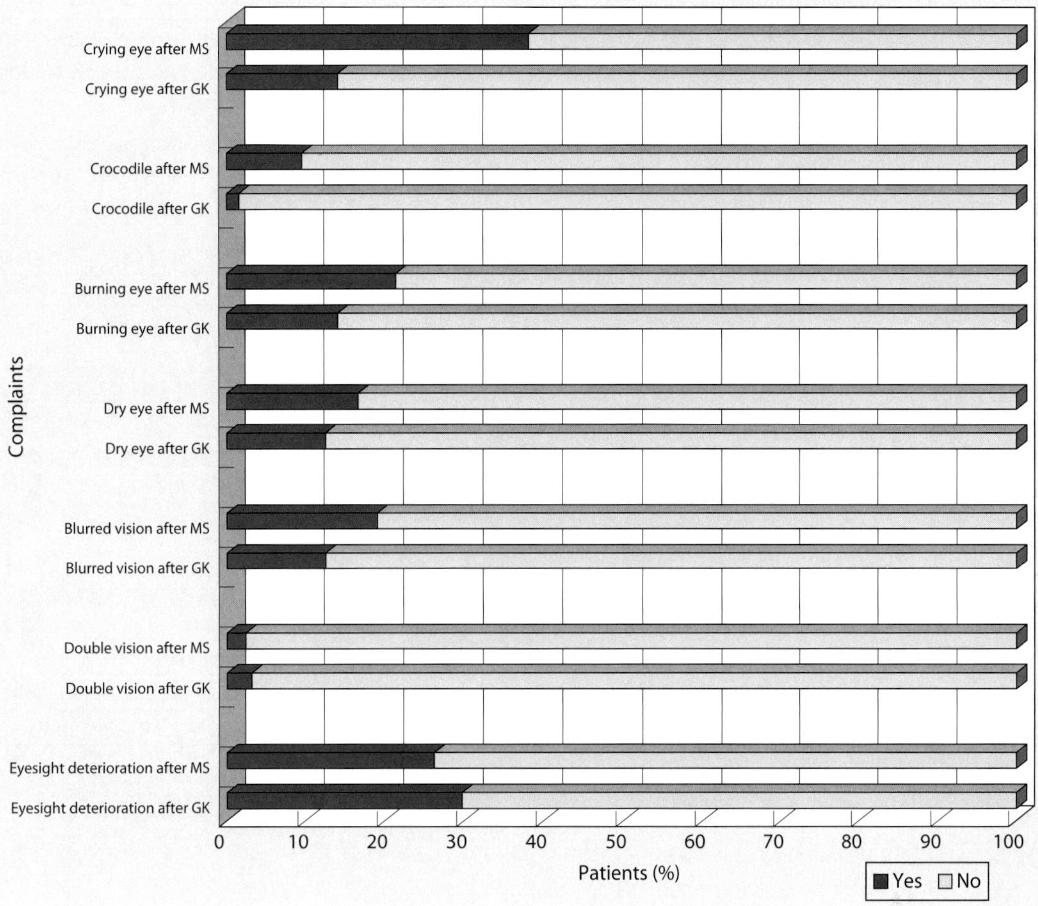

Fig. 2. Patient self-assessed functional outcome for items related to the eyes after MS and GKS (only cases without facial motor nerve dysfunction).

lower as compared to before GKS (fig. 3; χ^2, p = 0.025). For the purpose of statistical analysis, we compared worsened patients with the others. We found that in the group of abnormal lacrimation after GKS, 10 of 15 (66.7%) had already the symptom before GKS and in the normal group, 17 of 51 (33.3%) patients had already a dry eye (table 1). If one suffers injuries of the lacrimal component of the intermedius nerve before GKS, one will have also a higher possibility to suffer from dry eye after GKS (χ^2, p = 0.021). Among the patients filling out the 'eye discomfort' questionnaire, 27 have also been investigated with the Schirmer test before and after GKS. As already pointed out, in the global population the rate of eye discomfort is lower after GKS than after MS for the following items: crying eye, dry eye, burning eye and crocodile tear syndrome (table 2).

The risk of dry eye and burning eye is much higher in patients operated on using MS compared to patients operated on using GKS due to the high incidence of facial motor nerve dysfunction (FD) in the former (57/99) and its absence in the later (0/68). In the population operated on

Table 1. Lacrimation normalization and deterioration after RS according to the Shirmer test

	Lacrimation after GKS (n = 66)	
	normal (n = 51)	abnormal (n = 15)
Lacrimation before GKS (n = 66)		
Normal (n = 39)	34	5
Abnormal (n = 37)	17	10

The initial lacrimal deficit normalized after GKS in 63.0% of cases. The initial normal lacrimation deteriorated after GKS in 12.8% of cases.

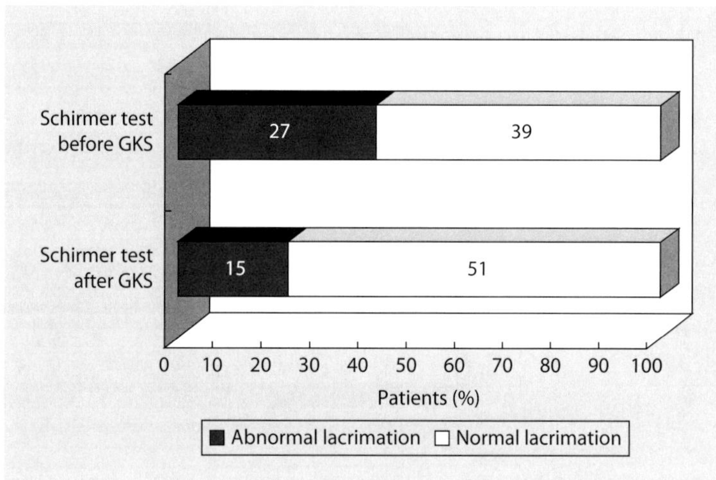

Fig. 3. Lacrimation deficit before and after RS according to the Shirmer test. The overall percentage of patients with lacrimation deficit is significantly decreased after RS (χ^2 test = 0.041).

microsurgically, the presence of a permanent facial motor nerve dysfunction (57 patients among 99 responding to the questionnaire) is, of course associated with a high rate of complaint, with burning eye in 27 and crying eye in 39 (fig. 1). In patients with no facial motor nerve deficit from the two arms, a dry eye is reported in 8/64 after GKS and 7/42 after MS (nonsignificant) and a burning eye in 9/64 after GKS and 9/42 after MS (nonsignificant; table 3). Thus, patients with no clinical signs of impairment of the VIIth motor nerve (fig. 2) present eye complaints in 14% of cases, indicating the injury of the intermedius nerve with the same probability whatever the kind of surgery.

Discussion

General Consideration (Facial Motor Nerve Dysfunction)

Because facial weakness is a physically and psychologically devastating sequel after resective surgery of VSs, the literature has mainly focused the attention on the injury of the motor component of the facial nerve. In MS, all operators try to find the interface between the facial nerve and tumor and keep the nerve morphology intact. Actually, the results of facial nerve preservation rate [House-Brackmann (H-B) 1 or 2] were above 60% in surgically treated patients. However, the rate of temporary facial motor nerve weakness

Table 2. Comparison of the ocular symptoms after MS and GKS (total population)

Ocular symptom	After MS, %	After GKS, %	p value
Eyesight deterioration	31.3	30.9	0.9529
Double vision	5.1	7.4	0.7762
Blurred vision	20.2	13.2	0.3372
Dry eye	25.3	13.2	0.0893
Burning eye	27.3	14.7	0.0547
Crocodile tears	12.1	1.5	0.0080
Crying eye	39.4	14.7	0.0006

Table 3. Comparison of the ocular symptoms after MS and GKS in the group with no facial motor nerve dysfunction

Ocular symptom	After MS, %	After GKS, %	p value
Eyesight deterioration	26.2	29.7	0.6958
Double vision	2.4	3.1	0.4389
Blurred vision	19.0	12.5	0.5198
Dry eye	16.7	12.5	0.7512
Burning eye	21.4	14.1	0.4964
Crocodile tears	9.5	1.6	0.0707
Crying eye	38.1	14.1	0.0089

after MS is still high and it takes at least 6 months to recover a normal or near-normal facial function [15]. We also summarized the rate of facial motor nerve preservation comparing the results of MS, RS, LINAC, fraction stereotactic radiotherapy and proton stereotactic RS (table 4). These results indicate that the facial motor nerve preservation is lower with MS than with GKS. In the modern area of RS, treatment refinements have been sought in order to provide maximum tumor control and minimum complication for the initial management of patients with VSs [16]. Especially facial nerve neuropathy could be expected in patients who received a marginal tumor dose of 14 Gy or more [16]. Nowadays, reduction of peripheral doses allows a decrease in facial nerve toxicity with a satisfactory rate of tumor control, which is an advantage of GKS compared to MS. Moreover, the paradigm shift created by RS has increased dramatically the interest of the medical community for postsurgical quality of life assessment [10, 17–22]. The nervus intermedius aggregates the special visceral atterent (for taste) and general somatic sensory atterent components of the facial nerve, and its fibers are found in close relation to the motor part of the facial nerve in the cerebellopontine cistern (fig. 4). This nerve includes preganglionic

Table 4. Facial motor nerve preservation (literature)

First author	Method	Publication date	FU	Period of FU months	Facial nerve pres1rv2tion, % (HB 1 or 2)/ tumor size	Total FP %	Permanent FP %	Temporary FP %
Ebersold [25]	MS	1992	161	1–12	64.1	35.9	ND	ND
Fischer [26]	MS	1992	99	24	65.7	34.3	ND	ND
Pellet [8]	MS	1993	178		66.0	34.0	ND	ND
Gormley [27]	MS	1997	173[1]	3–12	76.9	23.1	ND	ND
Samii [9]	MS	1997	830[1]	1–2	56.6	43.4	ND	ND
Koos [13]	MS	1998	113	12–18	87.6 (Koos I or II)	12.4	ND	ND
Anderson [15]	MS	2005	71[2]	1–12	73.2 (over 30 mm)	26.8	26.8	61.3
Prasad [28]	RS	2000	129	12–120	100	2.3	0	2.0
Flickinger [16]	RS	2001	192	30 (median)	99.0	1.0	ND	ND
Régis [10]	RS	2002	104	36 (minimum)	100 (Koos II or III)	1.9	0	1.9
Kondziolka [29]	RS	2003	124[1]	122 (median)	95.2	4.8	ND	ND
Spiegelman [30]	LINAC	2001	37	12–60	91.9	24.3	8.1	16.2
Sawamura [31]	Fraction SRT	2003	101	6–128	99.0	4.0	0.9	3.0
Harsh [32]	Proton SRS	2002	64	8–102	95.3	14.1	4.7	9.4
Weber [33]	Proton SRS	2003	79[1]	1–60	91.1	13.9	8.9	5.1

FP refers to the newly acquired worse symptoms (severe).
ND = Not described; SRT = stereotactic radiotherapy; SRS = stereotactic RS.
[1]For the patients in HB grade with normal facial nerve function before treatment.
[2]The number of followed up tumors.

parasympathetic secretomotor fibers innervating the lacrimal gland in addition to the nasal and palatine mucosal glands and submandibular sublingual salivary glands. This nerve also contains the special sensory (taste) fibers originating from the taste buds of the anterior two thirds of the tongue [23, 24].

Taste Disturbance

Watanabe et al. [23] have demonstrated a quite high incidence of taste disturbance in patients presenting a VSs, increasing after resective surgery. Thus 29% of the patients with no taste disturbance before surgery were presenting with such deficit after microsurgical resection (mean onset 1.1 ± 1.7 months after surgery). Fortunately, this deficit which can deprive the patient of any enjoyment of food (one of the great pleasures and motivations of human life) resolved in 65% of patients with postoperative taste disturbance. In our experience, comparing tasting disturbance after MS with tasting disturbance after RS, the deficit presented in 45.5% patients after MS and in 8.1% after RS. RS does indeed induce taste

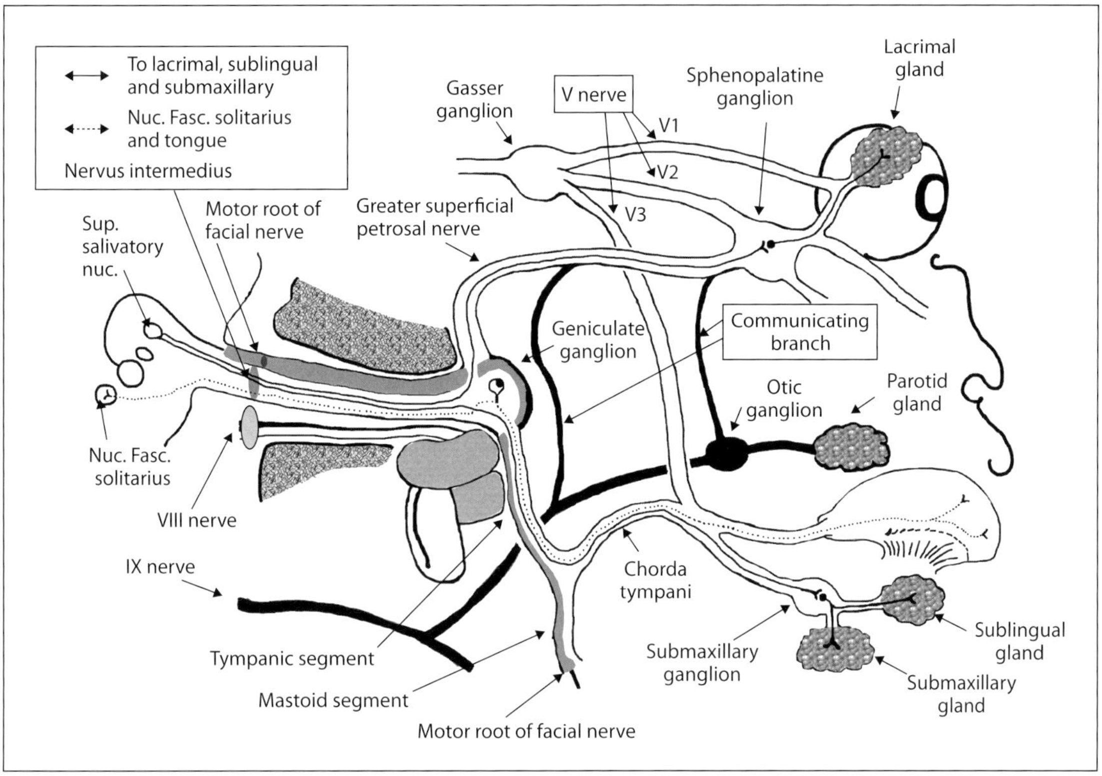

Fig. 4. Anatomy of the different components of the VIIth nerve.

disturbances, but less frequently than MS, as reported in the microsurgical literature.

Ocular Problems

When some years ago we used a questionnaire in order to compare the functional outcome and quality of life of patients undergoing resective surgery versus GKS [10], 47% of the patients operated on microsurgically and 0% operated on radiosurgically reported complaints related to any level of facial motor nerve dysfunction. The incidence of new hemifacial spasm was 27% after MS compared to 3% after RS. New ocular troubles were reported by 83% of the patients after MS and 27% after RS. This study demonstrated very clearly better functional preservation after RS. However, in both arms we observe undoubtedly a much higher rate of ocular problem than motor facial motor nerve dysfunction (ocular problem in 83% cases, and facial motor nerve dysfunction in 47% of cases after MS; ocular problem in 27% cases, and facial motor nerve dysfunction in 0% of cases after RS). This demonstrates that the mechanical consequences of the facial motor nerve dysfunction on the eye do not account for the totality of the disturbances induced by surgery, whatever the operative technique used. We can speculate that the fibers of the nervus intermedius are more sensitive than the motor fibers of the VIIth nerve both to MS and RS. In RS, it is commonly observed that sensory nerve fibers are more sensitive than motor nerve fibers. Taste disturbance was reported by 46% of the patients after MS and only 6% after RS. In this latter group of patients, 4 have developed hemifacial spasm, but in 2 of them this phenomenon disappeared

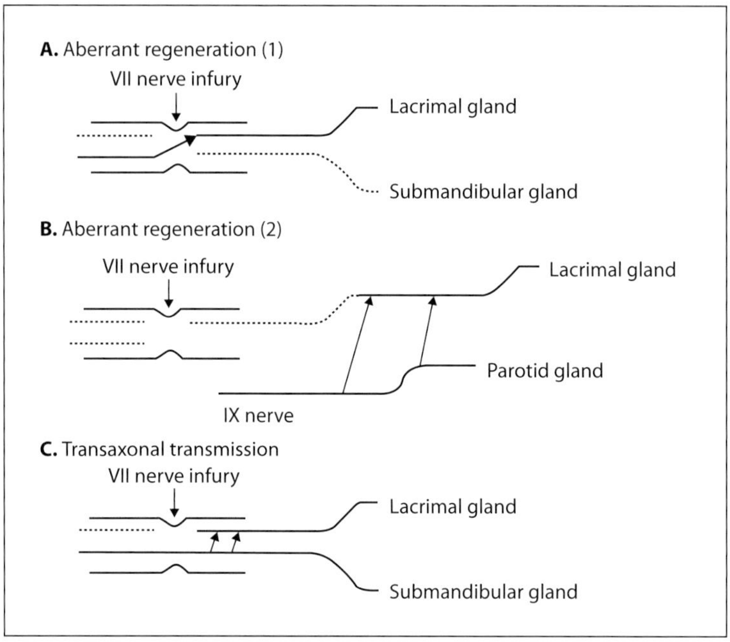

Fig. 5. Hypothesis supposed to account for the crocodile tear syndrome.

before the control at 3 years. No taste or ocular symptom was reported in any of these 4 patients. The relation between occurrence of hemifacial spasm and facial sensory nerve disturbance (lacrimation and taste) is unclear.

Dry eye is a commonly reported symptom, but it results not only from the decrease in the quantity of tears produced but also from the reduction in the frequency of blinking. It is important to note that in the study of Irving et al. [1] the deficit of lacrimation changed with time. These authors reported an absence or a significant reduction in the production of tears in 72% of their 224 patients operated on microsurgically, in contrast to the crocodile tears phenomenon which occurred in 44% of the patients and where recovery is rare. Interestingly, they found an overall rate of recovery of normal tearing in 27% of the patients with a mean delay of recovery of 7 months. In the subgroup of patients with a House grade between 1 and 3, recovery of normal tearing even occurred in almost half the patients. Consequently, based on this experience we can suspect in our study an underestimation of the immediate postoperative lacrimation deficit. Like us, Irving et al. [1] found a higher incidence in patients with poor motor function. In our material at 3 years after MS, the rate of dry eye was 25.3% in patients with facial motor nerve deficit and only 16.7% in patients with no facial motor nerve deficit.

Facial Nerve Plasticity

When no permanent facial motor nerve dysfunction is observed, crocodile tear syndrome is more frequently observed after MS (4/42 versus 1/64; p = 0.07). This suggests an early lesion of the motor component of the VIIth and intermedius nerves and a subsequent abnormal regrowth (fig. 4 and 5). The only patient reporting crocodile tear syndrome after GKS turned out to have a transient mild deficit of the orbicular muscle signing a transient partial facial nerve injury. In the absence of facial motor dysfunction, a 'crying eye' was reported more frequently after MS (16/42 versus 9/64; p = 0.01), leading us to suspect a frequent subclinical injury of the VIIth nerve in the patients operated on using MS with no obvious facial motor nerve dysfunction (FD). Patients with FD and dry eye are supposed to have a lesion proximal to the geniculate ganglion and patients with FD and 'crying eye' distal to this structure. The patients tested with the Schirmer test before and more than 2 years after RS were improved in 27.3%, stable in 56.1% and worse in 16.7%. Moreover, we observed that 63% of the patients who had abnormal lacrimation before GKS normalized their lacrimation after GKS. Without the reason for mechanical decompression on the nervus intermedius, what would explain the recovery of the facial nerve function? Plasticity of the facial nerve component would be induced with an axonal regeneration by the radiation effect; however, we have no evidence to show a neuroprotective reaction of radiation during the axonal change.

Conclusion

Whatever the treatment for VS (MS or RS), the risk of facial nerve surgical injury is unavoidable. We have firstly demonstrated that RS can induce nervus intermedius injury in a small percentage of cases (14%). These patients have been treated 12 years ago with what we can consider as primitive GKS technology compared to today's radiosurgical devices. Influence of modern GKS on the nervus intermedius is currently under evaluation in our group. However, symptoms related to the eye and taste either due to the injury of the nervus intermedius or the VIIth motor nerve or both are much more frequent after MS than after RS.

References

1 Irving RM, Viani L, Hardy DG, Baguley DM, Moffat DA: Nervus intermedius function after vestibular schwannoma removal: clinical features and pathophysiological mechanisms. Laryngoscope 1995;105:809–813.

2 Grey PL, Moffat DA, Palmer CR, Hardy DG, Baguley DM: Factors which influence the facial nerve outcome in vestibular schwannoma surgery. Clin Otolaryngol 1996;21:409–413.

3 Hardy DG, Macfarlane R, Baguley DM, Moffat DA: Facial nerve recovery following acoustic neuroma surgery. Br J Neurosurg 1989;3:675–680.

4 Moffat DA, Croxson GR, Baguley DM, Hardy DG: Facial nerve recovery after acoustic neuroma removal. J Laryngol Otol 1989;103:169–172.

5 Moffat DA, Hardy DG, Grey PL, Baguley DM: The operative learning curve and its effect on facial nerve outcome in vestibular schwannoma surgery. Am J Otol 1996;17:643–647.

6 Bruzzo M, Broder L, Chays A, Magnan J: [Our current results with acoustic neurinoma surgery]. Ann Otolaryngol Chir Cervicofac 2000;117:110–117.

7 Pellet W, Cannoni M, Pech A: Oto-neuro-surgery. Berlin, Heidelberg, Springer Verlag, 1993.

8 Pellet W, Emram B, Cannoni M, Pech A, Zanaret M, Thomassin M: [Functional results of the surgery of unilateral acoustic neuroma]. Neurochirurgie 1993;39:24–40; discussion 40–21.

9 Samii M, Matthies C: Management of 1000 vestibular schwannomas (acoustic neuromas): the facial nerve–preservation and restitution of function. Neurosurgery 1997;40:684–694; discussion 694–685.

10 Regis J, Pellet W, Delsanti C, Dufour H, Roche PH, Thomassin JM, Zanaret M, Peragut JC: Functional outcome after gamma knife surgery or microsurgery for vestibular schwannomas. J Neurosurg 2002;97:1091–1100.

11 Pollock B, Lunsford L, Kondziolka D, Flickinger J, Bissonette D, Kelsey S, Jannetta P: Outcome analysis of acoustic neuroma management: a comparison of microsurgery and stereotactic radiosurgery [published erratum appears in Neurosurgery 1995 Feb;36:427]. Neurosurgery 1995;36:215–224; discussion 224–219.

12 Regis J, Roche PH, Delsenti C, Soumare O, Thomassin JM, Pellet W: Stereotactic Radiosurgery for Vestibular Schwannoma, in Pollock BE (ed) Contemporary Stereotactic Radiosurgery: Thechnique and Evaluation. Armonk, New York, Futura Publishing Company, 2002, pp. 181–212.

13 Koos WT, Day JD, Matula C, Levy DI: Neurotopographic considerations in the microsurgical treatment of small acoustic neurinomas. J Neurosurg 1998;88:506–512.

14 House JW, Brackmann DE: Facial nerve grading system. Otolaryngology Head and Neck Surgery 1985;93:146–147.

15 Anderson DE, Leonetti J, Wind JJ, Cribari D, Fahey K: Resection of large vestibular schwannomas: facial nerve preservation in the context of surgical approach and patient-assessed outcome. J Neurosurg 2005;102:643–649.

16 Flickinger JC, Kondziolka D, Niranjan A, Lunsford LD: Results of acoustic neuroma radiosurgery: an analysis of 5 years' experience using current methods. J Neurosurg 2001;94:1–6.

17 Wiegand DA, Fickel V: Acoustic Neuroma The Patient 's Perspective: Subjective Assessment of Symptoms, Diagnosis, Therapy, and Outcome in 541 Patients. Laryngoscope 1989;99:179–187.
18 Nikolopoulos TP, Johnson I, O'Donoghue GM: Quality of life after acoustic neuroma surgery. Laryngoscope 1998;108:1382–1385.
19 Farace E, Marshall LF: Quality of life in acoustics. J Neurosurg 2003;99:807–808; discussion 808–809.
20 Da Cruz MJ, Moffat DA, Hardy DG: Postoperative quality of life in vestibular schwannoma patients measured by the SF36 Health Questionnaire. Laryngoscope 2000;110:151–155.
21 Hudgins WR: Patients' attitude about outcomes and the role of gamma knife radiosurgery in the treatment of vestibular schwannomas. Neurosurgery 1994;34:459–463.
22 Betchen SA, Walsh J, Post KD: Self-assessed quality of life after acoustic neuroma surgery. J Neurosurg 2003;99:818–823.
23 Watanabe K, Saito N, Taniguchi M, Kirino T, Sasaki T: Analysis of taste disturbance before and after surgery in patients with vestibular schwannoma. J Neurosurg 2003;99:999–1003.
24 Magliulo G, Cordeschi S, Sepe C, de Vincentiis M: [Taste and lacrimation after acoustic neuroma surgery]. Rev Laryngol Otol Rhinol (Bord) 1998;119:167–170.
25 Ebersold MJ, Harner SG, Beatty CW, Harper CM, Jr., Quast LM: Current results of the retrosigmoid approach to acoustic neurinoma [see comments]. J Neurosurg 1992;76:901–909.
26 Fischer G, Fischer C, Remond J: Hearing preservation in acoustic neurinoma surgery. J Neurosurg 1992;76:910–917.
27 Gormley WB, Sekhar LN, Wright DC, Kamerer D, Schessel D: Acoustic neuromas: results of current surgical management. Neurosurgery 1997;41:50–58; discussion 58–60.
28 Prasad D, Steiner M, Steiner L: Gamma surgery for vestibular schwannoma [see comments]. J Neurosurg 2000;92:745–759.
29 Kondziolka D, Nathoo N, Flickinger JC, Niranjan A, Maitz AH, Lunsford LD: Long-term results after radiosurgery for benign intracranial tumors. Neurosurgery 2003;53:815–821; discussion 821–812.
30 Spiegelmann R, Lidar Z, Gofman J, Alezra D, Hadani M, Pfeffer R: Linear accelerator radiosurgery for vestibular schwannoma. J Neurosurg 2001;94:7–13.
31 Sawamura Y, Shirato H, Sakamoto T, Aoyama H, Suzuki K, Onimaru R, Isu T, Fukuda S, Miyasaka K: Management of vestibular schwannoma by fractionated stereotactic radiotherapy and associated cerebrospinal fluid malapsorption. J Neurosurg 2003;99:685–692.
32 Harsh GR, Thornton AF, Chapman PH, Bussiere MR, Rabinov JD, Loeffler JS: Proton beam stereotactic radiosurgery of vestibular schwannomas. Int J Radiat Oncol Biol Phys 2002;54:35–44.
33 Weber DC, Chan AW, Bussiere MR, Harsh GRt, Ancukiewicz M, Barker FG, 2nd, Thornton AT, Martuza RL, Nadol JB, Jr., Chapman PH, Loeffler JS: Proton beam radiosurgery for vestibular schwannoma: tumor control and cranial nerve toxicity. Neurosurgery 2003;53:577–586; discussion 586–578.

Prof. Jean Régis
Service de Neurochirurgie Fonctionnelle et Stéréotaxique
Hôpital d'Adulte de la Timone, 264 bvd Saint Pierre
FR–13385 Marseille Cedex 05 (France)
Tel. +33 4 91 38 65 62, Fax +33 4 91 38 70 56, E-Mail jregis@ap-hm.fr

Régis J, Roche P-H (eds): Modern Management of Acoustic Neuroma.
Prog Neurol Surg. Basel, Karger, 2008, vol 21, pp 119–130

Surgical Treatment of Facial Nerve Schwannomas

Jan Frederick Cornelius[a] · Elisabeth Sauvaget[b] · Patrice Tran Ba Huy[b] · Bernard George[a]

Departments of [a]Neurosurgery and [b]Head and Neck Surgery, Lariboisiere Hospital, Paris, France

Abstract

Facial nerve schwannomas are rare. They occur all along the nerve's course from the cerebellopontine angle to the parotid region. Clinically, intracranial facial nerve schwannomas often present with facial nerve paralysis or hearing loss and may initially be misdiagnosed as vestibular schwannomas. Modern imaging techniques allow diagnosis and evaluate tumor location, size and extension. Functional tests evaluate facial nerve and hearing function. All this information results in an individual management plan. Microsurgery, stereotactic radiosurgery and observation are the therapeutic options. Surgery is planned depending on tumor features and the preoperative functional status. Subtemporal, transmastoid, translabyrinthine and retrosigmoid approaches are the principal routes. Preservation of facial nerve function is the main surgical difficulty. Anatomical nerve conservation, nerve resection with immediate grafting or delayed hypoglosso-facial nerve anastomosis are possible. The main predicting factors of postoperative facial function are the degree and duration of facial paralysis before surgery. Observation is an option for small tumors and asymptomatic patients. In these cases, a close follow-up is mandatory. The optimal timing for surgery is critical: waiting maximizes the time with good facial function, but increases the risk of hearing loss by cochlea erosion and lowers the chances of postoperative facial nerve recovery once paralysis has occurred. The role of radiosurgery is still to be determined: it seems suitable for inoperable patients and recurrent tumors.

Facial nerve schwannomas (also known as neuromas) are rare, benign slow-growing tumors arising from the Schwann cell sheath of the facial nerve. About 650 cases have been reported in the world literature [1]. The number of asymptomatic and thus undiagnosed tumors is estimated to be much higher [2]. The sex ratio is 1, the peak of presentation is in the 4th decade (range from 7 to 81 years, but very rare in children) [3]. The mean time to diagnosis is 3 years [4]. There is no preferential sidedness, bilateral location has never been reported and the association with neurofibromatosis is rare [4, 5].

Facial nerve schwannomas occur all along the nerve course and are often multisegmental [4, 5] (table 1). There is a predilection for the labyrinthine and tympanic segments, but even there they account for less than 1% of all intrapetrous mass lesions [4–7]. It has been speculated that the tumor origin is the sensory part of the facial nerve (intermedius nerve), because of the predilection of schwannomas for sensory nerve fibers [4, 5, 8]. However, only a few cases of authentic schwannomas of the intermedius nerve, along with 1 case of Jacobson's nerve and 5 cases of chorda tympani have been reported [4, 9]. The

Table 1. Overview of facial nerve segments involved in schwannoma

Segment	Patients (n = 438)
Cerebellopontine angle	82 (18.7%)
Canalicular segment	109 (24.9%)
Labyrinthine/geniculate segment	191 (43.6%)
Tympanic segment	185 (42.2%)
Mastoid segment	157 (35.8%)
Peripheral segment	64 (14.6%)
Chorda tympani	5 (1.1%)
Nerve to stapedius	4 (0.9%)

For a given patient, more than 1 segment may be involved. Adapted from Sherman et al. [4] by adding the cases of the present series.

diversity of possible tumor locations results in a variety of clinical presentations and the necessity of different management strategies. In order to work out rules, we analyzed the patients operated on in our institution and reviewed the literature.

Patients and Methods

We retrospectively reviewed the medical records of 10 patients operated on during 1992–2005 in the Departments of Neurosurgery and Otorhinolaryngology of Lariboisiere Hospital for an intracranial facial nerve schwannoma. Patients with a facial nerve schwannoma distally of the foramen stylomastoideum were excluded, because the management problems are different. Patients for whom the diagnosis of facial nerve schwannoma was only suspected and not proven histologically or by surgical exploration were also excluded. In total, there were 4 females and 6 males, with a mean age of 37 years (ranging from 18 to 54 years). The charts were reviewed for clinical presentation, pre- and postoperative facial nerve and hearing status, neuroradiological data, surgical technique and tumor recurrence. Preoperative computed tomography (CT) and magnetic resonance imaging (MRI) were analyzed to determine location, size and extension of tumor. Postoperative MRI was reviewed for tumor recurrence. Follow-up time ranged from 1 to 14 years, with a mean of 5.1 years (median 6 years).

Results

Patients' characteristics, presenting symptom, tumor location and extension, tumor size, surgical approach, degree of resection, type of anastomosis (if performed), pre- and postoperative facial and hearing status and recurrence-free follow-up duration are presented in table 2. The most common presenting symptom was hearing loss (4 cases, 40%), which was sudden in 3 patients and progressive in 1. The second most frequent symptom was facial paralysis (3 cases, 30%), 2 being sudden and 1 progressive. Tinnitus was the presenting symptom in 2 cases (20%). One facial nerve schwannoma was diagnosed incidentally in a patient after a seizure; this patient also had a frontal cavernoma (patient 1).

Most tumors were multisegmental (80%), only 1 tumor exclusively involved the cerebellopontine angle (CPA) and another solely the labyrinthine segment of the facial nerve. Besides, the CPA was involved in 6 cases (60%), the internal auditory canal (IAC) and the labyrinthine segment in 7 cases (70%), the geniculate ganglion in 3 cases (30%), the tympanic segment in 2 cases (20%) and extension to the middle fossa was observed in 1 case (10%). The size varied between 8 × 13 mm for the smallest tumor and 51 × 25 mm for the largest lesion. Generally, the largest tumor diameter was measured in the orthogonal axis to the IAC, rarely in the parallel axis.

A variety of surgical routes were used, including the retrosigmoid, subtemporal, translabyrinthine and transmastoid approaches. A total of 13 operations were performed in 10 patients: in 7 patients (70%), a unique surgical approach allowed satisfactory surgical resection, for 1 patient

Table 2. Surgical series of facial nerve schwannomas of Lariboisiere Hospital

Patient No., sex, age	Presenting symptom	Tumor location	Tumor size[1] mm	Surgical approach	Res	Ana	Facial H-B		Hearing		FU years
							preoperatively	postoperatively	preoperatively	postoperatively	
1, F, 32	incidental	CPA, IAC	40×20	RS[2]	ST	0	1	2	NS	NS	14
			42×25	RS	ST	0	6	6			
			48×26	ST	T	XII	6	4			
2, F, 44	FP sudden	LAB, MF	51×25	ST	T	XII	6	5	NS	NS	1
3, F, 52	HL progressive	CPA	25×20	RS	ST	0	1	2	NS	NS	6
4, F, 54	tinnitus	CPA, IAC	23×22	RS	T	XII	1	3	S	NS	6
5, M, 29	HL sudden	CPA, IAC, GG	30×25	TL	T	XII	1	3	NS	NS	7
6, M, 18	FP sudden	GG, TYMP	25×15	ST+TM	T	VII	3	3	S	S	2
7, M, 28	HL sudden	LAB	8×13	ST	Ex	0	1	1	NS	NS	1
			20×13	TL[2]	T	XII	1	3	NS	NS	
8, M, 35	tinnitus	CPA, IAC	11×20	RS	Ex	0	1	1	S	S	7
9, M, 47	HL sudden	CPA, IAC	19×16	RS	Ex	0	1	1	S	S	6
10, M, 29	FP progressive	GG, TYMP	30×20	ST	T	XII	4	6	S	S	0.3

FP = Facial paralysis; HL = hearing loss; S = serviceable; NS = nonserviceable; LAB = labyrinthine segment of the facial nerve; MF = middle cerebral fossa; GG = ganglion geniculi; TYMP = tympanic segment of the facial nerve; RS = retrosigmoid; ST = sub-temporal; TL = translabyrinthine; TM = transmastoid; Res = degree of resection; ST = subtotal; T = total; Ex = exploration; Ana = type of facial nerve repair; XII = hypoglosso-facial anastomosis; VII = facio-facial anastomosis; Facial H-B = facial function expressed in House-Brackman grade; FU = follow-up without recurrence.

[1]Tumor size as measured on the same axial MRI image showing maximal global tumor extension (T_1WI after gadolinium injection): the first number is the diameter measured orthogonally to the IAC and the second the diameter measured parallel to the IAC.

[2]More than 1 surgery: the pre- and postoperative facial nerve and hearing status on a given line correspond to the operation on the same line (type specified under approach).

a combined subtemporal/transmastoid approach was used. Two patients had multiple surgical procedures: Thus, in patient 1, a total of 3 operations were performed: 1st subtotal resection followed by radiosurgery and after some years of stabilization a 2nd surgery for regrowth, immediately followed by a 3rd operation for a remnant which could not be reached by the previous approach (see 'Illustrative Case'; fig. 1). In patient 7, a facial nerve schwannoma was discovered perioperatively; it was thought to be a vestibular schwannoma as the patient presented with sudden hearing loss and no facial paralysis. Perioperatively, it was decided not to resect the tumor and to observe. Tumor progression occurred 2 years later and the tumor was then resected.

Tumor removal was total in 7 of 13 operations (54%), subtotal in 3 operations (23%) and surgical exploration without tumor resection was done 3 times (23%). After total tumor resection, facial nerve repair consisted of hypoglosso-facial anastomosis in 6 cases and in facio-facial anastomosis with sural nerve interposition graft in 1 patient. In cases of subtotal tumor removal, the

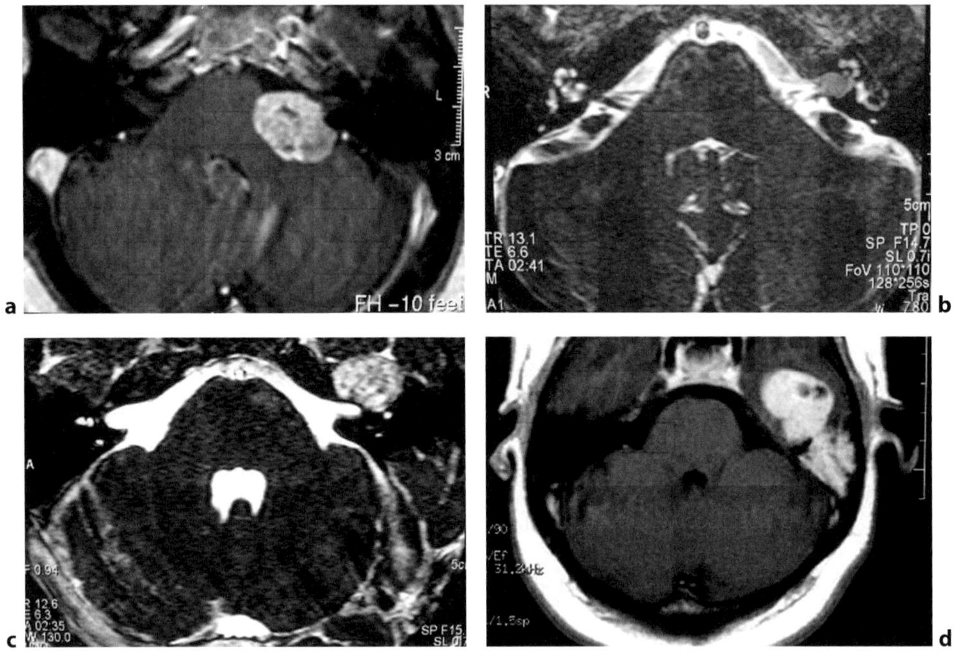

Fig. 1. Overview of typical locations of facial nerve schwannoma on MRI: CPA and IAC (**a**); IAC and labyrinthine segment (**b**); geniculate ganglion and tympanic segment (**c**); labyrinthine segment and temporal fossa extension (**d**).

anatomical continuity of the facial nerve was always preserved (n = 3). In 3 patients (7–9), surgery was interrupted when a facial nerve schwannoma was encountered instead of a presumed vestibular schwannoma ('surgical exploration').

Serviceable preoperative hearing (5 cases, 50%) was preserved postoperatively using hearing-sparing approaches, except in 1 case; this patient had already a preoperative hearing loss of −40 dB.

Concerning facial nerve function, this remained unchanged after simple exploration in previously asymptomatic patients (patients 7–9). A slight deterioration [from House-Brackmann grade (H-B) 1 to 2] after subtotal resection in patients without preoperative facial paralysis was noted (patients 1 and 3). After complete tumor resection and hypoglosso-facial anastomosis in beforehand asymptomatic patients, the functional result was H-B 3 after at least 1 year of waiting (patients 4, 5 and 7). After complete tumor removal and hypoglosso-facial anastomosis in a patient with a preoperatively existing facial paralysis (H-B 4, patient 2), this only recovered partially (H-B 5). One patient with a preoperative H-B 3 (patient 6) had complete tumor removal and received a facio-facial anastomosis resulting in H-B 3. Another patient with a preoperative facial paralysis who underwent a hypoglosso-facial anastomosis has not yet reached the 1 year follow-up consultation (patient 10).

Concerning tumor growth, there were 2 patients showing progression of their lesions during observation time (20%). In patient 1, tumor growth was observed during a 1-year observation period and then subtotal resection was performed. Tumor growth was observed 4 years later and then radiosurgery was done. The tumor involuted and stabilized for some years. Regrowth was significant 7 years after radiosurgery; at that time, total removal was performed and the patient

Table 3. Presenting symptoms of facial nerve schwannomas

Symptom/sign	Patients (n = 437)
Facial weakness	273 (62.5%)
Hearing loss	220 (50.3%)
Tinnitus	90 (20.6%)
Vestibular symptoms	61 (14.0%)
Ear canal mass	47 (10.8%)
Pain	35 (8.0%)
Otorrhea	15 (3.4%)
Loss of taste	12 (2.8%)
Parotid mass	12 (2.8%)
Facial spasm	9 (2.1%)

For a given patient more than 1 symptom/sign may be present.
Adapted from Sherman et al. [4] by adding the patients of the present series.

is recurrence free after 1 year. The other patient showing tumor growth (patient 7), was a patient in whom the tumor grew significantly 3 years after a simple surgical exploration; the lesion was finally totally resected. The 2 other patients who were only explored (8 and 9) remained asymptomatic and did not show any significant growth after 7 and 6 years, respectively. All the patients who underwent total resection (n = 7) were free of recurrence at the last follow-up consultation.

Discussion

Clinical Presentation

Clinical presentation depends on the tumor location on the nerve course. Typically, it presents with a spectrum of symptoms of compression of the VIIth and VIIIth cranial nerves (table 3). The mode of installation is generally progressive, but may sometimes be abrupt or recurrent. As a rule, for a proximal location (i.e. CPA/IAC and labyrinthine segment) vestibular symptoms and a sensorineural hearing loss dominate, whereas more distally (i.e. geniculate, tympanic and mastoid segment) signs of facial nerve compression and eventually associated conductive hearing loss occur. To a varying degree, other symptoms like tinnitus, vertigo, facial tics or spasms, dysgeusia, otalgia or otorrhea may be present. Often, the clinical picture of facial schwannomas is indistinguishable from that of vestibular schwannomas, for which they are often mistaken. In contrast, extratemporally located facial schwannomas, present as indolor preauricular mass associated with facial paralysis and without hearing loss [4, 8, 10, 11–13]. Another very typical clinical presentation is encountered for the subgroup of chorda tympani schwannomas: sensation of fullness of the ear, a conductive hearing loss and often absence of facial paralysis [14]. Brain stem compression is rarely reported.

Diagnostics

Imaging

The advent of MRI has significantly affected the management of facial schwannomas, because its sensitivity is higher than that of CT and makes detection of much smaller lesions possible. Also the specificity of MRI is higher and thus distinction from a vestibular schwannoma is facilitated.

On MRI, tumor tissue is well enhanced after gadolinium injection. Even a slight tumor infiltration along the facial nerve course may be documented where a smooth bony erosion on CT has raised the suspicion of a lesion. Furthermore, tumor tissue is well distinguishable from normal brain parenchyma, especially in the CPA and in the middle fossa, if there is an extension above the petrous bone. Some radiological features that allow to distinguish facial from vestibular schwannoma are an ex-centric attachment of the facial schwannoma on the IAC, rather than a symmetrical, central position as for vestibular schwannoma. Also involvement of the geniculate ganglion, the tympanic and mastoid segments are good indicators of a facial nerve tumor.

High resolution CT is complementary to MRI. Fine-cut bone windows with sagittal and coronal reconstructions of the petrous bone should be realized. This allows to visualize tumor within the IAC (sharp anterosuperior erosion), the geniculate ganglion and the different segments of the facial canal (smooth enlargement). Especially erosion of the cochlea, the semicircular canals and middle ear involvement can be evaluated. In case of extension into the middle fossa, the surface of the petrous bone may be completely destroyed; bony flakes may then be visible within a soft tissue mass. Tumoral tissue is strongly enhanced on CT after intravenous contrast injection. Moreover, CT permits to assess the pneumatization of the bones preoperatively and helps to estimate possible routes of CSF leakage.

Functional Tests

Topographical tests are of little value since the advent of MRI.

Electroneurography may help to predict the prognosis of postoperative facial paralysis [15]. Electromyography evaluates the residual motor function and helps to predict the postoperative recovery of a facial nerve after grafting [16]. Tone audiometry and speech discrimination should be performed to determine the type and degree of hearing loss. In the case of sensorineural hearing loss, brain stem-auditory evoked potentials may estimate the degree of involvement of the cochlear nerve. For pragmatic reasons, hearing should be qualified as servicable or nonserviceable in order to decide about a hearing-sparing surgical technique. Electronystagmography quantifies the impact of the tumor on the vestibular nerve and labyrinth function.

Fine Needle Aspiration Biopsy

Fine needle aspiration biopsy allows to differentiate chorda tympani schwannoma from other tumors of the external auditory canal [17]. For intracranial locations, the diagnosis is often only possible during surgery. The exact identification of the nerve from which the tumor arises is important, because facial and vestibular schwannomas are histologically identical.

Management

Since the advent of MRI, the discovery of asymptomatic facial schwannoma has become more likely. However, sometimes the distinction from vestibular schwannoma remains impossible until surgical exploration. Asymptomatic tumors preclude radical surgical resection which would leave the patient with irreversible facial paralysis and hearing deficits. Complete surgical resection which has long been the mainstay of treatment has to be compared with less invasive options such as subtotal resection, stereotactic radiosurgery or simple observation [4, 5].

Observation

In asymptomatic patients, the optimal management is not evident [3, 5, 18]. In fact, after surgery the patients must expect at least a partial facial paralysis (H-B 2 or worse), while conservatively treated patients may have a normal facial function for years without significant tumor growth. On the other hand, waitful watching may deteriorate sensorineural hearing by erosion of the cochlea. Thus, the timing of surgical resection is critical.

In some cases, the diagnostic of a facial nerve schwannoma is only done intraoperatively in a patient who was wrongly thought to have a vestibular schwannoma. Then, closure without tumor resection and further observation may be an option if the tumor is small and the patient has a facial function of H-B 3 or better.

Stereotactic Radiosurgery

The experience is not large regarding number of cases and follow-up time. Sparing of hearing and facial function with radiological stabilization have been reported in some cases [4]. In our experience (see 'Illustrative Case'), stereotactic radiosurgery was done in 1 case of tumor regrowth 4 years after a subtotal resection. This complementary treatment could stabilize tumor growth for another 7 years after which the tumor started regrowing and forming large cysts. The combined modalities of subtotal resection and radiosurgery may prolong the time with acceptable facial function for the patient. However, this treatment has not yet proven its long-term effectiveness and innocuity. Especially in young patients it can therefore not be recommended as first treatment choice. It may be an alternative, if progression occurs after a subtotal resection or if patients are old or inoperable.

Surgical Treatment

The best timing for surgery is controversial: it depends on facial and hearing function, size and intracranial mass effect of the tumor and last but not least patient's choice. The broadest consensus exists if the tumor is large and/or the patient has a moderate to severe facial paralysis (H-B ≥4); then, total resection with nerve grafting should be offered. Some authors also recommend total resection for smaller and less symptomatic tumors (H-B ≤3). The rationale is that a delay in resection increases the risk of hearing loss and that the outcome of facial nerve grafting is best with no or only a slight facial paralysis [6, 13]. Along with others, we think that if hearing remains good and there is no threat from intracranial mass effect, observation until H-B 3 is possible and radical tumor excision may be performed then. The reason is that even for good preoperative facial function (H-B 1 or 2) and regardless of the grafting technique, no better postoperative result than H-B 3 can be expected.

If surgery is decided for an H-B <3 (e.g. patient's choice or mass effect), we think that only a subtotal tumoral removal with nerve sparing technique should be performed. This preserves a good facial function (H-B 1 or 2) for a longer time, but tumor growth must be followed carefully.

Presurgical Considerations. Because facial nerve schwannomas occur at the intersection of the neurosurgical and ENT sphere, an interdisciplinary team work provides the best working conditions. Anesthesiology should be performed with nonparalyzing agents to permit perioperative facial nerve stimulation. Frameless guided surgical techniques are helpful to approach the region of interest quickly and safely. As the tumor is typically in close relationship to bony structures, the preciseness of navigation systems there is high. Cranial nerve monitoring and stimulation give real-time information about the facial and hearing function and add useful data to distinguish facial from vestibular schwannoma.

Depending on the surgical approach, the patient is installed in supine, park-bench or sitting position with a Mayfield head holder. Attention must be paid to preparation of potential nerve donor sites depending on the needed graft length (i.e. greater auricular nerve or sural nerve).

Surgical Approaches. The surgical approach depends on the tumor location, volume and extension to surrounding structures. Furthermore, it depends on the preoperative functional status of the facial and vestibulocochlear nerve. A well chosen approach should allow a good exposure with best possible conservation of normal anatomical structures and thus of function. Possible routes are: subtemporal, transmastoid, translabyrinthine or retrosigmoid.

The subtemporal approach allows access to the nerve between IAC and the proximal tympanic segment (i.e. IAC, labyrinthine segment, geniculate ganglion and proximal tympanic segment). The facial nerve may be reached at the brain stem, but if a large tumor mass is present in the CPA, this will hardly be resectable. Hearing preservation is possible by this route.

The transmastoid approach gives access to facial nerve segments between geniculate ganglion down to the stylomastoid foramen (i.e. geniculate ganglion, tympanic segment/chorda tympani, mastoid segment).

The combined subtemporal/transmastoid approach exposes the entire nerve from the IAC to the stylomastoid foramen. It is indicated for large tumors when an intracranial-intratemporal anastomosis [19] seems necessary and when serviceable hearing must be preserved (inner ear and ossicles). Sometimes primary/secondary ossicular chain reconstruction may be necessary.

The translabyrinthine approach also gives access to the entire nerve course from the brainstem down to the stylomastoid foramen. Even large masses in the CPA can be controlled by sacrificing the semicircular canals and the cochlea for large exposure. The access to the geniculate ganglion and the middle ear can be improved by removal of the external auditory canal, the tympanic membrane and the ossicles, needing closure of the external ear meatus. This approach may only be chosen if hearing is not serviceable or if tumor volume or inner ear erosion make hearing preservation impossible. The possibility for facial nerve grafting is good.

The retrosigmoid approach permits access to the nerve from brainstem to the IAC and allows management of large tumors in the CPA. It gives no access to the lateral IAC or the intratemporal facial nerve. Hearing preservation is possible.

Tumor Dissection and Handling of the Facial Nerve. As facial nerve schwannomas originate only from some nerve fibers pushing the others aside, it may sometimes be feasible to open the tumor capsule and dissect the tumor from the main part of the nerve without sacrificing it completely. This fascicle-sparing technique allowing total tumor resection is often not possible (about 20% of the cases), but if applied results in less severe postoperative facial nerve dysfunction than complete nerve sacrifice. The recurrence rate seems not to be higher than usual [1, 4, 12]. However, most often the affected nerve segment is invaded by tumor and must be completely resected. Then, immediate repair by an interposition nerve graft or delayed repair by a hypoglosso-facial anastomosis is indicated. Regardless of the type and timing of repair, the best possible recovery after complete facial nerve resection is a partial recovery (H-B 3) [5, 16, 18]. In patients who do not accept to wait for a possible facial nerve recovery, subtotal tumor resection may be indicated sparing the anatomical continuity of the facial nerve. This allows a better and quicker recovery of facial nerve function postoperatively, but requires a very close follow-up for regrowth.

Facial Nerve Repair. Primary nerve repair is rarely possible [1]. In a translabyrinthine approach, a short segment (1–2 cm) may be rerouted and directly anastomosed. Interpositional nerve grafts (e.g. sural nerve or greater auricular nerve) are helpful to bridge greater distances. Hypoglossal-facial anastomosis is useful if a short nerve stump near the brainstem precludes any interposition nerve graft [20]. It may be considered for long-standing facial paralysis up to 4 years. For desperate cases with distal neural fibrosis and muscle atrophy, other procedures as dynamic temporalis transfer or free muscle flap may be considered.

Postoperative Care. As some degree of postoperative facial paralysis is inevitable, prevention of corneal ulcus must be rigorous (hourly artificial teardrops, nocturnal vitamin A ointment and occlusion with Steristrips®). In cases of present ulcus, tarsoraphy may be indicated temporarily. Postoperative rehabilitation should only be started when tone and movements return in order to maximize function and minimize bothering synkinesis. Surgical correction of lagophtalmus (e.g. lower eyelid shortening and upper eyelid gold implants) should only be done if facial nerve resuscitation techniques have failed. A long enough time must be given for nerve regrowth (6 months for a lesion distal to the mastoid segment and 12 months for a lesion close to the brainstem).

The most common complications after this type of surgery are CSF liquorrhea and meningitis which are classically managed by draining techniques and antibiotic treatment.

Prognosis

Nowadays, surgical mortality is low. The outcome for facial nerve function depends on the duration and degree of preoperative facial paralysis as well as the surgical technique. After subtotal tumor resection in a patient without former facial paralysis, the facial nerve function may return to nearly normal (H-B 2) within 3 months. A moderate recovery (H-B 3) may be achieved after total resection and interposition nerve graft even if the preoperative function was worse (H-B 4 or 5). Less good recovery (H-B 4) is observed after total resection and hypoglosso-facial anastomosis which is usually done in large tumors with longstanding facial paralysis. Preservation of hearing is achievable, if serviceable hearing is present preoperatively and a hearing-sparing technique employed. In the case of conductive hearing loss, even postoperative improvement has been reported [4]. Concerning tumor regrowth after subtotal resection, this has to be expected within some years and may be further stabilized by radiotherapy. In totally resected tumors, no recurrence was observed during a mean follow-up of 5.1 years in our patients. In another series of 9 patients who underwent total resection, no recurrence was reported after a mean follow-up of 44 months [4].

Illustrative Case

A 32-year-old female patient presenting with multiple seizures since several months underwent an MRI in 1993 which showed a frontal cavernoma and a small lesion in the right IAC and cerebellopontine cistern without contact to the brainstem (fig. 2). At that time, the patient had no facial symptoms and a normal corneal reflex; hearing was subnormal and a vestibular areflexia was present. The patient had a café au lait spot on the left arm. That year, the cavernoma was resected because of medically intractable seizures. The patient was then followed by audiogram and MRI. In 1994, a significant increase in size was demonstrated; the tumor had a central necrosis and reached the brain stem (fig. 3). The audiogram showed a loss of −40 dB and the loss of speech discrimination (no serviceable hearing), but no facial paralysis. The tumor was resected subtotally by a retrosigmoid approach with an opening of the IAC and anatomical and electrophysiologic preservation of the facial and vestibulocochlear nerves. Postoperatively, the patient had a partial facial paralysis (H-B 2). A postoperative liquorrhea (without meningitis) resolved after surgical repair (fig. 4). In 1998 (4 years later), the patient complained of increasing tinnitus and dizziness; the hearing was completely lost. The facial function was assessed as H-B 3 with facial spasms. The MRI showed a significant tumor regrowth (fig. 5). The patient

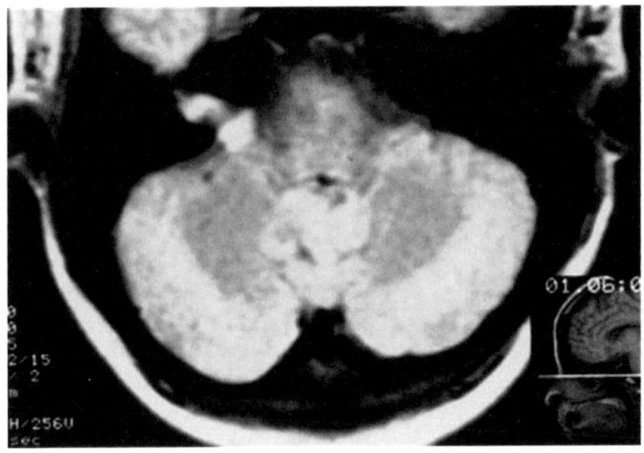

Fig. 2. MRI scan taken in 1993 showing enlargement of the right IAC due to a facial nerve schwannoma extending into the cerebellopontine cistern not compressing the brainstem; patient was nearly asymptomatic; she had no facial paralysis, but beginning of sensory hearing loss (audiogram); observation was decided.

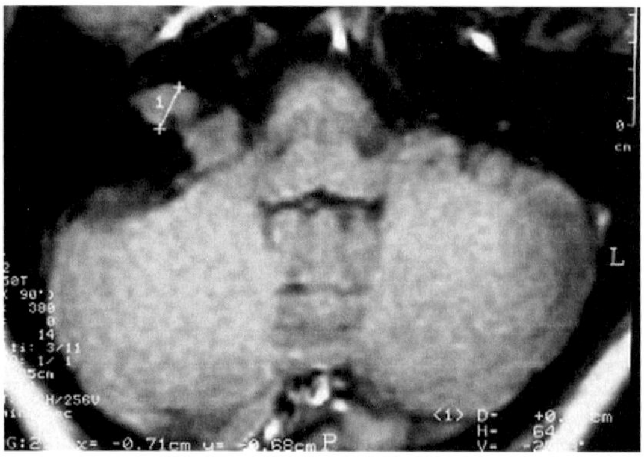

Fig. 3. MRI scan taken in 1994 showing significant tumor growth within 1 year of observation; note the enlargement in the geniculate ganglion region and extension in the cerebellopontine cistern with beginning mass effect on the brainstem; the patient had nonserviceable hearing but no facial paralysis; decision was taken to perform subtotal resection by a retrosigmoid approach sparing the facial nerve.

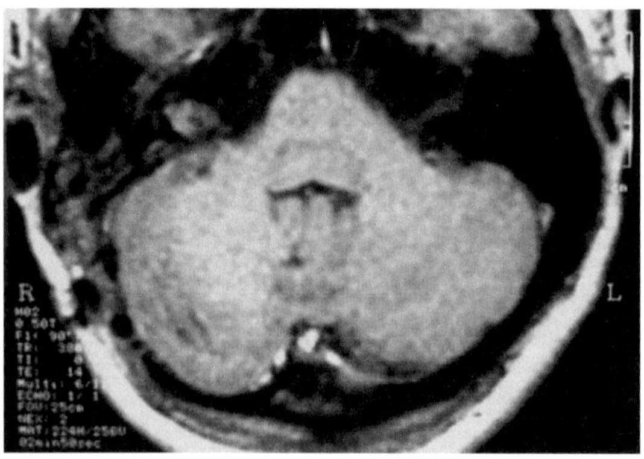

Fig. 4. MRI scan taken in 1995, 1 year after subtotal tumor resection sparing the facial and the vestibulo-cochlear nerves. Clinically, the patient had partial facial paralysis (H-B 2) and no amelioration of the hearing.

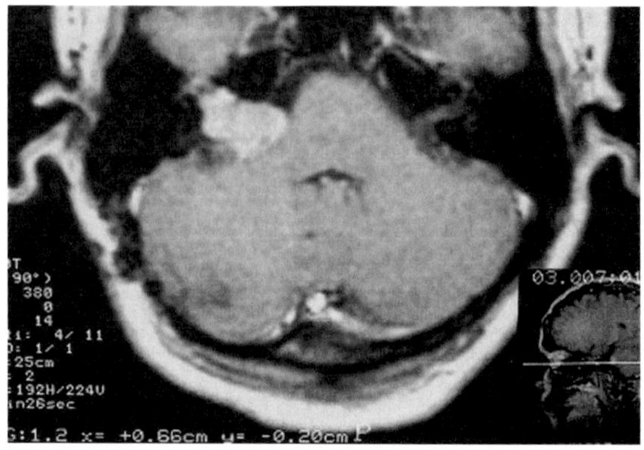

Fig. 5. MRI scan taken in 1998. Lesion was stable over 3 years after subtotal resection, but showed a significant regrowth in the 4th year; clinically, the patient had developed tinnitus and dizziness and had become deaf; facial function had deteriorated (H-B 3) and there occurred bothering facial spasms; decision to perform stereotactic radiosurgery was taken.

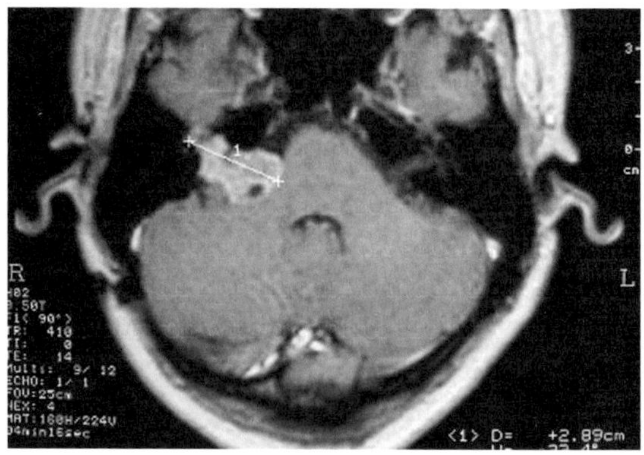

Fig. 6. MRI scan taken in 1998, 6 months after radiosurgery, showing size stabilization; note: medial tumor part became cystic; otalgia and synkinesia were clinically present.

was sent for stereotactic radiosurgery (Gamma Unit). 6 months later, the patient had otalgia and synkinesia (during eye closing); on MRI the size was the same, but the portion in the CPA had become cystic (fig. 6). In 1999 (1 year after radiosurgery), there was tumor extension to the geniculate ganglion and complementary radiosurgery was proposed. Meanwhile, the tumor had shown involution, and radiosurgery was finally not performed. Up to 2001, the lesion exhibited small growth, especially the cystic part of the lesion was concerned (fig. 7). This radiological evolution continued progressively until 2005 with significant regrowth within the CPA; clinically, the facial paralysis became complete (H-B 6) and bothering paresthesias of the face

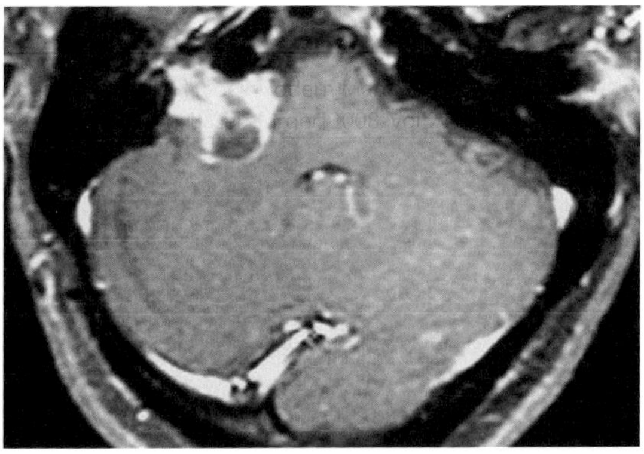

Fig. 7. MRI scan taken in 2001, 3 years after radiosurgery, showing moderate increase in size, especially in the cystic part of the lesion; facial paralysis was nearly complete (H-B 5).

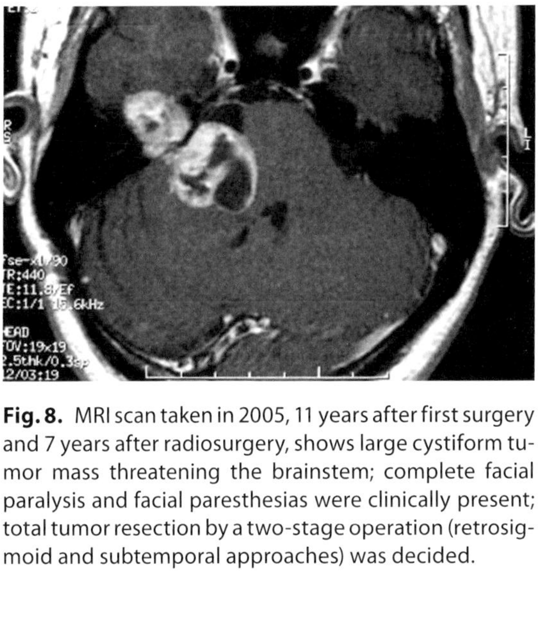

Fig. 8. MRI scan taken in 2005, 11 years after first surgery and 7 years after radiosurgery, shows large cystiform tumor mass threatening the brainstem; complete facial paralysis and facial paresthesias were clinically present; total tumor resection by a two-stage operation (retrosigmoid and subtemporal approaches) was decided.

were present (fig. 8). A retrosigmoid approach was performed again allowing near total resection. 1 month later a remnant was resected by a subtemporal approach allowing complete tumor removal (fig. 9). The patient received a hypoglosso-facial anastomosis 2 months after tumor resection. At the 1-year follow-up, no evidence of tumor recurrence was present and facial nerve function had partially recovered (H-B 4).

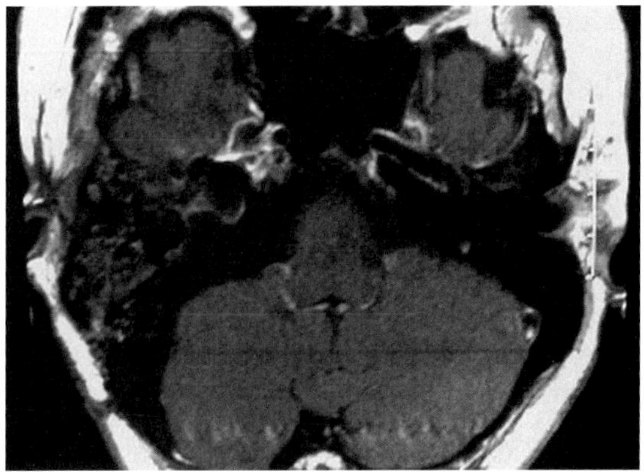

Fig. 9. MRI scan taken in 2005, 3 months after two-stage reoperation resulting in total tumor resection with facial nerve sacrifice and consecutive hypoglosso-facial nerve anastomosis.

Conclusion

Facial nerve schwannomas may be clinically and radiologically indistinguishable from vestibular schwannomas. Although, they are less frequent than the latter, they must always be considered as main differential diagnosis. The treatment depends on patient and tumor characteristics. If the patient is asymptomatic and the tumor small, observation and a close follow-up are recommended. If the tumor has mass effect or the patient is already functionally disabled, radical surgical resection with nerve repair is indicated. If the patient shows slight deterioration on functional tests or the tumor threatens nearby anatomical structures, subtotal surgical resection is best. This results in longer conservation of good facial nerve function than radical tumor resection with reconstruction. The drawbacks are a closer follow-up and probable reoperation. Stereotactic radiosurgery should be reserved for inoperable patients or recurrence after subtotally resected tumors. Undoubtedly, facial nerve schwannomas need an interdisciplinary team of neurosurgeons, ENT surgeons and radiosurgeons that discusses each individual case to provide the optimal management.

References

1 Nadeau DP, Sataloff RT: Fascicle preservation surgery for facial nerve neuromas involving the posterior cranial fossa. Otol Neurotol 2003;24:317–325.
2 Saito H, Baxter A: Undiagnosed intratemporal facial nerve neurilemomas. Arch Otolaryngol 1972;95:415–419.
3 Van Den Abbeele T, Viala P, Francois M, Narcy P: Facial neuromas in children: delayed or immediate surgery? Am J Otol 1999;20:253–256.
4 Sherman JD, Dagnew E, Pensak ML, van Loveren HR, Tew JM Jr: Facial nerve neuromas: report of 10 cases and review of the literature. Neurosurgery 2002;50:450–456.
5 Minovi A, Vosschulte R, Hofmann E, Draf W, Bockmuhl U: Facial nerve neuroma: surgical concept and functional results. Skull Base 2004;14:195–200; discussion 200–191.
6 Lipkin AF, Coker NJ, Jenkins HA, Alford BR: Intracranial and intratemporal facial neuroma. Otolaryngol Head Neck Surg 1987;96:71–79.
7 Pulec JL: Facial nerve neuroma. Ear Nose Throat J 1994;73:721–722, 725–739, 743–752.
8 O'Donoghue GM, Brackmann DE, House JW, Jackler RK: Neuromas of the facial nerve. Am J Otol 1989;10:49–54.
9 Kudo A, Suzuki M, Kubo N, Kuroda K, Ogawa A, Iwasaki Y: Schwannoma arising from the intermediate nerve and manifesting as hemifacial spasm. Case report. J Neurosurg 1996;84:277–279.
10 Fagan PA, Misra SN, Doust B: Facial neuroma of the cerebellopontine angle and the internal auditory canal. Laryngoscope 1993;103:442–446.
11 Lee KS, Britton BH, Kelly DL Jr: Schwannoma of the facial nerve in the cerebellopontine angle presenting with hearing loss. Surg Neurol 1989;32:231–234.
12 Sataloff RT, Frattali MA, Myers DL: Intracranial facial neuromas: total tumor removal with facial nerve preservation: a new surgical technique. Ear Nose Throat J 1995;74:244–246, 248–256.
13 Symon L, Cheesman AD, Kawauchi M, Bordi L: Neuromas of the facial nerve: a report of 12 cases. Br J Neurosurg 1993;7:13–22.
14 Kirazli T, Oner K, Bilgen C, Ovul I, Midilli R: Facial nerve neuroma: clinical, diagnostic, and surgical features. Skull Base 2004;14:115–120.
15 Angeli SI, Brackmann DE: Is surgical excision of facial nerve schwannomas always indicated? Otolaryngol Head Neck Surg 1997;117:144–147.
16 Yamaki T, Morimoto S, Ohtaki M, Sakatani K, Sakai J, Himi T, et al: Intracranial facial nerve neurinoma: surgical strategy of tumor removal and functional reconstruction. Surg Neurol 1998;49:538–546.
17 Magliulo G, D'Amico R, Varacalli S, Ciniglio-Appiani G: Chorda tympani neuroma: diagnosis and management. Am J Otolaryngol 2000;21:65–68.
18 Liu R, Fagan P: Facial nerve schwannoma: surgical excision versus conservative management. Ann Otol Rhinol Laryngol 2001;110:1025–1029.
19 Draf W, Samii M: Intracranial-intratemporal anastomosis of the facial nerve (author's transl). Laryngol Rhinol Otol (Stuttg) 1980;59:282–287.
20 Asaoka K, Sawamura Y, Nagashima M, Fukushima T: Surgical anatomy for direct hypoglossal-facial nerve side-to-end 'anastomosis'. J Neurosurg 1999;91:268–275.

Jan Frederick Cornelius, MD
Department of Neurosurgery, Lariboisiere Hospital
2, rue Ambroise Pare
FR–75010 Paris (France)
Tel. +33 1 49 95 81 44, Fax +33 1 49 95 81 55, E-Mail jfcornelius@yahoo.com

Régis J, Roche P-H (eds): Modern Management of Acoustic Neuroma.
Prog Neurol Surg. Basel, Karger, 2008, vol 21, pp 131–135

Gamma Knife Surgery for Facial Nerve Schwannomas

C.F. Litré · G. Pech Gourg · M. Tamura · P.-H. Roche · J. Régis

Stereotactic and Functional Neurosurgery, Timone University Hospital, Marseille, France

Abstract

Radical resection of facial nerve schwannomas classically implies a high risk of severe facial palsy. Due to the rarity of facial palsy following Gamma Knife surgery (GKS) of vestibular schwannomas, functional evaluation after GKS in this specific group of patient appears rational. Clinical management due to the specificity and heterogeneity of this group of patients has required the development of an original classification of 4 anatomical subtypes presenting different clinical and surgical difficulties. Among 1,783 schwannomas of the cerebellopontine angle treated by GKS in Timone University Hospital between July 1992 and May 2003, 11 were diagnosed as originating from the facial nerve. Criteria for this diagnosis were: the involvement of the tympanic or mastoid segment of the facial nerve (9 patients); and/or preoperative observation of a facial nerve deficit that had occurred during previous microsurgery (2 patients). The rare occurrence of facial palsy after vestibular schwannoma radiosurgery, usually occurring within 18 months of treatment, has been considered only in the patients with more than 2 years of follow-up (9 patients). At last follow-up examination, no patients had developed a new facial palsy or experienced deterioration of a pre-existing facial palsy; 3 patients had improvement of a preoperative facial palsy. Ten of 11 tumors were stable, or decreased in size; in the remaining case, microsurgical resection of the tumor had been recommended due to the development of a cyst. This first study demonstrates that radiosurgery allows treatment of these patients while preserving normal motor facial function. Such an advantage should lead to the consideration of GKS as a first treatment option for small- to middle-sized facial nerve schwannomas.

Facial nerve schwannomas (FNSs) represent less than 1% of intrapetrous tumors [1], while vestibular schwannomas (VSs) [2, 3] represent 8% of intracranial tumors (10 per 1 million inhabitants). The complete tumor resection generally needs to sacrifice the facial nerve. With successful interposition of a nerve graft or hypoglossofacial anastomosis, facial nerve recovery never reaches more than House-Brackmann grade 3 with obvious psychosocial consequences [4].

In this context, any therapeutic alternative, which can lead to a better preservation of the facial functions, must be studied. Stereotactic radiosurgery has demonstrated its efficiency in the treatment of intracranial benign tumors especially for VSs. Since facial nerve palsy [5, 6] is an exceptional event after Gamma Knife surgery (GKS) treatment (less than 0.5%), facial nerve functional preservation after GKS appears to be an interesting approach for FNS patients.

The diagnosis is not always obvious. FNS is a rare tumor affecting people from both genders. Tumor may be diagnosed at any age, but middle-aged people are predominantly affected. Clinical manifestations are heterogeneous, depending on the tumor origin and extension. Main symptoms are linked to the facial nerve dysfunction, whatever the location of the tumor on the facial nerve.

Hemifacial weakness or hemifacial spasm of sudden or progressive onset is the major symptom. Transient and recurrent deficit is typical of the disease. Isolated dry eye or dysguesia may happen in the case of isolated involvement of the geniculate ganglion or geniculate supra-petrous nerve. Otologic and vestibular manifestations are also frequently encountered. Imbalance and vertigo indicate that the tumor affects the vestibular system, in the case of cerebellopontine angle (CPA) or internal auditory canal (IAC) involvement. Sensorial hearing deficit or tinnitus implies a cochlear nerve dysfunction in the CPA or IAC, while the cochlea is generally not directly affected by the tumor. Conductive hearing loss or sensation of filled ear is typical of middle ear invasion. Such symptoms are encountered when the tympanic or the vertical segment of the nerve are affected by the disease. Diagnostic is based upon high-resolution neuroimaging. Bone window CT scan and T_1-weighted MR imaging sequences are both valuable for an early diagnosis. The CT shows an enlargement of a segment of the fallopian canal with homogeneous bone erosion, while the MRI shows the enhanced tumor mass on a segment of the nerve. In cases of geniculate fossa invasion, the tumor may extend upward in the middle fossa and sometimes displays cystic transformation.

Topological classification is important. In an extensive review of the literature conducted over more than 3 decades [7], the tumor location was described as follows: labyrinthine 43.5%, tympanic 42.8%, vertical segment 36.7% and CPA 17.8%. Owing to these imaging refinements, the diagnosis is performed earlier and the origin of the tumor is more accurately defined.

It has been recently postulated that FNS predominantly develops from the geniculate ganglion and petrosal nerves [8]. Taken collectively, data obtained from the clinical presentation and from the neuroimaging workup led us to establish an original topological classification of FNSs (fig. 1). Type I: the tumor is localized on the geniculate ganglion. Type II: the tumor is a dumbbell-shaped lesion on the geniculate ganglion, labyrinthine segment, IAC and CPA cistern. Type III: the tumor develops in the tympanic and/or vertical segments of the facial nerve. Type IV: the tumor develops in the IAC or the CPA without invasion of the fallopian canal or the geniculate ganglion. This category is difficult to distinguish from VS with radiologic criteria. In this group, the diagnosis was usually based on a previous microsurgical attempt.

Conversely, FNS must be described each time as a lesion resembling VS with facial palsy as the main symptom.

'Wait and see' and microsurgical approaches are traditionally discussed. FNS are benign tumors that are supposed to display slow growth but little is known about their natural history. In a recent study [9], a cohort of 13 patients have been followed conservatively. Facial nerve deterioration was observed in 38.5% of cases during a median follow-up time of 6 years (range 1–19 years). This information is important to take into account in the treatment decision process. Microsurgical radical removal used to be traditionally considered as the treatment of reference (table 1). Technical aspects of the removal depend on tumor origin, extension, hearing level and preexisting deficits. The main consequence of tumor extirpation is facial nerve palsy. Facial nerve anastomosis using an interposed cable graft or hypoglossofacial anastomosis partially reduces the deficit but even in best cases, the level of recovery that can be reached is never better than grade 3. In rare cases of extra fascicular growth of the nerve or in the case of geniculate supra-petrous nerve involvement, the nerve may be preserved [7], but this situation cannot be planned before the operative time. Consequently, several authors propose a 'wait and see' strategy and recommend radical resection after facial motor nerve function deterioration.

Radiosurgical alternative is in this context an appealing approach. Thus, it has been shown in a

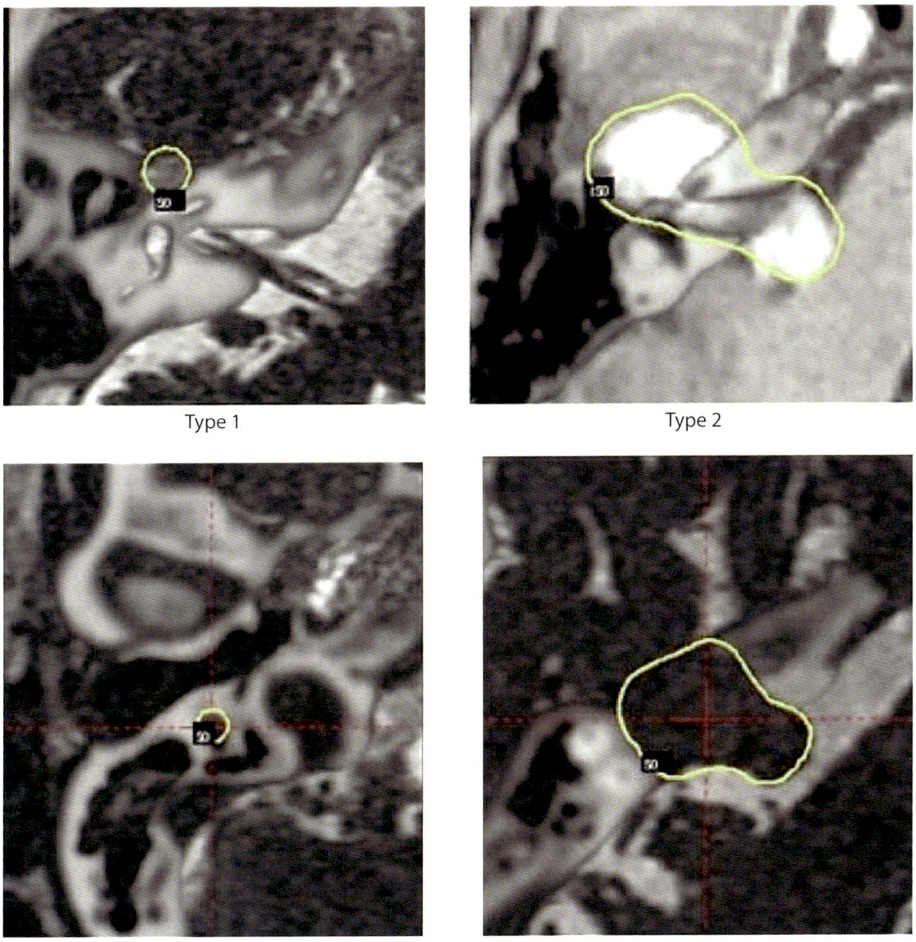

Fig. 1. Topographic classification of FNSs. Images are obtained from a fused bone window CT scan with MR sequences. The tumor margin is delimited by the yellow line.

recent report that the occurrence of facial nerve palsy never exceeded 0.5% after Gamma Knife radiosurgical treatment of VS [10], with a 97% rate of long-term tumor control while the facial nerve was always in close relationship with the tumor that was exposed to radiation (table 1). Taken collectively, these observations led us to consider that radiosurgery could bring an efficient and safe alternative to conventional microsurgical removal of FNS. Mabanta et al. [11] have reported in 1999 the absence of short-term facial motor function worsening in 2 patients treated with LINAC-based radiosurgery, but no definitive conclusion could be drawn from these reports. Our team has recently published the first report that focuses on a series of patients that have been treated homogeneously with a state of the art technique.

Among 1,783 schwannomas of the CPA treated by GKS in Timone University Hospital between July 1992 and May 2003, 11 have been diagnosed as originating from the facial nerve [12]. The follow-up was of 39.4 months (range: 18–84). The last follow-up examination revealed that none of these patients had developed facial

Table 1. Comparison of the series from the literature

Series	Cases	Therapy	Evolution	Hearing facial function	Follow-up months	Recurrence/ tumoral progression
Sherman et al., 2002	10	microsurgery	Ag: 2 St: 7 Am: 1	Ag: 2 St: 5 Am: 3	39.8	1
Lejeune et al., 2006	7	microsurgery	Ag: 6 Am: 1	Ag: 7		
Hasegawa et al., 1999	2	radiosurgery Gamma Knife	Am: 1 St: 1	St : 2	42.5	0
Mabanta et al., 1999	2/6 schwannomas	radiosurgery LINAC	St: 2	St: 2	32	0
Ulku et al., 2004	4	surgery	not detailed	St: 1 Ag: 1 Am: 2	38.6	0
Regis et al., 2006	11 (2 with surgery)	radiosurgery Gamma Knife	St: 11	Am: 3 St: 8	39.4	1[1]

Ag = Worsening; Am = enhancement; St = stabilization.
[1]Patient already operated (evolution with a cyst).

palsy; preoperative facial palsy had improved in 3 patients and worsened in none. All the tumors have been controlled until now, except one where a cyst developed.

The length of follow-up is still too short to give definitive data about tumor control but 50% of patients have been followed for more than 3 years and showed no tumor growth. Notwithstanding, this period is of enough length to provide reliable functional results. Facial nerve motion did not worsen in any patient, which compares favorably to microsurgery. This result is also interesting because most patients presented with facial nerve deficit before radiosurgery, and it should have been expected that radioinduced neuropathy may occur more often in cases where the nerves had already been weakened. This situation is comparable to what has already been observed for meningiomas affecting oculomotor nerves. In these cases, it is usual to observe a recovery of the oculomotor palsy after GKS [13], which can be interpreted as a neuroprotective effect of radiosurgery on several cranial nerves. It would have been of interest to correlate the severity and the duration of facial palsy with the benefit of GKS, but there is a need for treatment of additional patients to provide new insights into this field. Of particular interest is to know if complete palsy may recover after GKS since restorative microsurgery of the nerve is able to improve the motion up to grade 3. Hearing level was also preserved in all cases of the present series, while the intrapetrous neuro-otologic structures are jeopardized by open microsurgery.

To conclude, surgical management of FNS carries the risk of severe and permanent deficit of cochleovestibular and facial nerves. Our experience demonstrates that Gamma Knife radiosurgical treatment is an interesting option to achieve tumor control and functional preservation in small-to middle-sized tumors. Treatment of additional patients with longer follow-up after GKS should confirm these preliminary data. The decision to provide an early proactive treatment remains debatable. If tumor diameter exceeds 3 cm or if the facial nerve deficit is severe and permanent, it may be more valuable to recommend microsurgical removal and nerve reconstruction.

References

1 Lapena JF, Chiong CM: The tip of the iceberg: not all that palsies is bell's. A case series of five facial nerve neurilemmomas in the Philippines. First Prize of the Philippine Society of Otolaryngology-Head and Neck Surgery, Inc. Descriptive Research Contest, September 26, 1997.

2 Deen HG, Ebersold MJ, Harner SG, Beatty CW, Marion MS, Wharen RE, et al: Conservative management of acoustic neuroma: an outcome study. Neurosurgery 1996;39:260–264; Discussion 4–6.

3 Jackler RK, Pitts LH: Acoustic Neurinoma. Neurosurgery Clinics of North America 1990;1:199–223.

4 Irving R, Jackler R, Pitts L: Hearing preservation in patients undergoing vestibular schwannoma surgery: comparison of middle fossa and retrosigmoid approaches [see comments]. J Neurosurg 1998;88:840–845.

5 Lunsford LD, Niranjan A: Gamma Knife Radiosurgery for Acoustic Tumors. Techniques in Neurosurgery 2003;9:128–135.

6 Regis J, Roche PH, Delsenti C, Soumare O, Thomassin JM, Pellet W: Stereotactic Radiosurgery for Vestibular Schwannoma; in Pollock BE (ed): Contemporary Stereotactic Radiosurgery: Thechnique and Evaluation. Armonk, New York, Futura Publishing Company, 2002, pp 181–212.

7 Sherman JD, Dagnew E, Pensak ML, van Loveren HR, Tew JM Jr: Facial nerve neuromas: report of 10 cases and review of the literature. Neurosurgery 2002;50:450–456.

8 Wiggins RH 3rd, Harnsberger HR, Salzman KL, Shelton C, Kertesz TR, Glastonbury CM: The many faces of facial nerve schwannoma. AJNR Am J Neuroradiol 2006;27:694–699.

9 Perez R, Chen JM, Nedzelski JM: Intratemporal facial nerve schwannoma: a management dilemma. Otol Neurotol 2005;26:121–126.

10 Regis J, Delsanti C, Roche PH, Thomassin JM, Pellet W: [Functional outcomes of radiosurgical treatment of vestibular schwannomas: 1,000 successive cases and review of the literature]. Neurochirurgie 2004;50(2–3 Pt 2):301–311.

11 Mabanta SR, Buatti JM, Friedman WA, Meeks SL, Mendenhall WM, Bova FJ: Linear accelerator radiosurgery for nonacoustic schwannomas. Int J Radiat Oncol Biol Phys 1999;43:545–548.

12 Litre CF, Gourg GP, Tamura M, Mdarhri D, Touzani A, Roche PH, et al: Gamma knife surgery for facial nerve schwannomas. Neurosurgery. 2007;60:853–859; Discussion –9.

13 Roche PH, Pellet W, Fuentes S, Thomassin JM, Regis J: Gamma knife radiosurgical management of petroclival meningiomas results and indications. Acta Neurochir (Wien) 2003;145:883–888; Discussion 8.

Dr. C.F. Litré
Service de Neurochirurgie Fonctionnelle et Stéréotaxique
Hôpital d'Adulte de la Timone, 264 bvd Saint Pierre
FR–13385 Marseille Cedex 05 (France)
Tel. +33 4 91 38 70 58, Fax +33 4 91 38 70 56, E-Mail fabien.litre@mac.com

Régis J, Roche P-H (eds): Modern Management of Acoustic Neuroma.
Prog Neurol Surg. Basel, Karger, 2008, vol 21, pp 136–141

Hearing Preservation after Complete Microsurgical Removal in Vestibular Schwannomas

M. Samii · V. Gerganov · A. Samii

International Neuroscience Institute, Hannover, Germany

Abstract

Aim: To evaluate and present the treatment strategy and hearing preservation in a recent series of vestibular schwannoma cases. **Materials and Methods:** A retrospective analysis of 200 patients operated consecutively over a 3 year period was performed. Patient records, operative reports, including data from the electrophysiological monitoring, follow-up audiometric examinations, and neuroradiological findings were analyzed. **Results:** The anatomical integrity of the cochlear nerve was preserved in 75.8% of the cases. When only patients with preserved preoperative hearing were included, the rate was 84%. The overall rate of functional hearing preservation was 51%. It was highest in small tumors – 60% in class T1 and 72% in class T2. In tumors extending to and compressing the brain stem, preservation of some hearing was possible in up to 43%. **Conclusions:** Vestibular schwannomas are benign lesions whose total removal leads to definitive healing of the patient. The goal of every surgery should be functional preservation of all cranial nerves. Using the retrosigmoid approach with the patient in the semi-sitting position, hearing preservation is possible even for large schwannomas.

Hearing preservation is an important prerequisite for achieving good quality of life after vestibular schwannoma (VS) surgery. Thanks to the widespread use of modern neuroimaging, VSs are detected at earlier stages and hearing preservation becomes a realistic goal. In the 21st century, surgery of VS should be functional sparing.

Since 1968, the senior author (S.M.) has operated on more than 3,000 patients with VS. The hearing function of his first 1,000 patients was presented in 1997 [1]. Several years later, hearing function was analyzed in a series of 1,800 cases [2]. The goal of the present study was to evaluate the evolution of his treatment strategy and to present hearing preservation outcome in the last 200 consecutively operated cases at the INI-Hannover.

Materials and Methods

Patient records, operative reports, including data from the electrophysiological monitoring, follow-up audiometric examinations, and neuroradiological findings were analyzed. The main outcome measures were hearing preservation, MRI imaging, and neurological status.

Hearing was classified according to the New Hannover Classification [1, 2]. Tumors larger than 30 × 20 mm were defined as large. The Hannover Tumor Extension System was applied [3]: T1 – purely intracanalicular VS; T2 – intra-extrameatal; T3A – filling the CPA cistern; T3B – reaching the brain stem; T4A – compressing the brain stem; T4B – severe compression and dislocation of the brain stem and of the fourth ventricle.

Operative Technique
The retrosigmoid approach was applied in all cases. Anatomical, and if possible, functional preservation of the cochlear nerve was the goal in each case. The details of the technique applied have been presented in detail previously [1–3], so only those steps, crucial for hearing preservation, are outlined: (1) Continuous electrophysiological monitoring of auditory evoked potentials was performed in all cases. In selected cases, direct brainstem recording of auditory evoked potentials by placing a retractor with electrodes was used. (2) The preferred position of the patient is the semi-sitting position. (3) Cerebrospinal fluid is allowed to drain by opening of the lateral cerebellomedullary cistern. Thus, the cerebellum relaxes away from the petrous bone. (4) The intrameatal tumor portion is exposed initially. The internal auditory canal (IAC) is drilled under constant irrigation over 180° of its circumference. Less radical exposure of the IAC leads to a greater risk of either incomplete removal of the most lateral part of the tumor or of worse functional outcome. On the other hand, if hearing is to be preserved, the inner ear structures should not be damaged. (5) Once the facial and vestibulocochlear nerves are identified in the region of the fundus due to their constant relation to the bony structures, the tumor is piecemeal removed. (6) The dissection of the capsule from the surrounding neural structures should begin only after adequate internal decompression of the tumor portion has been achieved. The dissection of the tumor is performed by strictly gripping the tumor capsule and dissecting in the level of the arachnoid plane under continuous saline irrigation. (6) If the arachnoid plane does not exist, the 'onion skin technique' of tumor removal could be applied. Each layer of the lesion is removed from inward to outwards until the most outer layer is reached and removed piecemeal. This dissection technique allows preservation of the cochlear nerve integrity and function. (7) Bipolar coagulation is reduced to a minimum. The tumor part just medial to and inside the porus is removed at the end with great care.

Results

The mean age of the patients in the study group was 46.8 years, ranging from 18 to 73 years. Nineteen patients had undergone previous surgery at another institution. Tumor regrowth after previous radiosurgical treatment was observed in 5 patients. Almost half of the tumors (46%) were large, corresponding to class T4.

Clinical examination preoperatively revealed that the cochlear was the most frequently affected cranial nerve. Only 12 of the patients (6%) presented with normal hearing. Complete hearing loss was observed in 10% and hypacusis – 84%. Functional hearing (pure tone average up to 60 dB, and speech discrimination of 50%) was present in 63% of the patients before the operation.

Surgical Outcome
Total tumor removal was achieved in 196 patients (98%). Subtotal removal was performed in 4 patients with class IV schwannomas in order to preserve the anatomical integrity of the facial nerve.

In 75, 8% the anatomical integrity of the cochlear nerve was preserved. When only patients with preserved preoperative hearing were included, the rate was 84%. The rate of preservation was highest in class 1 VS (94%) and gradually decreased with the increase in tumor size – 89, 82 and 65% in class T2, T3 and T4, respectively. The overall rate of functional hearing preservation was 51%. It was highest in small tumors – 60% in class T1, 72% in class T2, 56% in class T3A, and 54% in class T3B. In tumors extending to and compressing the brain stem (class T4), preservation of hearing was possible in up to 43% (fig. 1 and 2).

Discussion

The first reported case of hearing preservation after removal of a VS was presented by Elliott and McKissock in 1954 [4]. The rapid development of neuroanesthesia, neurophysiology, and microsurgery, as well as the introduction of new technologies, led to significant changes in the treatment of VS during the last decades. The focus of treatment has changed to preservation of functional hearing and this is being achieved at increasing rates [5].

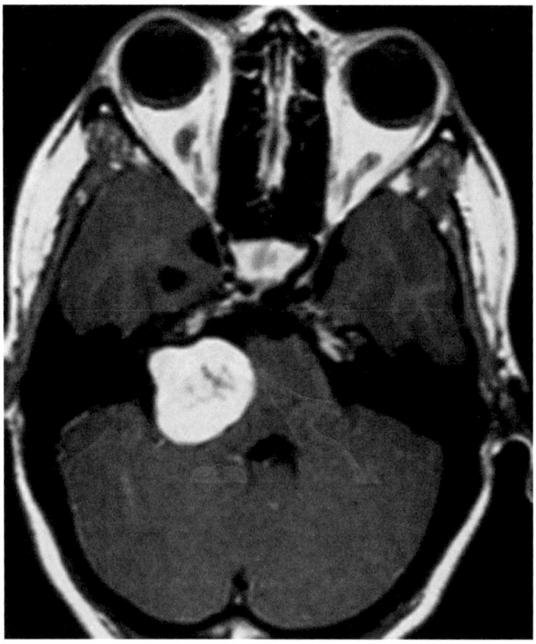

Fig. 1. Preoperative MRI of a patient demonstrating a large (class T4) right-sided VS.

Treatment strategies of VS include observation, radiosurgery, combined surgical excision and radiosurgery of the tumor remnant and microsurgery. Observation could be a short-term option for a subgroup of patients but a regular neuroimaging follow-up is obligatory. In experienced hands, radiosurgical treatment leads to tumor control in up to 93–98%. The rate of hearing preservation in the recently published series is 40–74% [6], but there have been no studies that focused on long-term hearing preservation in such patients [5].

Another treatment option for large tumors, elderly patients, surgery on the only hearing side, or tight adhesion of the cochlear nerve to the tumor, is the staged therapy [7]. At the first stage, the tumor is removed partially. The remnant is being observed or treated radiosurgically at a second stage. Long-term follow-up of tumor remnants indicates that further growth is observed in 20–44% [8]. VSs are benign tumors. Their total removal in one stage with hearing preservation is an attainable goal and leads to a definite healing of the patient. The only exception to total removal should be the attempt to preserve function, as in patients with bilateral VS with real risk of bilateral deafness if normal or good preoperative hearing is present.

The two hearing-preserving surgical approaches are the middle fossa and the retrosigmoid. The rate of hearing preservation is similar with both approaches [9, 10]. The analysis of the published results indicates that outcome is mainly related to the experience of the surgeon with a particular approach.

High rates of hearing preservation with the middle fossa approach have been reported. In selected cases (small tumor size and good preoperative hearing level) hearing preservation is achieved in 52–60% [4, 9, 10–14]. If larger tumors are included, the rates are significantly worse. In the series of Yates et al. [12] the rate falls from 72 to 34% for VSs extending more than 1 cm in the CPA.

With the retrosigmoid approach, similar rates of hearing presentation are achieved for small tumors. The main advantage of the approach is that it is the only hearing-preserving surgical option for large tumors [4, 10, 15–17].

The most important predictive factors for hearing preservation are the tumor size and preoperative hearing level [1, 2, 18]. Among the surgical factors, the experience of the surgeon and the operative technique applied are of utmost importance [19]. Detailed knowledge of the anatomy of the CPA is especially important. Early identification of cranial nerves due to their constant relationship to other anatomical structures, both in their lateral and proximal parts, facilitates their preservation. The cochlear nerve enters the brain stem in the lateral part of pontomedullary sulcus, 1–2 mm anterior to the exit site of the facial nerve [20]. In the most lateral part of the IAC, the nerve occupies the anteroinferior quadrant of the fundus – below the transverse plate and anterior to the vertical crest. In the CPA, the location of

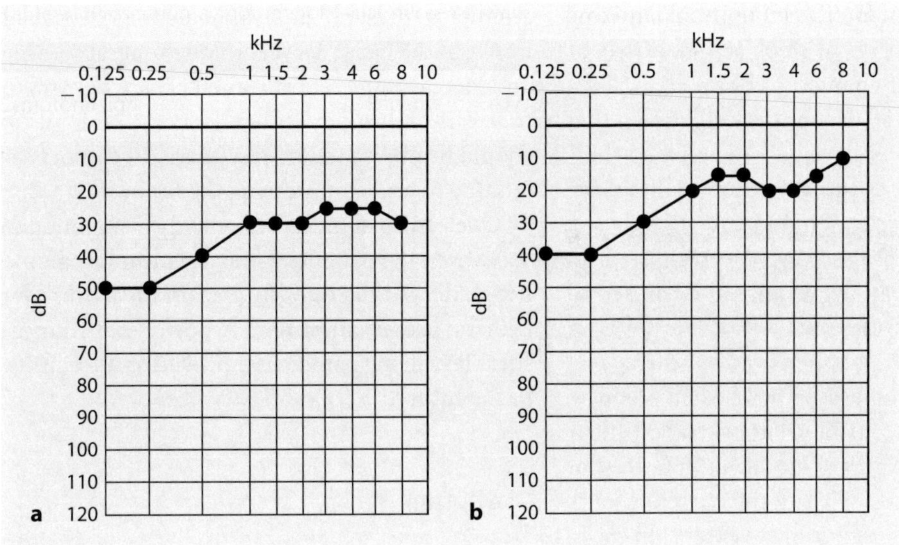

Fig. 2. Preoperative (**a**) and postoperative (**b**) audiograms of the same patient demonstrating improved auditory function after total tumor removal.

the cochlear nerve is less variable than that of the facial nerve. It is found most frequently on the anterior-inferior tumor surface [21].

Intraoperative monitoring of auditory brain stem responses is to be done on a regular basis [15, 18, 22]. It provides a constant feedback information on the function of hearing pathways at every 30–90 s. Changes due to traction or injury to the cochlear nerve, interruption of its vascular supply or compression of the brain stem, are readily detected [15]. A loss of wave V is most frequently associated with deafness, temporary or permanent [22]. The disappearance of wave V is usually preceded by changes of waves I and III. Applying the direct brainstem recording of the auditory evoked potentials, greater reliability of the results is achieved. The potentials are recorded by placing a retractor with electrodes attached to its tip at the cerebellomedullary junction [23].

The retrosigmoid approach with the patient in the semi-sitting position offers the best chances of good functional outcome, according to our experience. This position allows the so-called 'three hands technique' to be used. The assistant is irrigating continuously with saline. This obviates the need of coagulation during tumor removal. The surgeon is free to use both of his hands for tumor dissection because there is no need of constant suction. The morbidity related to the position is insignificant if the procedure is carefully planned and immediate measures at the first sign of venous air embolism are undertaken. During the drilling of the IAC, the structures of the inner ear have to be preserved. The endoscopic inspection of the fundus could be helpful if the location of the labyrinth obviates the wide opening of the IAC.

The cochlear nerve could be damaged if excessive retraction of the cerebellar hemisphere is applied. Experimental evidence suggests that this mechanical traction destroys the nerve fibers at their weakest point – the Obersteiner-Redlich zone. The self-retaining retractor should gently support and protect the hemisphere, instead of compressing it. The dissection technique is of critical importance. It should proceed from known to unknown structures. The dissection is alternated from different directions and stretching of neural structures in one direction for a long time is avoided. Microsurgical steps are modified or even interrupted if changes of brain stem auditory evoked potential occur. It is well known that the cochlear nerve is extremely sensitive to thermal injury. Bipolar coagulation, especially in the proximity of the nerve, should be restricted.

Using this surgical strategy, we achieved an increase in cochlear nerve anatomic preservation from 68% in our first 1,000 cases (79% in patients with preserved preoperative hearing) [1] to 75.8% in the current series (84% when preoperative hearing was available). Functional cochlear nerve preservation was achieved in 46% in that series and improved to 51% in the current group. In smaller VSs, corresponding to extension classes T1–T3A, the rate of functional hearing preservation was 60, 72 and 56%, respectively.

The indications for hearing-preserving surgery are a matter of debate [13]. The low chance of hearing preservation in cases of large VS is the reason for the preference by some surgeons of the translabyrinthine approach. They point that the attempt to preserve hearing increases the risk of injury to the facial nerve, prolongs operative time and increases the rate of recurrences. Contrary to that, our philosophy is that hearing preservation should be attempted in every case. In tumors extending to and compressing the brain stem (class T4), we achieved preservation of hearing in up to 43%. Even the patients with larger tumors should not be denied the opportunity for an attempt for hearing preservation [19]. A postoperative measurable hearing could be improved to serviceable in the future.

Conclusion

VSs are benign lesions whose total removal leads to definitive healing of the patient. The goal of every surgery should be functional preservation of all cranial nerves. Using the retrosigmoid approach with the patient in the semi-sitting position, hearing preservation is possible even in patients with large VSs.

References

1 Samii M, Matthies C: Management of 1,000 vestibular schwannomas (acoustic neuromas): hearing function in 1,000 tumor resections. Neurosurgery 1997;40:248–262.

2 Matthies C, Samii M: Vestibular schwannomas and auditory function: options in large T3 and T4 tumors? Neurochirurgie 2002;48:461–470.

3 Samii M, Matthies C: Management of 1,000 vestibular schwannomas (acoustic neuromas): surgical management and results with an emphasis on complications and how to avoid them. Neurosurgery 1997;40:11–21.

4 Irving RM, Jackler KR, Pitts LH: Hearing preservation in patients undergoing vestibular schwannoma surgery: comparison of middle fossa and retrosigmoid approaches. J Neurosurg 1998;88:840–845.

5 Betchen SA, Walsh J, Post KD: Long-term hearing preservation after surgery for vestibular schwannoma. J Neurosurg 2005;102:6–9.

6 Kondziolka D, Lunsford LD, Flickinger JC: Gamma knife radiosurgery for vestibular schwannomas. Neurosurg Clin North Am 2000;11:651–658.

7 Iwai Y, Yamanaka K, Ishiguro T: Surgery combined with radiosurgery of large acoustic neuromas. Surg Neurol 2003;59:283–289.

8 Thomassin JM, Pellet W, Epron JP, Brachinni F, Roche PH: Recurrent acoustic neurinoma after complete surgical resection. Ann Otolaryngol Chir Cervicofac 2001;118:3–10.

9 Staecker H, Nadol JB, Ojeman R, Ronner S, McKenna MJ: Hearing preservation in acoustic neuroma surgery: middle fossa versus retrosigmoid approach. Am J Otol 2000;21:399–404.

10 Briggs RJ, Fabinyi G, Kaye AH: Current management of acoustic neuromas: review of surgical approaches and outcomes. J Clin Neurosc 2000;7: 521–526.

11 Slattery WH, Brackmann DE, Hitselberger WE: Middle fossa approach for hearing preservation with acoustic neuromas. Am J Otol 1997;18: 596–601.

12 Yates PD, Jackler RK, Satar B: Is it worthwhile to attempt hearing preservation in larger acoustic neuromas? Otol Neurotol 2003;24:460–464.

13 Gjuric M, Wigand ME, Wolf SR: Enlarged middle fossa vestibular schwannoma surgery: experience with 735 cases. Otol Neurotol 2001; 22:223–230.

14 Rowed DW, Nedzelski JM: Hearing preservation in the removal of intracanalicular acoustic neuromas via the retrosigmoid approach. J Neurosurg 1997;86:456–461.

15 Fischer G, Fischer C, Remond J: Hearing preservation in acoustic neuroma surgery. J Neurosurg 1992;76:910–917.
16 Koos WT, Diaz Day J, Matula C, Levy DI: Neurotopographic considerations in the microsurgical treatment of small acoustic neurinomas. J Neurosurg 1998;88:506–512.
17 Tonn JC, Schlake HP, Goldbrunner R, Milewski C, Helms J, Roosen K: Acoustic neuroma surgery as an interdisciplinary approach: a neurosurgical series of 508 patients. J Neurol Neurosurg Psychiatry 2000;69: 61–166.
18 Mohr G, Sade B, Dufour JJ, Rappaport JM: Preservation of hearing in patients undergoing microsurgery for vestibular schwannoma: degree of meatal filling J Neurosurg 2005;102: 1–5.
19 Yamakami I, Uchino Y, Kobayashi E, Yamaura A, Oka N: Removal of large acoustic neurinomas (vestibular schwannomas) by the retrosigmoid approach with no mortality and minimal morbidity. J Neurol Neurosurg Psychiatry 2004;75:453–458.
20 Rhoton AL Jr: The cerebellopontine angle and posterior fossa cranial nerves by the retrosigmoid approach. Neurosurgery 2000;47:S93–S129.
21 Sampath P, Rini D, Long DM: Microanatomical variations in the cerebellopontine angle associated with vestibular scwhannomas (acoustic neuromas): a retrospective study of 1,006 consecutive cases. J Neurosurg 2000;92:70–78.
22 Matthies C, Samii M: Management of vestibular schwannomas (acoustic neuromas): the value of neurophysiology for evaluation and prediction of auditory function in 420 cases. Neurosurgery 1997;40:919–929.
23 Matthies C, Samii M: Direct brainstem recording of auditory evoked potentials during vestibular schwannoma resection: nuclear BAEP recording. J Neurosurg 1997;86: 1057–1062.

Prof. M. Samii, MD, PhD
Rudolf Pichlmayrstrasse 4
DE–30625 Hannover (Germany)
Tel. +49 511 27092 700, Fax +49 511 27092 706, E-Mail samii@ini-hannover.de

Régis J, Roche P-H (eds): Modern Management of Acoustic Neuroma.
Prog Neurol Surg. Basel, Karger, 2008, vol 21, pp 142–151

Hearing Preservation in Patients with Unilateral Vestibular Schwannoma after Gamma Knife Surgery

Jean Régis · Manabu Tamura · Christine Delsanti · Pierre-Hugues Roche · William Pellet · Jean-Marc Thomassin

Groupe d'Otoneurochirurgie de l'Hôpital Universitaire de la Timone, Marseille, France

Abstract

Introduction: The majority of patients still lose the functionality of their hearing in spite of the technical advances in microsurgery. Our aim was to evaluate the hearing preservation potential of Gamma Knife Surgery. We have reviewed our experience and the literature in order to evaluate the probability to obtain such functional preservation and the factors influencing it. **Methods:** Since July 1992, 2,053 patients have been operated on by Gamma Knife Radiosurgery in Timone University Hospital. This population included 184 unilateral schwannoma patients with functional preoperative hearing (Gardner-Robertson 1 or 2) treated by first intention radiosurgery with a marginal dose lower than 13 Gy. The population included 74 patients with subnormal hearing (class 1). All have been studied with a follow-up longer than 3 years. Univariate and multivariate analyses have been carried out. **Results:** Numerous parameters greatly influence the probability of functional hearing preservation at 3 years, which is globally 60%. The main preoperative parameters of predictability are limited hearing loss that is Gardner-Robertson stage 1 (vs. 2), presence of tinnitus, young age of the patient and small size of the lesion. The functional hearing preservation at 3 years is 77.8% when the patient is initially in stage 1, 80% in patients with tinnitus as a first symptom and 95% when the patient has both. In these patients, the probability of functional preservation at 5 years is 84%. Comparison of these results with the main series of the literature confirms the reproducibility of our results. Additionally, we have demonstrated a higher chance of hearing preservation when the dose to the cochlea is lower than 4 Gy. **Conclusion:** We report a large population of patients treated by radiosurgery with functional preoperative hearing. These results demonstrate the possibility to preserve functional hearing in a high percentage of selected patients. Radiosurgery offers them a higher chance of functional hearing preservation than microsurgery or simple follow-up.

Since the development of vestibular schwannoma surgery by Sir Walter Dandy [1] at the beginning of the 20th century, the management of those tumors has changed a lot. Mortality has decreased dramatically. Facial palsy is less frequent and less severe and even hearing preservation has become a realistic challenge. Modern imaging allows diagnosis of tumors at an earlier stage when tumors are paucisymptomatic and still small not yet compressing the brainstem. The attempt to preserve functional hearing in these patients makes a lot of sense.

Gamma Knife Surgery (GKS) is one of the possible neurosurgical approaches, and its potential role in hearing function sparing must therefore be investigated.

Material and Methods

Since July 1992, 2,053 vestibular schwannomas have been operated on using GKS in Marseille. Among those, 184 patients presented with unilateral vestibular schwannoma (no neurofibromatosis type 2, NF2) with no previous surgery and functional hearing at time of radiosurgery (Gardner–Robertson, GR, 1 or 2). Their follow–up was longer than 3 years. According to the Koos classification [2], 23 were in stage I, 108 stage II, 46 stage III, 7 stage IV. Among these 184 patients, 74 were classified as GR1 (subnormal hearing) and 110 as GR2 (useful hearing) [3].

All the patients have been investigated preoperatively (the day before radiosurgery) with tonal and vocal audiometry, auditory evoked potentials and vestibular testing.

All radiosurgical procedures were carried out in the same center (Hôpital Timone, Marseille, France) using the Leksell 201-source Cobalt 60 Gamma Knife (Elekta Instruments, Stockholm, Sweden). The patient enters hospital the night before the operation to undergo preoperative evaluation procedures consisting of a clinical examination with House-Brackmann grading, tonal and vocal audiometry, auditory evoked potentials, caloric and pendular tests and a Schirmer test. Additionally, a baseline magnetic resonance (MR) performed several months before radiosurgery provided some information on the preoperative growing pattern. We perform radiosurgery under local anesthesia, and patients are discharged from the hospital within 24 h after treatment. Patients return to their preoperative level of function or employment within 3–10 days after treatment. On the morning of the treatment, we apply an imaging-compatible Leksell stereotactic co-ordinate frame (Elekta Instruments) to the patient's head using local anesthesia. We then perform a high-resolution contrast-enhanced CT scan with 3-mm axial cuts and sagittal/coronal reconstruction to localize the target, define its boundaries and localize surrounding radiosensitive structures. MR imaging is now always required, but for the first patients of our experience (before 1994) MR imaging was used only for tumors close to the brainstem. Total dose, number of isocenters, and treatment time were calculated using the Kula System on a MicroVax II computer during the first period and presently with GammaPlan software (since July 1997). The 50% isodose line was used to match the tumor margin in most patients. We use low peripheral doses according to Norén teaching. The choice of the margin dose is mostly determined by the treatment volume.

Follow-Up Methods

Patients are reviewed with MR imaging and with tonal and vocal audiometry (in cases where they were not deaf before surgery) at 6 months, 1, 2, 3, 5, 7, and 10 years. After more than 3 years, a complete evaluation is carried out identical to the preoperative one as described above.

Univariate and multivariate analysis (χ^2 test, Fisher exact test and Mann-Whitney test) have been done testing the influence of several preoperative parameters (age, sex, initial symptoms, GR class, size of the lesion, Koos stages, Ohata classification, tumor volume, tumor volume in the canal) and perioperative parameters (dose rate, dose to the cochlea, mean dose to the tumor, mean dose to the intracanalicular part of the tumor, integrated dose to the tumor, integrated dose to the intracanalicular part of the tumor, marginal dose, number of isocenters, number of isocenters by cm^3).

Results

All the 184 patients have been followed for more than 3 years (mean 7, range 3–13 years). Mean age was 52 (range 17–82) years. Young age was associated with a higher chance to preserve functional hearing ($p = 0.006$). Among those 184 patients, 60% have kept functional hearing at 3 years. GR2 is related to a high probability of functional hearing loss ($p < 0.001$). Preoperatively, 74 patients (41.2%) were GR1. Among those, 78.4% have kept functional hearing. When the first symptom was not a sudden hearing loss and especially when it was tinnitus, the probability of hearing preservation was higher ($p < 0.004$). The first symptoms most frequently reported by the patients were hypoacousia (46.8%) and tinnitus (26.3%). The probability to preserve functional hearing at 3 years in a patient presenting first with tinnitus was 80% or even 95% if the initial hearing was subnormal (GR1). Using logistic regression modeling, we have identified independent predictors and classified them according to their power of prediction: the first is GR1 ($p = 0.001$), the second is tinnitus as the first clinical symptom ($p = 0.003$), the third is age (for 1 year more $p = 0.03$), the fourth is largest diameter (for 1 cm more $p = 0.03$). Actually, at 3 years the probability to

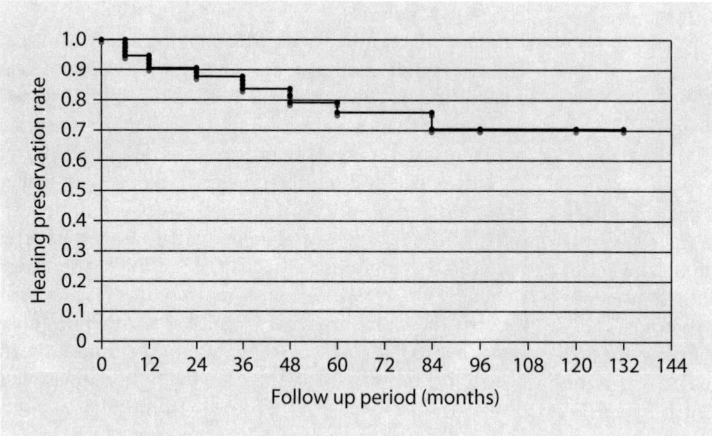

Fig. 1. Long-term functional hearing preservation (GR1 or 2 hearing).

preserve functional hearing is more likely if GR is 1, first symptom is tinnitus, age is young and diameter small. The probability to preserve functional hearing can be calculated according to the following formula:

$$\text{Log odd} = (-5.38) + X + Y + 0.04\,(\text{age} - 52.41) + 0.15\,(D - 8.08)$$

The term related to the initial quality of hearing is X = 1.01 (if GR2) or 0 (if GR1). The term related to the first clinical symptom is Y = 1.56 if hypoacousia, 1.20 if other, 0 if tinnitus. The number 52.41 represents the mean age of the population and 8.08 the mean of the maximum diameter (D). The probability to preserve functional hearing thus varies from 23.5 to 100%, according to the value of these 4 terms.

When functional hearing preservation is evaluated subjectively by the patients, 78.5% turn out to be satisfied (84.2% in Koos I, 77.3% in Koos II, 81.3% in Koos III and 70.6% in Koos IV). The suddenness of the initial hearing loss is here a significant predictor ($p = 0.002$). When the patient started with a sudden hearing loss, the probability to be satisfied and consider having preserved or improved the functionality of his/her hearing at 3 years is 82.3% (instead of 56.3% in the opposite case).

If we look at the group of 74 patients with initially GR1 at the 3-year follow-up, 78.4% have kept functional hearing, 50% were still GR1 and 8.1% became deaf. In the long-term, hearing stabilizes at 84 months (fig. 1) with 70% of patients still presenting functional hearing. In this group of patients, among the preoperative parameters those demonstrating a negative influence are: hearing loss as a first initial symptom, larger tumor according to Koos classification or maximum diameter, and larger extent of the tumor toward the lateral part of the canal according to the Ohata classification (table 1). Among the perioperative parameters, those that lower the risk of losing the functionality of hearing are: lower dose rate, lower dose to the cochlea, lower mean dose to the tumor, lower integrated dose to the tumor, lower integrated dose to the intracanalicular part of the tumor, and lower number of isocenters.

Discussion

The concept of useful hearing is ambiguous [4]. Being able to hear a sound at certain intensity does not mean that a word can be understood at the same intensity. Thus, vocal audiometry must be used as well as tonal audiometry. GR1 and 2 correspond to functional hearing and are

Table 1. Monovariate analysis of the influence of pre- and perioperative parameters on the probability to lose functional hearing

	Tendency	p value	
		monovariate	multivariate
Parameters related to patient features			
Sex	male > female	0.351 (χ)	0.157
Tumor side	right > left	0.480 (χ)	0.816
Initial sign: hearing loss	other sign > hearing loss	0.002 (χ)	0.007
Previous facial palsy	H-B class 2 > class 1	0.179 (Fisher)	0.875
Koos classification	stage 1 > other stage	0.131 (Fisher)	0.041
Ohata classification	less lateral extent > more	0.062 (χ)	0.013
Age	young > old	0.115 (t test)	0.212
TT volume	large > small	0.766 (M-W)	0.035
ICT volume	large > small	0.841 (M-W)	0.685
Parameters related to treatment			
Dose rate	low > high	0.608 (M-W)	0.025
Dose to cochlea	low > high	0.009 (t test)	0.037
Mean dose to tumor (TT)	low > high	0.636 (t test)	0.036
Mean dose to tumor (ICT)	high > low	0.773 (t test)	0.168
Integrated dose (mJ) to TT	high > low	0.650 (M-W)	0.048
Integrated dose (mJ/cm^3) to TT	low > high	0.417 (M-W)	0.004
Integrated dose (mJ) to ICT	high > low	0.638 (M-W)	0.694
Integrated dose (mJ/cm^3) to ICT	low > high	0.918 (M-W)	0.124
Number of isocenters	more	0.593 (M-W)	0.177
Number of isocenters to ICT	more	0.717 (M-W)	0.023

TT = Total tumor; ICT = Intracanalicular tumor; M-W = Mann-Whitney test; H-B = House-Brackmann grading.

equivalent to the Los Angeles stages A and B from the American Academy of Otolaryngology-Head and Neck Surgery classification [5]. Finally, the quality of hearing in the contralateral ear is of great importance at the individual scale (fig. 2).

Comparing hearing preservation from one series to another is especially difficult. Even when the classification parameters are the same, heterogeneity of the population is frequently a major bias. Our series, like others, demonstrates well the influence of parameters related to the population like tumor size, patient age, quality of his/her hearing before operation. Of course, NF2 patients must not be mixed due to a very different

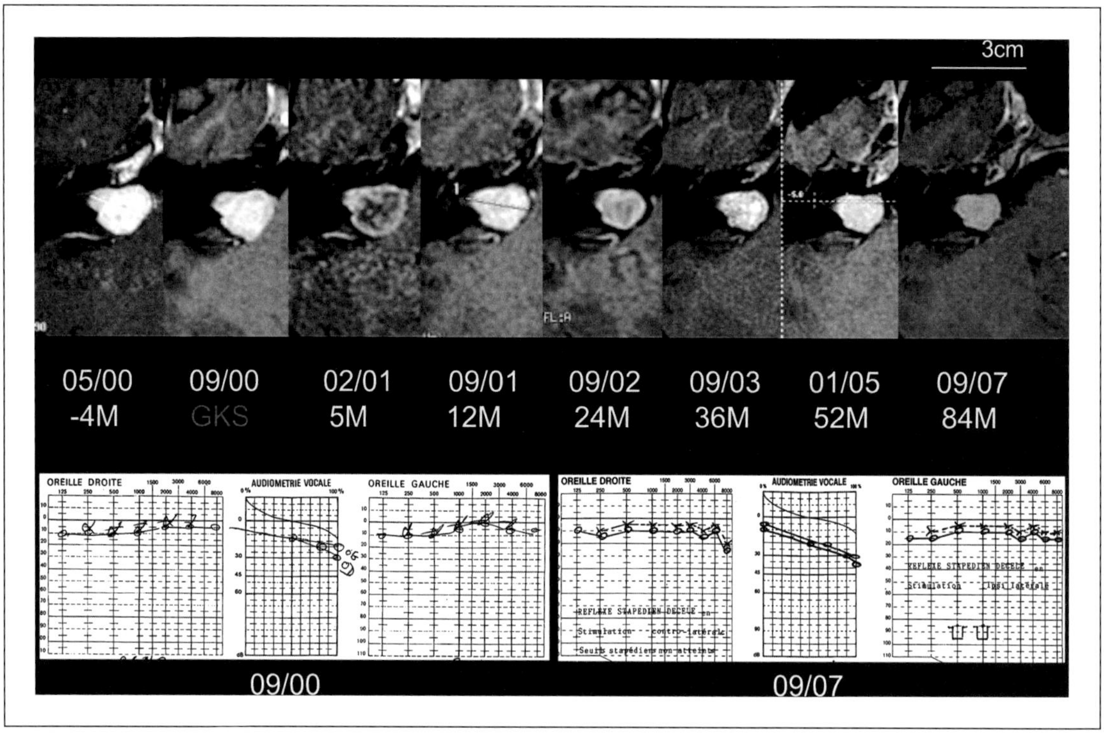

Fig. 2. Example of long-term hearing preservation. Tonal and vocal audiometry the day before radiosurgery and 7 years later demonstrates in this patient a perfect preservation of the hearing in addition to the progressive regression of the lesion.

rate of hearing preservation. By the way, the only acceptable strategy for comparing results from different series is to stratify these results according to the population-related parameters having demonstrated their impact on the hearing preservation rate. An additional extremely important parameter is follow-up length. Authors claiming to have obtained a high rate of preservation with a minimum follow-up not longer or equal to 3 years are just not serious.

Literature analysis demonstrates that the rate of functional hearing preservation after radiosurgery varies from 33 to 73% [6–15]. Our global hearing preservation rate is 60% at 3 years. Ogunrinde et al. [16] reported a 55% rate of functional hearing preservation at 2 years. Foote using LINAC [17] and Forster [18] reported a quite low rate of functional hearing preservation of 33% at 3 and 4 years, respectively. Noren et al. [19] reported a high rate of preservation (77%) but apparently relying only on pure tone average and not vocal audiometry. Poen et al. [20] reported a rate of 77% (10/17 patients) with fractionated stereotactic radiotherapy. Unfortunately, due to the very small size of the population and the very short follow-up the report is of very low value. Niranjan et al. [21], in a series of 29 Koos stage I vestibular schwannomas, found a 73% rate of hearing preservation (11/15 patients).

We have summarized in table 2 studies reporting their results with audiometric evaluation, a minimum follow-up of 2 years and large enough populations. We have found only 10 papers.

Our rate of functional hearing preservation is in the range of the best series of the literature, especially considering the fact that our minimum

Table 2. Comparison of rates of hearing preservation in the radiosurgical literature

	Patients	Patients with GR ≤2	Follow-up years	Marginal dose, Gy	Useful hearing, %
Kobayashi et al., 1994 [7]	44		1	14.8	48
Noren, 1998 [6]	254		3	13.6	60 at 2 years
Lunsford et al., 1998 [10]	402		3		68
Thomassin et al., 1998 [28]	138		3		50
Kondziolka et al., 1998 [11]	162		5–10	16	47
Prasad et al., 2000 [9]	153	96	4.27	13	58
Flinckinger et al., 2001 [8]	198		2.5	13	71
Harsh et al., 2002 [12]	64		3.6	12	33
Unger et al., 2002 [13]	60	29	1–8	13	55
Régis et al., 2003	1,000	175	7	12.74	60 at 3 years

follow-up is 3 years (mean 7 years) [15]. These results are particularly good when compared to the results of the best series with retrosigmoid or translabyrinthine approach [22–27].

After microsurgical resection, the functional hearing preservation varies from 15 to 48% according to the literature [22–27] with two papers surprisingly out of range. Haines and Levine [29] reported extraordinary results compared to the best large series of the literature (82%). Their results are based on 14 operated patients, but it has to be stressed that large series with high quality methodology are extremely rare. Here, also the reliability of the series is highly varying, and in fact there are very few high-level contributions reporting large series of operated patients followed with a strict methodology and a long-term follow-up. We can even say that such a series does not exist, and we have to stop referring to series with serious methodological limitations.

For Koos I tumors, the most enthusiastic authors report a rate of hearing preservation between 12 and 66% in the short-term [30]. In the subgroups of patients selected for an attempt of hearing preservation by Samii and Matthies [30], the rate of hearing preservation is 40% (47% in the more recent cases). This rate is 38% (48% for the smaller lesions) for Gormley et al. [27], 24% (50% for the smaller lesions) for Ebershold et al. [25], 32% (50% for intracanalicular) for Nadol et al. [31], and 1% for Wigand and Fickel [32].

In fact, these comparisons are false. A small subgroup of patients is selected for microsurgery according to predictors of hearing preservation and compared with the total group of patients with serviceable hearing treated by radiosurgery. In spite of this major bias, the probability of hearing preservation is much higher after GKS than microsurgery in the best hands.

The physiopathogenesis of hearing deterioration after microsurgery is explained either by ischemia (of the cochlea or cochlear nerve) or by a mechanical injury of the nerve inducing immediate deafness. Hearing loss induced by an ischemic phenomenon can be delayed by several weeks or months. Thus, microsurgical series evaluating hearing loss only immediately after microsurgery do not present a realistic estimate of the functional hearing preservation probability. Rare cases of acute hearing loss after radiosurgery have been reported.

Steven et al. [33] reported 2 cases of sudden hearing loss within the 24 h following fractionated stereotactic radiotherapy in NF2 patients.

Two hypotheses are proposed [34–36]: (1) vasogenic edema occurring in the tumor inducing a compression of the cochlear artery [37]; (2) local production of free radicals.

For Prasad et al. [9], the worsening of the hearing occurs within the 2 years following radiosurgery. A higher rate of hearing preservation is reported when marginal doses used are lower than 13–14 Gy [8, 21]. Since 1992, the doses used have always been is this range (mean 12.74 Gy). Classically, patients with Koos I tumors have a higher chance of hearing preservation [9, 16]. Our material is additionally demonstrating a higher chance of hearing preservation with a more limited lateral extent in the canal (according to the Ohata classification). Patients with tinnitus as a first symptom or younger age have been demonstrated to have a high probability of hearing preservation. The strong influence of these parameters leads to 2 major conclusions. First, due to the huge heterogeneity of chance according to these preoperative parameters, serious comparison of series requires stratification. Secondly, thanks to our model, the information delivered preoperatively to the patient can be enriched by an individual prediction of his or her probability of hearing preservation.

The discovery of the influence of some operative nuances (e.g. dose to the cochlea) has significantly influenced our technical strategy (fig. 3) and should allow improvement of the clinical results.

It is important to note the difference between functional preservation of the VIIIth and VIIth nerves. After radiosurgery, facial palsy is rare but can be related to the neurosurgical procedure due to the fact that spontaneous facial palsy in patients presenting with vestibular schwannomas is extremely rare. In contrast, spontaneous acute or progressive hearing worsening in patients presenting with VS are common: 13 dB/year for Ogawa et al. [38], 9 dB/year for Thomsen et al. [39], 6 dB/year for Nedzelski et al. [40] and this with no correlation to morphological evolution [41]. In our experience [3], this loss is 3–6 dB/year. At 3 years, patients not treated by Gamma Knife should have lost an average of 9–39 dB compared with an average loss of 2 dB at 3 years after radiosurgery with a preservation of hearing functionality in 60–75%. A better preservation of functional hearing in the long-term in patients with Koos I tumors operated on by Gamma Knife compared with patients not treated and only followed with MR has led us to change our strategy and to be more proactive in patients with intracanalicular vestibular schwannomas and functional hearing. A simple wait and see strategy is proposed only in patients presenting with an intracanalicular lesion and nonfunctional hearing [3].

Conclusion

All patients presenting with vestibular schwannoma must be proposed the 3 alternatives (wait and see, radiosurgery and microsurgical resection).

Safety and efficacy of radiosurgery has been well demonstrated [9, 42], in particular its low invasiveness and low rate of trigeminal or motor facial function worsening [9]. The possibility given to the patient to preserve in the long-term his/her hearing functionality is an additional major advantage (fig. 2). Globally, the hearing preservation in our hands is 60%. However, in patients with subnormal hearing at the time of radiosurgery this probability is higher (77.8%) especially if tinnitus was the first sign. There is a real rationale to treat more proactively younger patients with subnormal hearing.

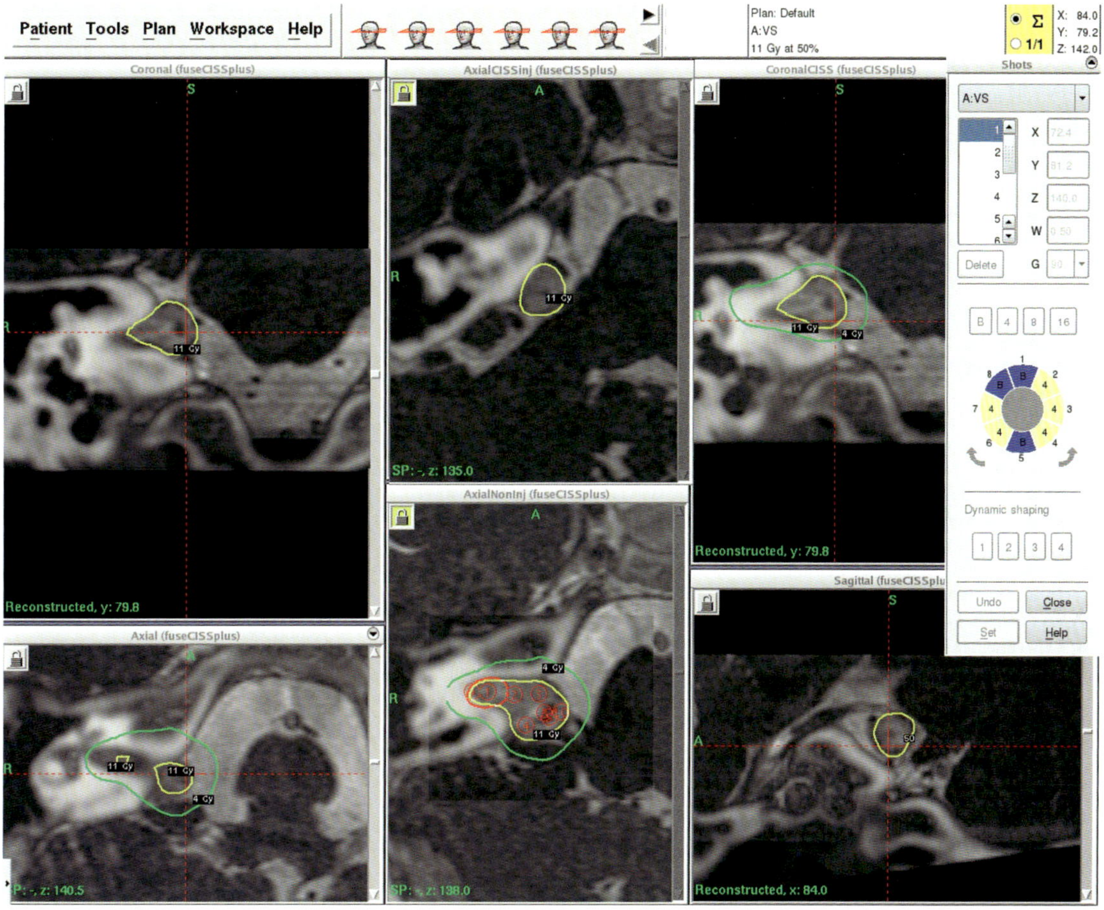

Fig. 3. Dose planning for Koos II vestibular schwannomas with Perfexion Gamma Knife. In order to maintain the dose to the cochlea lower than 4 Gy, dedicated sector occlusion strategy is used.

References

1 Dandy W: Operation for total removal of cerebellopontine (acoustic) tumors. Surg Gynecol Obstet 1925;41:129–148.
2 Koos WT, Day JD, Matula C, Levy DI: Neurotopographic considerations in the microsurgical treatment of small acoustic neurinomas. J Neurosurg 1998;88, 506–512.
3 Regis J, Roche PH, Delsenti C, Soumare O, Thomassin JM, Pellet W: Stereotactic Radiosurgery for Vestibular Schwannoma; in Pollock BE (ed): Contemporary Stereotactic Radiosurgery: Thechnique and Evaluation. Vol. Chap. 9. Futura Publishing Company, Armonk, New York, 2002;181–212.
4 Kanzaki J, Tos M, Sanna M, Moffat DA, Monsell EM, Berliner KI: New and modified reporting systems from the consensus meeting on systems for reporting results in vestibular schwannoma. Otol Neurotol 2003;24:642–648; discussion 648–649.
5 Comittee on Hearing and Equilibrium. Guidelines for the evaluation of hearing preservation in acoustic neuroma(vestibular schwannoma). Otolaryngol Head Neck Surg 1995;113: 179–180.
6 Noren G: Long-term complications following gamma knife radiosurgery of vestibular schwannomas. Stereotact Funct Neurosurg 1998;70(Suppl 1): 65–73.
7 Kobayashi T, Tanaka T, Kida Y: The early effects of gamma knife on 40 cases of acoustic neurinoma. Acta Neurochir Suppl (Wien), 1994;62:93–97.
8 Flickinger JC, Kondziolka D, Niranjan A, Lunsford LD: Results of acoustic neuroma radiosurgery: an analysis of 5 years' experience using current methods. J Neurosurg 2001;94:1–6.

9 Prasad D, Steiner M, Steiner L: Gamma surgery for vestibular schwannoma. J Neurosurg 2000;92:745–759.
10 Lunsford L, Kondziolka D, Flickinger J: Acoustic neuroma management: Evolution and Revolution. Basel: Karger, 1998.
11 Kondziolka D, Lunsford LD, McLaughlin MR, Flickinger JC: Long-term outcomes after radiosurgery for acoustic neuromas. N Engl J Med 1998;339: 1426–1433.
12 Harsh GR, Thornton AF, Chapman PH, Bussiere MR, Rabinov JD, Loeffler JS: Proton beam stereotactic radiosurgery of vestibular schwannomas. Int J Radiat Oncol Biol Phys 2002;54:35–44.
13 Unger F, Walch C, Schrottner O, Eustacchio S, Sutter B, Pendl G: Cranial nerve preservation after radiosurgery of vestibular schwannomas. Acta Neurochir Suppl 2002;84:77–83.
14 Pellet W, Regis J, Roche PH, Delsanti C: Relative indications for radiosurgery and microsurgery for acoustic schwannoma. Adv Tech Stand Neurosurg2003; 28: 227–282; discussion 282–224.
15 Regis J, Delsanti C, Roche P, Soumare O, Dufour H, Porcheron D, Peragut JC, Thomassin JM, Pellet W: Preservation of hearing function in the radiosurgical treatment of unilateral vestibular schwannomas. Preliminary results. Neurochirurgie 2002;48:471–478.
16 Ogunrinde OK, Lunsford DL, Kondziolka DS,Bissonette DJ, Flickinger JC: Cranial nerve preservation after stereotactic radiosurgery of intracanalicular acoustic tumors. Stereotact Funct Neurosurg 1995;64(Suppl 1): 87–97.
17 Foote RL, Coffey RJ, Swanson JW, Harner SG, Beatty CW, Kline RW, Stevens LN, Hu TC: Stereotactic radiosurgery using the gamma knife for acoustic neuromas. Int J Radiat Oncol Biol Phys 1995;32:1153–1160.
18 Forster DM, Kemeny AA, Pathak A, Walton L: Radiosurgery: a minimally interventional alternative to microsurgery in the management of acoustic neuroma. Br J Neurosurg 1996;10: 169–174.
19 Noren G, Greitz D, Hirsch A, Lax I: Gamma knife surgery in acoustic tumours. Acta Neurochir Suppl (Wien) 1993;58:104–107.
20 Poen JC, Golby AJ, Forster KM, Martin DP, Chinn DM, Hancock SL, Adler JR, Jr: Fractionated stereotactic radiosurgery and preservation of hearing in patients with vestibular schwannoma: a preliminary report. Neurosurgery 1999;45:1299–1305; discussion 1305–1297.
21 Niranjan A, Lunsford LD, Flickinger JC, Maitz A, Kondziolka D: Dose reduction improves hearing preservation rates after intracanalicular acoustic tumor radiosurgery. Neurosurgery 1999;45:753–762; discussion 762–755.
22 Pollock BE, Lunsford LD, Kondziolka D, Flickinger JC, Bissonette DJ, Kelsey SF, Jannetta PJ: Outcome analysis of acoustic neuroma management: a comparison of microsurgery and stereotactic radiosurgery. Neurosurgery 1995;36:215–224; discussion 224–219.
23 Glasscock ME, 3rd, Hays JW, Minor LB, Haynes DS, Carrasco VN: Preservation of hearing in surgery for acoustic neuromas. J Neurosurg 1993;78: 864–870.
24 Cerullo LJ, Grutsch JF, Heiferman K, Osterdock R: The preservation of hearing and facial nerve function in a consecutive series of unilateral vestibular nerve schwannoma surgical patients (acoustic neuroma). Surg Neurol 1993;39:485–493.
25 Ebersold MJ, Harner SG, Beatty CW, Harper CM, Jr, Quast LM: Current results of the retrosigmoid approach to acoustic neurinoma [see comments]. J Neurosurg 1992;76:901–909.
26 Fischer G, Fischer C, Remond J: Hearing preservation in acoustic neurinoma surgery. J Neurosurg 1992;76: 910–917.
27 Gormley WB, Sekhar LN, Wright DC, Kamerer D, Schessel D: Acoustic neuromas: results of current surgical management. Neurosurgery 1997;41:50–58; discussion 58–60.
28 Thomassin JM, Epron JP, Regis J, Delsanti C, Sarabian A, Peragut JC, Pellet W: Preservation of hearing in acoustic neuromas treated by gamma knife surgery. Stereotact Funct Neurosurg 1998;70(Suppl 1):74–79.
29 Haines SJ, Levine SC: Intracanalicular acoustic neuroma: early surgery for preservation of hearing. J Neurosurg 1993;79:515–520.
30 Samii M, Matthies C: Management of 1000 vestibular schwannomas (acoustic neuromas): Hearing function in 1000 tumor resections. Neurosurgery 1997;40:248–262.
31 Nadol JB, Jr, Chiong CM, Ojemann RG, McKenna M. J, Martuza RL, Montgomery WW, Levine RA, Ronner SF, Glynn RJ: Preservation of hearing and facial nerve function in resection of acoustic neuroma. Laryngoscope 1992;102:1153–1158.
32 Wigand DA, Fickel V: Acoustic Neuroma the patient's perspective: subjective assessment of symptoms, diagnosis, therapy, and outcome in 541 patients. Laryngoscope 1989;99: 179–187.
33 Steven D, Chang M, Poen J, Steven L, Hancock: Acute hearing loss following fractionated stereotactic radiosurgery for acoustic neuroma. J Neurosurg 1998;89:321–325.
34 Shirato H, Sakamoto T, Takeichi N, Aoyama H, Suzuki K, Kagei K, Nishioka T, Fukuda S, Sawamura Y, Miyasaka K: Fractionated stereotactic radiotherapy for vestibular schwannoma (VS): comparison between cystic-type and solid-type VS. Int J Radiat Oncol Biol Phys 2000;48:1395–1401.
35 Sims E, Doughty D, Macaulay E, Royle N, Wraith C, Darlison R, Plowman PN: Stereotactically delivered cranial radiation therapy: a ten-year experience of linac-based radiosurgery in the UK. Clin Oncol (R Coll Radiol) 1999;11: 303–320.
36 Smith MF, Miller RN, Cox DJ: Suboccipital microsurgical removal of acoustic neurinomas of all sizes. Ann Otol Rhinol Laryngol 1973;82:407–414.
37 Yamane H, Nakai Y, Takayama M: Appearance of free radicals in the guinea pig inner ear after noise-induced acoustic trauma. Eur Arch Otorhinolaryngol 1995;252:504–508.
38 Ogawa K, Kanzaki J, Ogawa S, Tsuchihashi N, Ikeda S: Progression of hearing loss in acoustic neuromas. Acta Otolaryngol Suppl 1991;487:133–137.
39 Thomsen J, Terkildsen K, Tos M: Acoustic neuromas. Progression of hearing impairment and function of the eighth cranial nerve. Am J Otol 1983;5:20–33.

40 Nedzelski JM, Canter RJ, Kassel EE, Rowed DW, Tator CH: Is no treatment good treatment in the management of acoustic neuromas in the elderly? Laryngoscope 1986;96:825–829.

41 Clark WC, Moretz WH, Jr, Acker JD, Gardner LG, Eggers F, Robertson JH: Nonsurgical management of small and intracanalicular acoustic tumors. Neurosurgery 1985;16:801–803.

42 Kondziolka D, Levy EI, Niranjan A, Flickinger JC, Lunsford LD: Long-term outcomes after meningioma radiosurgery: physician and patient perspectives. J Neurosurg 1999;91:44–50.

Prof. Jean Régis
Service de Neurochirurgie Fonctionnelle et Stéréotaxique
Hôpital d'Adulte de la Timone, 264 bvd Saint Pierre
FR–13385 Marseille Cedex 05 (France)
Tel. +33 4 91 38 65 62, Fax +33 4 91 38 70 56, E-Mail jregis@ap-hm.fr

Régis J, Roche P-H (eds): Modern Management of Acoustic Neuroma.
Prog Neurol Surg. Basel, Karger, 2008, vol 21, pp 152–157

Surgical Removal of Vestibular Schwannoma after Failed Gamma Knife Radiosurgery

Pierre-Hugues Roche[a] · Muhamad Khalil[a] · Jean-Marc Thomassin[b] · Christine Delsanti[c] · Jean Régis[c]

[a]Service de Neurochirurgie, Hôpital Sainte-Marguerite, [b]Fédération d'Oto-rhino-laryngologie, et [c]Service de Neurochirurgie stéréotaxique et fonctionnelle, Hôpital la Timone, Assistance Publique-Hôpitaux de Marseille, Marseille, France

Abstract

One of the main criticisms of vestibular schwannoma (VS) radiosurgery is that the risk of surgical morbidity is increased for patients whose tumor progresses in cases of failed procedures. The authors reviewed the French neurosurgical experience of operated patients after failed Gamma Knife radiosurgery (GKR). From July 1992 to December 2000, 23 unilateral VS out of the 1,000 treated patients have undergone a microsurgical procedure after failed GKR. In order to analyze the difficulties observed during the surgery, a questionnaire was completed by the surgeons. The mean interval between radiosurgery and removal was 39 months (range: 10–92 months). The mean increasing volume was 389% (range: 37–1,600) and the median was 150%. Seven patients have been operated on for radiological tumor growth and 13 for clinicoradiological evolution. In 10 cases, the surgeon considered that he had to face unusual difficulties mainly because of adhesion of the tumor to neurovascular structures. Tumor removal was total in 15 cases, near total in 4 cases and subtotal in 4 cases. One case of venous infarction was noticed on the 2nd day following surgery and was responsible for hemiparesis and aphasia that gradually recovered. At the last follow-up examination, facial nerve was normal or near normal (House-Brackmann grades 1 and 2) in 12 cases (52%) while it was grade 3 in 9 cases and grades 4 and 5 in 2 cases. Our results show that the quality of removal and of facial nerve preservation might be impaired after GKR in half of cases. However, these results do not support a change in our policy of first intention radiosurgical treatment of small- to medium-sized VSs.

It is now widely accepted that radiosurgery is an interesting therapeutic option for small- to middle-sized vestibular schwannomas (VSs). After the early period of pioneering radiosurgery, the trend has been to decrease the doses delivered on the tumor volume in order to decrease the incidence of neuropathies. Such low doses protocol has been used from the beginning of our experience in Marseille, and has helped to provide satisfactory functional results [1]. However, a part of the scientific community postulated that low doses could bring more failures, thereby requiring tumor resection. The same authors also asserted that previous radiosurgery may significantly complicate this resection and lead to additional morbidity. In order to clarify these assertions, we have conducted a French cooperative study about microsurgery after failed radiosurgery of the whole group of VSs that have been treated in our center.

Material and Methods

Patient Population

The study retrospectively analyzed the follow-up of the 1,000 patients who underwent radiosurgery between July 1992 and March 2000. We excluded from the present analysis cases of bilateral VSs and cases of facial nerve schwannomas. The median patient age at the time of radiosurgery was 51 years (range 34–70 years). Hearing level and facial nerve grading were given following Gardner and Roberston [2] and House and Brackmann [3], respectively.

Radiosurgical Technique

Radiosurgery was performed using a 201-source ^{60}Co Gamma Knife system. In all cases, radiosurgery was done as the primary treatment of the VS. Technical details of this procedure are provided in a previous chapter. The Gammaplan working station was available since September 1997. The median number of isocenters used for dose planning was 8 (range 3–35 isocenters). The 50% isodose line covered the tumor margin in all patients. The median radiation dose to the tumor margin was 12 Gy (range 9–14 Gy). The median tumor volume was 1.2 cm^3 (range 0.2–6.6 cm^3). These treatment parameters are not different from those used in the successful cases.

Follow-Up Review

The clinical characteristics and radiosurgical parameters of all patients were prospectively entered into a computer database at the time of radiosurgery. Clinical examination and imaging were requested at 6, 12, 24, 48, and 96 months after radiosurgery. Measurements of the tumor were made on follow-up MR and compared with the stereotactic imaging study performed on the day of radiosurgery. Five measurements were used, but we also calculated the tumor volume and provided a tumor grading following the Koos classification [4].

We established a questionnaire about the criterions of failure, the operative difficulties and the postoperative status of the patient. The corresponding surgeons were asked to fill out this questionnaire and also to send us the radiological chart and the pathological slides of the VS they removed.

Results

The median time from radiosurgery to surgical resection was 39 months (range 10–92 months). The indications for microsurgical removal were tumor enlargement with stable symptoms in 10 cases and tumor enlargement with new or increased symptoms in 13 cases – 1 trigeminal neuralgia, 1 hemifacial spasm, 3 symptomatic hydrocephalus requiring a VP shunt before resection (patients 6, 14, 21), VIII nerve symptoms. The mean increasing volume was 389% (range: 37–1,600) and the median was 150%.

Surgery

Ten of the 23 patients have been operated on in our and 13 in other centers. The translabyrinthine approach was used in 18 cases, and the retrosigmoid approach in 5 cases.

Quality of Resection

Total removal could be achieved in 15 cases and near-total resection (some tumor remnants no thicker than 2 mm, and nothing clearly identified on the MR control) in 4 cases. In 4 cases, subtotal removal was done. Two of the patients from this later group were referred for a second radiosurgical procedure at our institution; no additional complications resulting from this procedure have been observed so far.

Difficulties of Resection

Following the answers of the questionnaire, the surgeons estimated that surgery was more difficult in 10 out of 23 cases (43.5%, CI 23–66). These additional difficulties were mainly due to more adhesion to the brain stem and/or cranial nerves (8 cases), modification of shape and consistency (4 cases), lack of dissection plane (2 cases), arachnoid thicknening (3 cases), and hypervascularization (1 case).

Functional Outcome

No attempt to preserve hearing was done due to the poor hearing level and to the size of the tumor. Facial nerve was anatomically preserved in all cases but functional preservation was considered as satisfactory (8 gd 1 and 4 gd 2) in 12 cases (52%, CI 31–73). The motor facial nerve function was moderately impaired in 9 cases (9 gd 3) and severely impaired in 2 cases (1 gd 4 and 1 gd 5). As for quality of life, all patients could go back to their previous professional and daily life activities.

Pathology

We could obtain the histological confirmation of the benign nature of the removed schwannomas in all cases. An independent pathologist examined the fixed pathological specimens from 17 cases. The results have been published elsewhere [5]. Briefly, the basic histopathologic pattern consisted in an outer capsule zone (vigorous neoplastic cells) covering a middle transitional zone (containing loosened tissue structure of shrunken tumor cells) and an inner necrotic core.

Complications

We have observed one case of cerebral infarction. A 51-year-old man underwent radiosurgery in November 1999 for a left stage IV schwannoma. An asymptomatic continuous tumor growth was observed on sequential MRI, requiring a surgical removal in February 2003. The translabyrinthine total removal of the tumor was uneventful but at 48-hour follow-up the patient's level of consciousness worsened. A left hemiparesis with aphasia was then observed, and the computed tomography (CT) scan showed a left temporoparietal hypodensity with a significant mass effect. Nothing remarkable was observed in the operative field. The angiogram did not show any arterial or venous occlusion from the vein of Labbé; the transverse and sigmoid sinuses were patent. However, as we still suspected a venous infarction, anticoagulating doses of heparin were administrated and the patient's clinical status improved. Six months after surgery, the patient was independent in his daily life activities, and had moderate speech difficulties. The CT scan showed a small well-circumscribed left temporal hypodense sequela.

Other complications could be attributed to the facial nerve deficit (one hemifacial spasm and one keratitis). In another case, a postoperative cerebrospinal fluid leak had to be managed using a lumbar drainage, and another patient displayed an asymptomatic cerebellopontine hematoma that was diagnosed on the systematic postoperative CT scan before discharge and resolved spontaneously. Two patients died during the follow-up from problems that were not directly linked to the surgery. In one case, an ipsilateral temporal glioblastoma was diagnosed 8 years and 4 months after radiosurgery. This patient died from a local recurrence 1 year after tumor removal [6]. The other patient committed suicide 6 months after surgery despite the medical management of his depressed status that he attributed to the surgery.

Discussion

From the beginning of radiosurgery of VS, the problem of failure has been a continuous matter of debates particularly about the criterions of failure and about the difficulties to surgically manage these patients. We report the largest experience of failed cases after radiosurgery of unilateral sporadic VS in patients that have undergone a homogeneous low doses protocol of treatment in the same center. Although the study is retrospective and despite the fact that the totality of patients have not been followed and operated on by us, we received continuous information from their referral surgeons, providing reliable data about the pattern of volumetric modifications in the years following the treatment.

Failure of Radiation or Unusual Patterns of Volume Change after Gamma Knife Radiosurgery?

In the years following radiosurgery, the subsequent MR images can show an unexpected pattern of increasing tumor volume. Careful clinical and MR imaging follow-up of these patients allow the description of three different final outcomes. The first situation that is reported in most of the patients from the present cohort is the occurrence of a continuous and significant tumor growth over a more than 2- or 3-year period. This pattern corresponds to the definition of failure and requires a secondary therapeutic procedure, preferentially surgical resection. From our own experience of low doses protocol, this long-term failure risk is estimated at 3% of cases [7]. Apart from the regular pattern of middle-term failure, we observed 2 cases of delayed tumor growth while the tumor volume remained stable in the first 3 years. Even though exceptional (less than 10% of the failed cases), this situation justifies a long-term sequential MR control of all patients.

A second subgroup of patients followed after Gamma Knife radiosurgery (GKR) will maintain their tumor volume stable at a higher level than before radiosurgery but the tumor will not threaten the brain stem and will not require an additional procedure. In this situation, the percentage of tumor volume growth remains moderate, usually less than 70% of the initial volume [7]. This particular pattern of volume change has been rarely mentioned in the literature but also deserves careful watching in the long term and represents around 5% of the Marseille experience.

The third growing pattern that can be observed consists in transient tumor growth. This growth pattern is usually encountered in the 6–12 months that follow the treatment and has been observed in 15% [7] of the patients that have been treated in our center. The true incidence of this pattern has been underestimated in the early studies, between 2 and 5% [8], while Prasad et al. [9] described this event in 31% of cases. The description of these three distinct patterns of tumor growth is now well established and should be explained to the patient and to the referral physician in order to avoid unnecessary early resection. The lack of information may have led to an inappropriate resection in one patient of the present series and also in the Pittsburgh series [8].

Difficulties of Microsurgery after Failed Gamma Knife Radiosurgery

This issue is difficult to analyze because of evident methodological bias. Microsurgical teams collect information from patients treated by different radiosurgical protocols with different tools but operated on in the same center [10–13], while radiosurgical teams provide information for patients homogeneously irradiated but operated on in various centers [8]. Of course, we could not avoid the latter bias in our own study because among all the patients treated in our center for GKR, more than half were operated elsewhere. Still, the variable level of expertise of the surgeons from different centers suggests some weakness regarding the issue of technical difficulties. At the same time, the averaging of opinions coming from different surgeons coming from several centers that are not directly involved in radiosurgery may provide some impact to the study.

One attempt to solve the problem of difficulties is to design case-control studies. In a recent paper from Baltimore [11], the authors conducted a retrospective case-control study. Patients were matched for clinical and radiological characteristics. However, in the 'failed irradiation group', patients had previously undergone a radiation therapy that consisted in GKR in 3 cases and fractionated technique in 6 cases. Criterions for failure and interval between irradiation and surgery were not assessed. In the control group of the study, tumor resection was done as a primary treatment. Conversely, the Pittsburgh team [8] gave details about a group of patients treated homogeneously in the same center. They brought all the data about the timing of resection after Gamma Knife, the reasons for resection and the range of volumetric changes. However, in 6 of the 13 failed cases at least one resection had been attempted prior to radiosurgery, which may have contributed to additional difficulties for radiosurgery and of course the secondary microsurgical procedure.

From a subjective point of view, surgeons explained that tumors were more difficult to remove in 43% of cases in comparison with size-matched tumors. Severe facial nerve or brainstem adherences were the main difficulties that were encountered during surgery. Less frequently, arachnoiditis, high vascularization and modification of the consistency were at the source of the problems. Same conclusions were stressed in the other groups. It should be observed that some of these features might happen without any previous radiation therapy. Moreover, even if present, these modifications may not systematically add difficulties. These data should be put in perspective with objective results, namely the ability to remove the tumor and to preserve the facial nerve.

Analysis of the Objective Results

Analysis of the Facial Nerve Deficit
In the present series, 52% of patients could keep their facial motion normal or near normal, which is quite similar to nonirradiated patients with large tumors. The study from the House clinic indicated 50% of House-Brackmann gd 1–2 compared to 72% in the nonirradiated group, with no statistically significant difference. This result is quite better than in the Pittsburg series, but we have already underlined the problems linked to this selected population.

Radicality of the Surgical Removal
Gross total removal was achieved in 15 out of 23 patients in our study, and was obtained in 78.9% of patients in the Los Angeles study [10]. Completeness of tumor removal was uncertain in 5 of 8 cases of the Baltimore group [11], but gross tumor removal was achieved in all cases. In this series, no information was provided about postoperative MR control. In most cases, the justification for incomplete resection was the difficulties encountered during surgery to remove the tumor safely and preserve the facial nerve. There is a trend to consider that in the modern surgical management of large VS, radical resection is not the primary goal and that priority should be given to preserve the facial nerve function [14].

Conclusion

According to the data brought by this study, we can summarize the information that should be given to patients and doctors. (1) Failure of treatment is a rare and unpredictable situation after radiosurgery, once the treatment has been done for reasonable indications. (2) Evidence of a significant and continuous augmentation of the tumor volume is an indispensable criterion to affirm the failure. Indeed, such recommendation should avoid the misinterpretation of a transient growth that frequently occurs in the year that follows radiosurgery. (3) Failure is generally diagnosed between the 2nd and 4th years that follow GKR, but occurrence of late failure is a possible situation that justifies a long-term survey of this population. (4) Failure may render the surgery more difficult in less then half of these cases, particularly with regard to the facial nerve preservation. These potential additional difficulties should be put in balance with the well-recognized difficulties that are expected by the surgeons after a previous failed microsurgical procedure.

References

1 Régis J, Pellet W, Delsanti C, Dufour H, Roche PH, Thomassin JM, Zanaret M, Péragut JC: Functional outcome after gamma knife surgery or microsurgery for vestibular schwannomas. J Neurosurg 2002;97:1091–1100.

2 Gardner G, Robertson JH: Hearing preservation in unilateral acoustic neuroma surgery. Ann Otol Rhinol Laryngol 1988;97:57–66.

3 House JW, Brackmann DE: Facial nerve grading system. Otolaryngol Head Neck Surg 1985;93:146–147.

4 Koos WT, Day JD, Matula C, Levy DI: Neurotopographic considerations in the microsurgical treatment of small acoustic neurinomas. J Neurosurg 1998;88:506–512.

5 Szeifert GT, Figarella-Branger D, Roche PH, Régis J: Histopathological observations on vestibular schwannomas after gamma knife radiosurgery: The Marseille experience. Neurochirurgie 2004;50:327–337.
6 Muracciole X, Cowen D, Régis J: Radiochirurgie et carcinogénèse radioinduite cérébrale. Le point actuel. Neurochirurgie 2004;50:414–420.
7 Delsanti C, Tamura M, Galanaud D, Régis J: Dynamique des résultats radiologiques, pièges et critères d'échec. Neurochirurgie 2004;50:312–319.
8 Pollock BE, Lunsford D, Kondziolka D, Sekula R, Subach BR, Foote RL, Flickinger JC: Vestibular schwannoma management. Part II. Failed radiosurgery and the role of delayed microsurgery. J Neurosurg 1998;89: 949–955.
9 Prasad D, Steiner M, Steiner L: Gamma surgery for vestibular schwannoma. J Neurosurg 2000;92:745–759.
10 Friedman RA, Brackmann DE, Hitselberger WE, Schwartz MS, Iqbal Z, Berliner KI: Surgical salvage after failed irradiation for vestibular schwannoma. Laryngoscope 2005;115:1827–1832.
11 Limb CJ, Long DM, Niparko JK: Acoustic neuroma after failed radiation therapy: challenges of surgical salvage. Laryngoscope 2005;115: 93–98.
12 Sekhar LN, Gormley WB, Wright DC: The best treatment for vestibular schwannoma (acoustic neuroma): Microsurgery or radiosurgery? Am J Otol 1996;17:676–682.
13 Slattery WH, Brackmann DE: Results of surgery following stereotactic irradiation for acoustic neuromas. Am J Otol 1995;16:315–321.
14 Roche PH, Lari N, Thomassin JM, Régis J: Facial nerve. J Neurosurg 2006;104:175–176.

Prof. Pierre-Hugues Roche
Service de Neurochirurgie de l'Hôpital Nord
Assistance Publique-Hôpitaux de Marseille
Chemin des Bourrelly
FR–13915 Marseille Cedex 20 (France)
Tel. +33 4 91 96 86 20, Fax +33 4 91 96 89 15, E-Mail proche@mail.ap-hm.fr

Régis J, Roche P-H (eds): Modern Management of Acoustic Neuroma.
Prog Neurol Surg. Basel, Karger, 2008, vol 21, pp 158–162

Microsurgical Removal of Vestibular Schwannomas after Failed Previous Microsurgery

Pierre-Hugues Roche[a] · Muhamad Khalil[a] · Jean-Marc Thomassin[b]

[a]Service de Neurochirurgie, Hôpital Sainte-Marguerite, et [b]Fédération d'Oto-Rhino-Laryngologie, Hôpital la Timone, Assistance Publique-Hôpitaux de Marseille, Marseille, France

Abstract

Recurrent and regrowing large vestibular schwannomas (VSs) may require another microsurgical procedure. Little is known about the incidence and the consequences of this second surgical procedure. We reviewed our own 10 reoperated cases during a 20-year period. Eight of them were supposed to have a radical surgery at the initial step, while 2 had experienced a subtotal resection. The mean interval between the 2 surgeries was 8.3 years with an ultra-late recurrent case at 20 years. Additional surgery was justified by a large-sized growing tumor in main cases and/or occurrence of new symptoms. We used a widened translabyrinthine approach in 9 cases and a retrosigmoid route in 1 case. Preservation of a good facial nerve motion (H-B gd I or II) was obtained in 3 out of the 6 cases who displayed this preoperative status. Excluding the facial nerve injury, no major complication was observed in these cases. These results confirm that the iterative surgical procedure for VS carries additional difficulties with respect to functional preservation. Assuming that radiosurgery is an effective tool to control small- to middle-sized VSs, priority was recently given to the facial nerve preservation during the surgical removal of recurrent and regrowing VSs.

In the recent literature, we found very scanty information about the incidence and the way to manage recurrent or regrowing vestibular schwannomas (VSs). Today, radiosurgery can be considered as a safe and effective treatment in this situation but microsurgical removal remains the unique option in case of large recurrent VS. Many surgeons advocate that microsurgery that is done after failed radiosurgery carries more risks than when undertaken as a first step treatment. However, they do not give any data about the difficulties encountered during microsurgery after a previous operation. In this perspective, we made the synthesis of our own experience and reviewed the literature.

Patients and Methods

From 1985 to 2005, among an experience of more than 700 operated cases in our team, we had to manage surgically 10 patients that have been previously operated on for a VS using various approaches. Nine of these cases came from our institution while one patient was initially managed in another center. This population does not exactly match our own recurrent or regrowing cases, since several patients have been treated with GKR and others that were lost to follow-up may have switched centers.

There were 4 females and 6 males, with age ranging from 37 to 72 at the time of the first procedure. Despite incomplete radiological follow-up data for 6 patients after initial surgery, tumor resection was considered as total in

8 patients and near total in 2 patients. The mean interval between the first surgery and recurrence was 8.3 years, ranging from 1 to 20 years (median: 7 years). The diagnosis of recurrence was based on new symptoms and neuroimaging in 9 cases and on images without symptom in 1 case. New symptoms at the time of recurrence were ataxia in 4 cases, tinnitus in 2 cases, diplopia in 1 case, trigeminal hypesthesia in 2 cases and hemifacial spasm in 1 case.

Radiological findings of recurrent cases showed that tumor size ranged from Koos [1] III in 4 cases to Koos IV in 6 cases. Seven tumors displayed a nodular shape and 3 lesions a macrocystic structure. The origin of recurrence was deduced from the operative chart and image data. The topography of recurrence was distributed as follows: lateral portion of the internal auditory canal in 1 case, lateral brain stem in 1 case, cerebellopontine angle (CPA) and porus acousticus in 6 cases and multifocal recurrence in 3 cases.

Results

The results of our personal experience have been partially published in a previous paper [2]. One patient was operated on using a retrosigmoid route and 9 using a widened translabyrinthine approach (WTA). The technical aspects of this latter approach have been detailed in a previous chapter of this volume. Clinical features and outcome of these patients are shown in table 1.

Operative Findings

Surgical difficulties that were encountered were mainly due to adhesion of the tumor capsule to adjacent structures. Adhesion to the brain stem and cerebellar hemisphere was observed in 5 cases. Adhesion to the facial nerve at the level of the porus acousticus and in its cisternal course was observed in 2 and 5 cases, respectively. Adhesion to the trigeminal nerve and to the lower cranial nerve was observed in 6 and 5 cases, respectively. Adhesion to the vessels involved the posteroinferior cerebellar artery in one case and the petrosal veins in 2 cases. In all cases, features of arachnoid thickening were observed, which brought significant difficulties of identification and preservation of adjacent neurovascular structures. Softness and vascularization of the tumor did not affect the operative steps in any case. Pathological features of the specimens confirmed typical benign schwannomas in all cases.

Tumor Removal

Gross total removal was obtained in 6 cases, near total removal in 1 case and subtotal removal in 3 cases. The decision of nonradical removal was justified by the high level of priority we put to preserve still functioning facial nerves. In the delayed follow-up, sequential radiological examinations did not allow to identify residual tumor in all but one case (case 9) in which an adjunctive radiosurgical treatment is scheduled.

Functional Results

Following the House-Brackmann (H-B) classification [3] and among the 6 patients who displayed a good (I and II) facial motion before the second procedure, 3 of them kept the same status. One patient experienced permanent severe facial nerve palsy. These results are shown in table 2. In the long-term follow-up one patient died from an unrelated cause 7 years after the second operation (case 5). None of the other patients experienced any major complication.

Case Illustration

This 55-year-old woman was initially managed for her large left-sided VS via a WTA. Radical removal was obtained and confirmed by a CT scan but a lack of recovery of her facial nerve function required an additional hypoglossal-facial nerve anastomosis. She could improve her facial nerve motion to an H-B grade 3 and had an uneventful outcome. At 10 years after surgery, a new MRI study could rule out any recurrent tumor (fig. 1a) and she was considered cured. At 20 years after surgery, she complained of a sudden-onset imbalance problem followed by a left-side facial numbness. Physical examination showed an obvious cerebellar ataxia and trigeminal hypesthesia. A new MRI indicated a recurrent cystic tumor in a left CPA and an additional microsurgical removal

Table 1. Summary of cases that have been surgically managed after postoperative recurrence

Case	Sex, age, tumor stage (Koos)	First surgery and postoperative VII gd (H-B)	Postoperative radiology	Time of recurrence, symptoms, tumor size	Second surgery, postoperative VII	Follow-up
1	F, 60, IV	1985 TL, TR, gd 4	TDM OK postoperatively	1994, ataxia, VS IV	TL, TR, gd 4	TDM 1 year normal
2	M, 37	1990 RS, TR, gd 2	ND	1994, hemispasm, VS III	TL, TR, gd 3	TDM 1 year normal
3	M, 38, IV	1982 TL, TR, gd 1	ND	1989, tinnitus, ataxia, III	TL, TR, gd 1	TDM 6 years normal
4	M, 72	1982 RS, gd 1	ND	1988, diplopia, III, evol. IV	TL, STR, gd 4	TDM 3 months normal
5	M, 55, IV	1979 TL, STR, gd 2	TDM: RT	1985, ataxia, IV	TL, STR, gd 6	Died at 7 years (unrelated problem)
6	M, 33	1971 RS, STR, gd 2	ND	1987, tinnitus, III	TL, TR, gd 2	TDM 6 years normal
7	F, 54	1979 RS, gd 1	TDM: no RT	1986, asymptomatic, III	TL, TR, gd 2	TDM 5 years normal
8	M, 49, IV	1993 TL, NTR, gd 3	ND	1994, facial hypesthesia, IV cyst	TL, NTR, gd 4	TDM 1 year normal
9	F, 45, IV	1998 TL, TR, gd 3	ND	2005, ataxia, MRI: IV cystic	TL, STR, gd 3	MRI 6 months: RT – GK planned
10	F, 55, IV	1986 TL, TR, gd 3 after VII–XII anastomosis	MRI 10 years: no RT	2006, ataxia and V numbness, MRI: IV cystic	RS, TR, gd 3	MRI 3 months normal

GK = Gamma Knife radiosurgery; H-B = House-Brackmann facial nerve grading system; ND = not documented; RS = retrosigmoid approach; RT = residual tumor; TDM = tomodensitometry; TL = translabyrinthine approach; TR = total removal; STR = subtotal removal; NTR = near-total removal.

was planned (fig. 1b). At the time of admission for surgery 3 months after the diagnosis of recurrence, a new MRI was given and showed additional tumor growth (fig. 1c). This tumor was removed via a retrosigmoid route. Adhesion to the petrosal vein and to the trigeminal and lower cranial nerves was observed, while dissection of the tumor capsule from the brain stem could be achieved without additional difficulties.

Discussion

Taken collectively, our experience and the few data extracted from the literature deserve several comments about the results.

Surgery is more difficult because of scarring and adhesion that compromise the identification and dissection of critical neurovascular structures that lay at the tumor boundaries. Of special

Table 2. Facial nerve motion before and after microsurgery of the recurrent tumor

H-B facial grading	Patients	
	before surgery	after surgery
I	3	1
II	3	2
III	3[1]	3
IV	1	3
V	0	0
VI	0	1

[1]This result was obtained after hypoglossal-facial anastomosis.

interest, the facial nerve function is jeopardized by the attempt of radical resection. Actually, even if the facial motion looks normal or near normal before the second procedure, the nerve and its vascularization may have been weakened during the first procedure. In our experience, 50% of patients with normal or near-normal facial nerve function kept this status, compared with only 33% in the series published by Beatty et al. [4]. In the 5 cases reported by Sterkers et al. [5], facial nerve had to be sacrificed in 3 cases, while 2 out of 4 facial nerves could not be anatomically preserved in the cases reported by Thedinger et al. [6], which is a rare event in a first-intention treatment. These observations have recently led us to change our policy. We now inform the patient that optimal subtotal resection with facial nerve preservation will be our first goal, considering that subsequent radiosurgical treatment of the remnant tumor will offer a good potential of long-term tumor control.

Technical Considerations

In cases of recurrent or regrowing tumor, microsurgery may be the unique option of treatment, particularly if the tumor is large. In such a situation, we consider that the use of the WTA is the most suitable route.

Scar tissues that spread against the cerebellum bed are overlooked if a retrosigmoid approach had been used as the initial route. The WTA allows the control of the whole CPA and internal auditory canal altogether. Considering the extreme variability of the site of recurrence, such wide exposure is of special interest. The facial nerve may be identified at the fundus. In case of unsuited facial nerve sacrifice, the WTA gives enough room to perform an anastomosis. The whole course of the intrapetrous facial nerve can be exposed after skeletonization of the Fallopian canal, and the nerve can be directly anastomosed in a tensionless end-to-end manner if the proximal stump is of sufficient quality. If not, it is possible to provide a hypoglosso-facial anastomosis during the same approach, and especially a lateroterminal anastomosis to avoid the tong atrophy [7]. In the case where a WTA has been used previously, it may be difficult to elevate the fat that plugged the petrous bone defect. The fat needs to be detached from normal bony limits but also from the previously dissected dura using a sharp instrument. Care is taken not to injure the sigmoid sinus while elevating this graft.

In some cases, the retrosigmoid approach may offer the advantage of a straightforward and faster approach. This option is of particular interest when an intracapsular debulking is planned in elderly and poor condition patients, or when recurrence is exclusively located inside the CPA.

Conclusion

Tumor recurrence after initial optimal surgery may require additional surgery in rare circumstances. The results obtained in the present study and those from the previous reports in the literature indicate that this subsequent surgery carries additional functional risks regarding facial nerve preservation when radical removal is attempted.

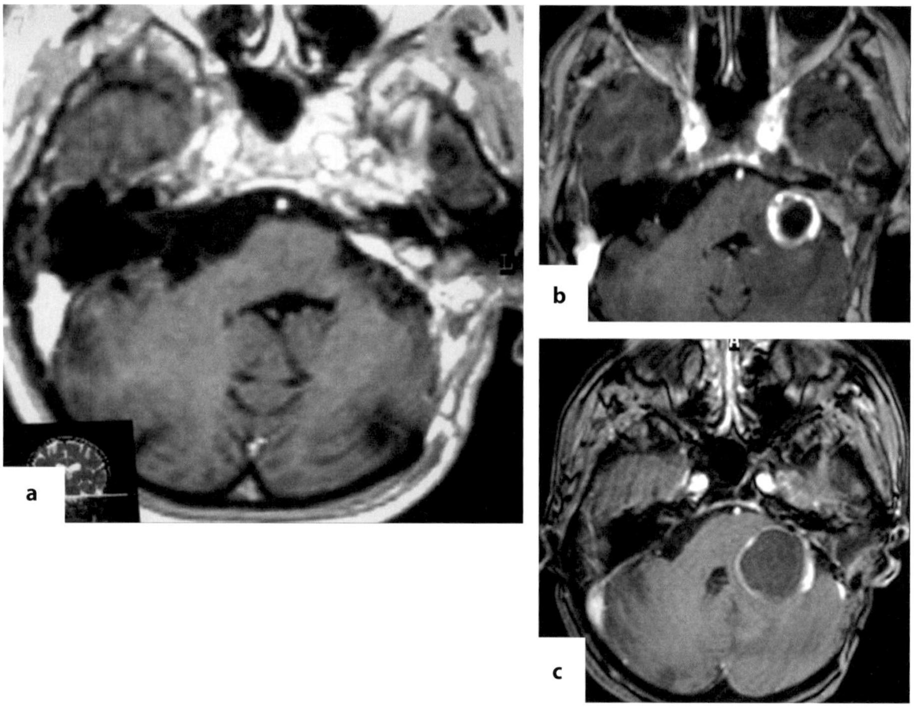

Fig. 1. Illustrative case of an ultra-late recurrence. **a** Axial post-gadolinium MRI done at 10 years after the left-sided translabyrinthine approach showing no sign of recurrence. **b** Same imaging study was done at 20 years after surgery because of new symptoms and showing cystic recurrence. **c** Two months later, the MRI confirms the growing potential of this tumor.

Since residual microfragments of the tumor cannot be definitively ruled out by a meticulous checking at the end of the operative procedure, we ask our patients to undergo sequential MR controls after the initial microsurgical treatment. In this way, recurrence is identified early and can be eligible for a noninvasive radiosurgical treatment.

References

1 Koos WT, Day JD, Matula C, Levy DI: Neurotopographic considerations in the microsurgical treatment of small acoustic neurinomas. J Neurosurg 1998;88:506–512.
2 Thomassin JM, Pellet W, Eron JP, Braccini F, Roche PH: Recurrent acoustic neurinoma after complete surgical resection. Ann Otolaryngol Chir Cervicofacial 2001;118:3–10.
3 House JW, Brackmann DE: Facial nerve grading system. Bull Am Acad Otolaryngol Head Neck Surg 1985;4:4.
4 Beatty CW, Ebersold MJ, Harner SG: Residual and recurrent acoustic neuromas. Laryngoscope 1987;97:1168–1171.
5 Sterkers JM, Viala P, Benghalem A: Recurrence of acoustic neurinomas. Rev Laryngol Otol Rhinol 1988;109:71–73.
6 Thedinger BS, Whittaker K, Luetje CM: Recurrent acoustic tumor after a suboccipital removal. Neurosurgery 1991;29:681–687.
7 Asaoka K, Sawamura Y, Nagashima M, Fukushima T: Surgical anatomy for direct hypoglossal-facial nerve side-to-end anastomosis. J Neurosurg 1999;268–275.

Prof. Pierre-Hugues Roche
Service de Neurochirurgie de l'Hôpital Nord, Assistance Publique-Hôpitaux de Marseille
Chemin des Bourrelly, FR–13915 Marseille Cedex 20 (France)
Tel. +33 4 91 96 86 20, Fax +33 4 91 96 89 15, E-Mail proche@mail.ap-hm.fr

Régis J, Roche P-H (eds): Modern Management of Acoustic Neuroma.
Prog Neurol Surg. Basel, Karger, 2008, vol 21, pp 163–168

Vestibular Schwannoma Radiosurgery after Previous Surgical Resection or Stereotactic Radiosurgery

Bruce E. Pollock[a,b] · Michael J. Link[a]

Departments of [a]Neurological Surgery and [b]Radiation Oncology, Mayo Clinic College of Medicine, Rochester, Minn., USA

Abstract

Objective: To evaluate radiosurgery outcomes in vestibular schwannoma (VS) patients who have undergone prior tumor treatment. **Methods:** Retrospective review of 55 consecutive VS patients having radiosurgery for recurrent (n = 22) or residual tumors (n = 33) after prior microsurgery. The median time from the patients' last surgery was 60 months (range, 2–463). Forty-seven patients (84%) had enlarging tumors at the time of radiosurgery. **Results:** The majority of patients (67%) had facial weakness prior to radiosurgery; 52 patients (95%) were deaf. The median tumor volume was 3.0 cm^3 (range, 0.1–18.1). The median tumor margin dose was 14 Gy (range, 12–20). Fifty patients had follow-up available at a median of 47 months (range, 5–148) after radiosurgery. The tumor control rate was 94%. Trigeminal deficits developed in 2 patients (4%). Four of 42 patients (10%) with normal to moderate facial nerve function before radiosurgery developed facial weakness. Three of these 4 patients received a tumor margin dose of 20 Gy. **Conclusion:** Radiosurgery is effective for patients with recurrent or residual VSs after prior surgical removal. Repeat radiosurgery after initial failed radiosurgery can be considered, but little information is available to evaluate this approach. Staged treatment involving subtotal tumor removal and radiosurgery is an option for patients with large VSs to facilitate both cranial nerve preservation and long-term tumor control.

Although there remains great debate about the best treatment for patients with newly diagnosed vestibular schwannomas (VSs) [1, 2], radiosurgery has emerged as the clear treatment of choice for patients with recurrent or enlarging tumors after prior surgical resection [3–5]. This chapter reviews the results of 55 patients having VS radiosurgery after prior surgical resection over a 15-year interval. In addition, the limited information available on repeat VS radiosurgery will be reviewed.

Materials and Methods

Patients

Three hundred and sixty-nine patients had VS radiosurgery at the Mayo Clinic, Rochester, Minn., USA, between March 1990 and December 2005. Fifty-five (18 males, 37 females, 15% of the total VS series) of these patients had undergone one or more previous tumor resections. The characteristics of these patients are outlined in table 1. The median patient age was 51 years (range, 18–79). Tumor resection was graded as gross total in 22 patients (40%). The median time from their last surgery to radiosurgery was 86 months (range, 24–463). Thirty-three patients (60%) had subtotal tumor resections. The

Table 1. Patient characteristics

Factor	Patients
Neurofibromatosis type 2	4 (7)
Operations	
1	50 (91)
2	3 (5)
3	2 (4)
Tumor removal (last surgery)	
Gross total resection	22 (40)
Subtotal resection	33 (60)
Prior VPS	4 (7)
Trigeminal deficit	15 (27)
Facial movement	
Normal	18 (33)
Weakness	28 (51)
Palsy	9 (16)
Deaf	52 (94)
Lower CN dysfunction	2 (4)
Ataxia	15 (27)

Figures in parentheses indicate percentages. CN = Cranial nerve; VPS = ventriculoperitoneal shunt.

median time from their last surgery to radiosurgery was 26 months (range, 2–252). Overall, 46 patients (84%) had enlarging tumors at the time of radiosurgery.

Radiosurgery
Radiosurgery was performed using the Leksell Gamma Knife® (Elekta Instruments, Norcross, Ga., USA) and magnetic resonance imaging (MRI) for dose planning in most cases. The median number of isocenters was 8 (range, 2–14). The median tumor volume was 3.0 cm^3 (range, 0.1–18.1). The median tumor margin dose was 14 Gy (range, 12–20); the median maximum radiation dose was 28 Gy (range, 24–40).

Follow-Up
Patients were requested to undergo clinical and MRI follow-up at 6, 12, 24 months, and bi-yearly thereafter. Fifty patients had follow-up available at a median of 47 months (range, 5–148) after radiosurgery.

Results

Tumor Control and Additional Surgery
The tumors were unchanged in 16 patients (32%), smaller in 29 patients (58%), and larger in 5 patients (10%). Two of these 5 patients underwent tumor resection at 6 and 18 months due to symptomatic enlargement. One patient showed tumor progression on serial MRI, and underwent tumor resection 26 months after radiosurgery. Two patients had initial tumor enlargement after radiosurgery, then no further evidence of tumor progression on subsequent imaging. Overall, the tumor control rate was 94%.

Neurologic Morbidity
Seven patients (14%) had complications after radiosurgery including trigeminal deficits (n = 2), facial weakness (n = 4), ataxia (n = 3), or diplopia (n = 1). Of note, three of the four patients developing new facial weakness received a tumor margin dose of 20 Gy. One of 3 patients with hearing before radiosurgery retained unchanged auditory function at last follow-up (speech reception threshold 65 dB, speech discrimination score, 16%).

Discussion

Radiosurgery after Failed Surgical Resection
A gross total resection of VSs is achieved for the vast majority of patients when experienced surgeons perform the operation. Tumor recurrence rates after complete tumor removal vary widely in the literature with recurrence rates ranging from <1% [6–8], to as high as 8–9% in the MRI era [9, 10]. However, it must be remembered that most of these estimates are based on clinical, not radiographic recurrences, and that VS

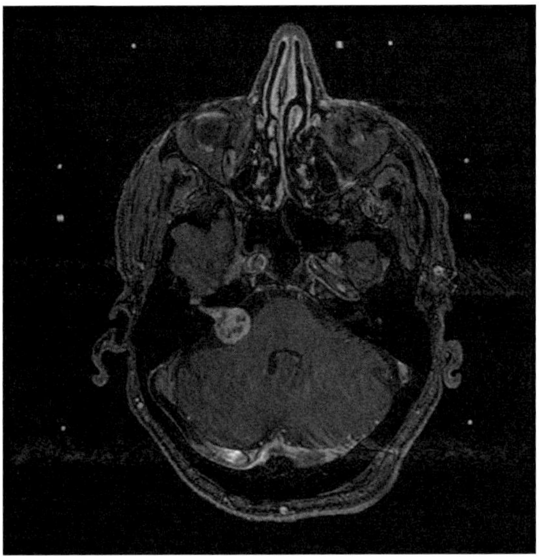

Fig. 1. MRI of a 73-year-old man who underwent complete resection of a VS via a middle fossa approach in 1965. MRI in 1990 showed no evidence of recurrent tumor. The patient had progressive right-sided hearing loss and repeat imaging showed a recurrent 2-cm tumor (38 years after surgery). The recurrent tumor was treated with radiosurgery.

regrowth may occur many years after surgery (fig. 1). Tumor progression after incomplete VS resection can also occur and likely relates to the amount of residual tumor. Bloch et al. [11] followed 52 VS patients after near-total (remnant ≤25 mm^2 or ≤2 mm thick) or subtotal (any larger remnant) resections. The tumor recurrence rate was 3% (1 of 33 patients) after near-total resection compared to 32% (6 of 19 patients). The mean time from surgery to detection of tumor recurrence was 3 years. The odds ratio for tumor recurrence was 12 times greater for patients with a subtotal resection. The treatment options for a patient having recurrent or progressing VS after prior surgery include repeat resection, fractionated radiation therapy, or stereotactic radiosurgery. Beatty et al. [12] reported on 23 patients having repeat VS resection. Although the number of patients is small, 4 of 10 patients with normal-to-moderate facial nerve function before surgery developed severe facial weakness after repeat surgery. In addition, 3 patients had worsened ataxia, and 1 patient required placement of a gastrotomy tube secondary to lower cranial nerve damage. No study on fractionated radiation therapy has specifically addressed outcomes for VS patients after failed surgical resection.

As an alternative to repeat resection or radiation therapy, radiosurgery has been performed for three decades for VS patients after prior surgical resection. Recent studies on VS radiosurgery have shown that between 15 and 39% of patients underwent previous surgery [13–15]. Our experience has been similar with 15% of the patients having VS radiosurgery at our center over the past 15 years having undergone one or more prior operations. Table 2 outlines the findings of papers focused on outcomes after VS radiosurgery in patients having prior surgical resection of their tumor. Pollock et al. [3] reported on 76 patients (78 tumors) having radiosurgery at the University of Pittsburgh from 1987 to 1995. Notable in this series were the pre-radiosurgical deficits for this group of patients. Half of the patients described trigeminal nerve deficits and only 30% had normal facial movement. Only 3 patients (4%) retained a speech discrimination score greater than 50% before radiosurgery. Seventy-three tumors (94%) showed no evidence of progression at a median follow-up of 43 months. Eleven of 47 patients with normal to moderate facial nerve function developed increased facial weakness. A clear relationship with radiation dose and new facial weakness was noted. For patients receiving tumor margin doses of 12–14 Gy, the incidence of facial weakness was 14%, whereas patients receiving 15–17 or 18 or greater Gy had worsened facial function in 22 and 57% of cases, respectively. Unger et al. [5] followed 50 patients for a median of 75 months after radiosurgery. The median tumor margin dose was 13 Gy; the tumor control rate was 96%. No patient developed a new permanent

Table 2. Published results for VS radiosurgery after prior surgical resection

Series	Patients	Median tumor margin dose, Gy	Median follow-up, months	Facial weakness, %	Tumor control, %
Pollock et al., 1998	76 (78 tumors)	15	43	23	94
Unger et al., 2002	50	13	75	10 (temporary) 0 (permanent)	96
Roche et al., 2004[1]	60	NS	52	0	93
Present study, 2006	50	14	47	10	94

NS = Not stated.
[1]Information gathered from abstract; paper not available in English.

trigeminal or facial nerve deficit. Roche et al. [4] managed 60 VS patients with radiosurgery after surgical resection from 1992 to 2002. At a median follow-up of 52 months, 7% of tumors progressed. No patient developed new or worsened trigeminal of facial nerve function.

Our results parallel these earlier studies. The median interval from patients' last surgery and radiosurgery was 60 months. The time to radiosurgery was significantly less for patients having subtotal resections (median, 26 months) compared to patients having prior complete resections (86 months). Roche et al. [4] noted a mean interval between resection and radiosurgery of 72 months. Before radiosurgery, only 18 patients (33%) had normal facial movement, and only 3 patients (6%) had any preserved hearing. Fifty patients had follow-up available at a median of 47 months (range, 5–148) after radiosurgery. The tumor control rate was 94%. Trigeminal deficits developed in 2 patients (4%). Four of 42 patients (10%) with normal to moderate facial nerve function before radiosurgery developed facial weakness. Three of these four patients received a tumor margin dose of 20 Gy. Consequently, a tumor margin dose of 13–14 Gy is recommended to limit the chance of trigeminal or facial nerve injury. Numerous studies have demonstrated that this dosing regimen is associated with long-term tumor control [13, 14, 16–18]. Patients with recurrent VS and a pre-existing facial palsy can be safely treated with slightly higher doses (15–16 Gy), although it remains unclear that this minimal dose increase provides any greater chance from tumor progression.

Repeat Radiosurgery after Failed Radiosurgery

Several recent studies have demonstrated that the cranial nerve outcomes for patients having surgical resection after prior radiosurgery are relatively poor [6, 19, 20]. Consequently, it may not be unreasonable to consider repeat VS radiosurgery if there is clear tumor progression, the tumor is not causing brainstem progression, and the patient is asymptomatic. Our center has discussed this option with several patients, but we have yet to perform a case of repeat VS radiosurgery. The only information on this topic comes from the father of VS radiosurgery, Dr. Georg Noren. Noren describes performing repeat VS for 8 patients between 1969 and 1994 [21]. To compensate for the dramatic changes in radiosurgical technique and different doses radiation used over this 25-year interval, the results were presented in three time intervals. Of note, 3 of the initial 8 VS patients had tumors which did not respond. Analysis of

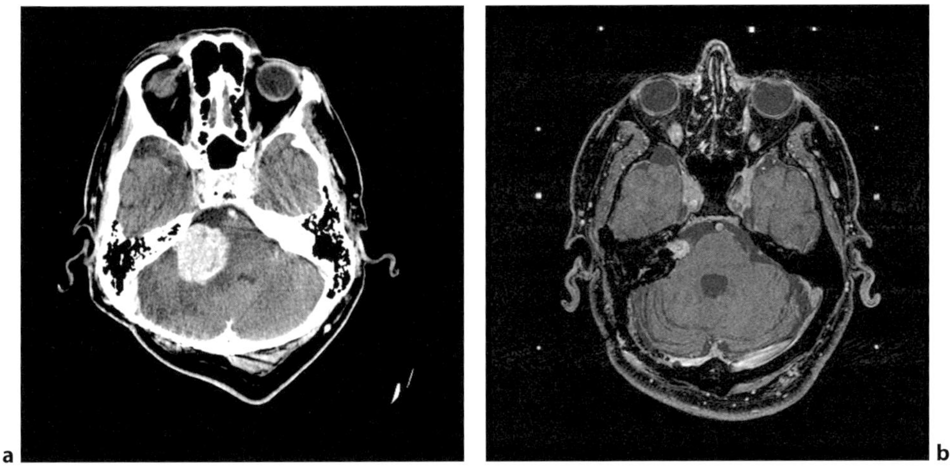

Fig. 2. Imaging of a 71-year-old man with a recurrent VS after two prior surgeries and placement of a ventriculoperitoneal shunt. **a** Axial postcontrast CT showing large (34-mm) recurrent tumor. His facial sensation and movement were intact; he was deaf on the right. The patient underwent a planned subtotal tumor resection via a translabyrinthine approach. **b** MRI 10 months later at the time of radiosurgery. The tumor was treated with a margin dose of 14 Gy. Thirty months after radiosurgery, the tumor has not progressed and the patient has normal facial movement.

their dose plans showed that despite an average maximum tumor dose of 56.7 Gy, the minimum tumor dose for these patients was <1 Gy. Overall, 7 of the 8 patients having repeat VS radiosurgery had tumor control and did not require additional tumor treatment. The dosimetry or clinical outcomes of these patients were not provided. Watanabe et al. [22] described a patient who underwent two radiosurgical procedures for a VS. The patient developed facial palsy 25 months after the second radiosurgery (56 months after the initial radiosurgery); the combined tumor margin dose was 24 Gy. The patient underwent complete tumor resection 27 months after repeat radiosurgery. Histologic and immunohistochemical examination of the excised facial nerve showed axonal degeneration, axonal loss, demyelination, and microvasculitis.

More information is needed to determine whether repeat VS radiosurgery is a viable option for patients who failed their initial radiosurgical procedure.

Staged Surgical Resection and Radiosurgery

There is a clear relationship between tumor size and the morbidity associated with VS resection [2, 7, 8]. For example, Sekhar et al. [2] noted moderate to severe facial weakness in 5% of patients with tumors less than 2.0 cm, 27% with tumors from 2.0 to 3.9 cm, and 65% with tumors greater than 4.0 cm. Unfortunately, patients with large VSs rarely are candidates for radiosurgery because of symptomatic mass effect. To minimize the morbidity of treatment for patients with large VSs, a strategy of combined surgical resection and radiosurgery has been proposed [4, 23]. In this approach, the goal of microsurgery is to perform a subtotal tumor removal to minimize the risk of cranial nerve injury, but still remove enough tumor to relieve the mass effect on the brainstem and cerebellum (fig. 2). Iwai et al. [23] managed 14 VS patients with large tumors using this planned approach from 1994 to 2000. The average tumor diameter before surgery was 42 mm. Patients then underwent radiosurgery at an average of 3 months later. The mean tumor margin dose was 12.1 Gy. At a mean follow-up of 32 months after radiosurgery, one patient required additional surgical resection. Twelve patients (86%) retained normal or near-normal movement at last follow-up. Therefore, a staged approach combining both micro- and radiosurgery may facilitate both cranial nerve preservation and long-term tumor control for patients diagnosed with large VSs.

References

1 Pollock BE, Lunsford LD, Noren G: Vestibular schwannoma management in the next century: a radiosurgical perspective. Neurosurgery 1998;43:475–483.
2 Sekhar LN, Gormley WB, Wright DC: The best treatment for vestibular schwannoma (acoustic neuroma): microsurgery or radiosurgery? Am J Otol 1996;17:676–682.
3 Pollock BE, Lunsford LD, Flickinger JC, Clyde BL, Kondziolka D: Vestibular schwannoma management. Part I. Failed microsurgery and the role of delayed stereotactic radiosurgery. J Neurosurg 1998;89:944–948.
4 Roche PH, Robitail S, Delsanti C, Marouf R, Pellet W, Regis J: Radiosurgery of vestibular schwannomas after microsurgery and combined radio-microsurgery. Neurochirurgie 2004;50:394–400.
5 Unger F, Walch C, Papaefthymiou G, Feichtinger K, Trummer M, Pendl G: Radiosurgery of residual and recurrent vestibular schwannomas. Acta Neurochir (Wein) 2002;144:671–676.
6 Friedman RA, Brackmann DE, Hitselberger WE, Schwartz MS, Iqbal Z, Berliner KI: Surgical salvage after failed irradiation for vestibular schwannoma. Laryngoscope 2005;115:1827–1832.
7 Samii M, Matthies C: Management of 1000 vestibular schwannomas (acoustic neuromas): hearing function in 1000 tumor resections. Neurosurgery 1997;40:248–260.
8 Sampath P, Holliday MJ, Brem H, Niparko JK, Long DM: Facial nerve injury in acoustic neuroma (vestibular schwannoma) surgery: etiology and prevention. Neurosurgery 1997;87:60–66.
9 Cerullo LJ, Grutsch JF, Heiferman K, Osterdock R: The preservation of hearing and facial nerve function in a consecutive series of unilateral vestibular nerve schwannoma surgical patients (acoustic neuroma). Surg Neurol 1993;39:485–493.
10 Mazzoni A, Calabrese V, Moschini L: Residual and recurrent acoustic neuroma in hearing preservation procedures: neuroradiologic and surgical findings. Skull Base Surg 1996;6:105–112.
11 Bloch DC, Oghalai JS, Jackler RK, Osofsky M, Pitts LH: The fate of the tumor remnant after less-than-complete acoustic neuroma resection. Otolaryngol Head Neck Surg 2004;130:104–112.
12 Beatty CW, Ebersold MJ, Harner SG: Residual and recurrent acoustic neuromas. Laryngoscope 1987;97:1168–1171.
13 Chung W, Kang-Du L, Shiau C, Wu H, Wang L, Guo W, Ho DM, Pan DH: Gamma knife surgery for vestibular schwannoma: 10-year experience of 195 cases. J Neurosurg (Suppl) 2005;102:87–96.
14 Lunsford LD, Niranjan A, Flickinger JC, Maitz A, Kondziolka D: Radiosurgery of vestibular schwannoma: summary of experience in 829 cases. J Neurosurg (Suppl) 2005;102:195–199.
15 Prasad D, Steiner M, Steiner L: Gamma surgery for vestibular schwannoma. J Neurosurg 2000;92:745–759.
16 Hasegawa T, Fujitani S, Katsumata S, Kida Y, Yoshimoto M, Koike J: Stereotactic radiosurgery for vestibular schwannomas: analysis of 317 patients followed more than 5 years. Neurosurgery 2005;57:257–264.
17 Iwai Y, Yamanaka K, Shiotani M, Uyama T: Radiosurgery for acoustic neuromas: results of low-dose treatment. Neurosurgery 2003;53:282–287.
18 Petit JH, Hudes RS, Chen TT, Eisenberg HM, Simard JM, Chin LS: Reduced-dose radiosurgery for vestibular schwannomas. Neurosurgery 2001;49:1299–1306.
19 Lee DJ, Westra WH, Staecker H, Long D, Niparko JK: Clinical and histopathologic features of recurrent vestibular schwannomas (acoustic neuroma) after stereotactic radiosurgery. Otol Neurotol 2003;24:650–660.
20 Roche PH, Regis J, Deveze A, Delsanti C, Thomassin JM, Pellet W: Surgical removal of unilateral vestibular schwannomas after failed gamma knife surgery. Neurochirurgie 2004;50:383–393.
21 Noren G: Gamma knife radiosurgery for acoustic neurinomas; in Gildenberg PL, Tasker RR (eds): Textbook of Stereotactic and Functional Neurosurgery. New York, McGraw-Hill, 1998, pp 835–844.
22 Watanabe T, Saito N, Hirato J, Shimaguchi H, Fujimaki H, Sasaki T: Facial neuropathy due to axonal degeneration and microvasculitis following gamma knife surgery for vestibular schwannoma: a histological analysis. Case report. J Neurosurg 2003;99:916–920.
23 Iwai Y, Yamanaka K, Ishiguro T: Surgery combined with radiosurgery of large acoustic neuromas. Surg Neurol 2003;59:283–289.

Bruce E. Pollock, MD
Department of Neurological Surgery, Mayo Clinic
Rochester, MN 55905 (USA)
Tel. +1 507 284 5317, Fax +1 507 294 5206, E-Mail pollock.bruce@mayo.edu

Régis J, Roche P-H (eds): Modern Management of Acoustic Neuroma.
Prog Neurol Surg. Basel, Karger, 2008, vol 21, pp 169–175

Microsurgery Management of Vestibular Schwannomas in Neurofibromatosis Type 2: Indications and Results

M. Samii · V. Gerganov · A. Samii

International Neuroscience Institute, Hannover, Germany

Abstract

Aim: To analyze the senior author's experience and strategy of treatment of patients with neurofibromatosis type 2 (NF2), with particular emphasis on vestibular schwannoma (VS) surgery. **Materials and Methods:** Over a period of more than 35 years, the senior author (M.S.) has operated on more than 165 patients with NF2. The total number of VS surgeries was 210. This retrospective analysis includes 145 consecutively operated patients. Medical records, operative reports, follow-up neurological, audiometric examinations, and neuroradiological findings were analyzed. **Results:** Total tumor removal was achieved in 85% of the operated tumors. In 15%, deliberately subtotal removal was performed for brain stem decompression and hearing preservation in the only hearing ear. The overall rate of hearing preservation was 35%. When only patients with preserved useful preoperative hearing were included, the rate was 65%. Bilateral hearing after surgery was preserved in 23% of the patients. The anatomical integrity of the facial nerve was preserved in 89%. **Conclusions:** The goal of VS surgery in patients with NF2 should be complete removal but not at the expense of functional impairment. Carefully individualized treatment strategy offers the possibility of prolongation of life and preservation of neurological functions.

Neurofibromatosis type 2 (NF2) is a rare autosomal dominant inherited disease [1]. Patients with NF2 have a predisposition to formation of multiple tumors of the central nervous system, characteristically bilateral vestibular schwannomas (VSs). Criteria for NF2 are bilateral VS or a parent, sibling, or child with NF2 and either unilateral vestibulocochlear nerve tumor or any one of the following: neurofibroma, meningioma, glioma, schwannoma, posterior capsular cataract or opacity at a young age [2]. About 5% of all patients with VS have NF2.

The lifelong tendency to formation of new central nervous system tumors predetermines the impossibility of definitive cure of these patients. Treatment is focused on life prolongation, maintenance of quality of life, preservation of cranial nerve function or auditory rehabilitation [3].

The goal of this study was to analyze the senior author's experience with the treatment of patients with NF2 and to present his treatment strategies, with particular emphasis on VS surgery.

Materials and Methods

Over a period of more than 35 years, the senior author (M.S.) has operated on more than 165 patients with NF2. The total number of VS surgeries in these patients was 210. This retrospective analysis includes 145

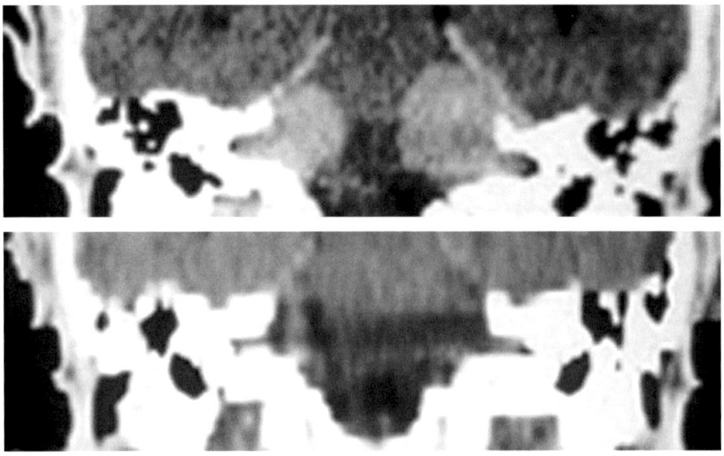

a

b

Fig. 1. a Preoperative CT with bone window of a patient with NF2, demonstrating large bilateral VS with severe brainstem compression. Intrameatal tumor extension is clearly visible bilaterally. **b** Postoperative CT. Total tumor removal with bilateral preservation of facial nerve function was achieved.

consecutively operated patients. The total number of surgeries for VS was 195. Medical records, operative reports, neurological, and neuroradiological findings were recorded. Audiometric examinations were performed both preoperatively and at follow-up examinations. Hearing was classified according to the New Hannover Classification [4]. Hearing levels according to classes 1 and 2 were accepted as useful.

Results

Total tumor removal was achieved in 85% of the operated tumors. In 15% (29 cases) deliberately subtotal removal was performed for brain stem decompression (6 cases) and hearing preservation in the only hearing ear (23 cases). The subtotal removal and internal auditory canal (IAC) decompression led to long-term hearing preservation in 15 cases. 24% of all patients were deaf preoperatively, with preserved unilateral hearing in 34% and with preserved bilateral hearing in 42%. The overall rate of hearing preservation in the series was 35% (fig. 1 and 2). When only patients with preserved useful preoperative hearing were included, the rate was 65%. 23% of the patients had bilateral hearing after surgery. The anatomical integrity of the facial nerve was preserved in 89%.

Discussion

The first case of bilateral VS was reported in 1922 by Wishart [5]. Recent developments led to significant progress of our knowledge of the molecular biology of the disease. NF2 is caused by a single germline mutation of the chromosome band 22q12 [6]. It is supposed that the normal allele is lost due to a somatic mutation in the cells giving rise to the tumor. In approximately 50%, NF2 is a sequence of a new germline mutation. In these patients, no evidence of other affected family members can be found. If a person inherits the abnormal gene, there is a 95% chance that he will develop bilateral VS. No differences have been reported between mutations detected in patients with NF2 and patients with sporadic tumors [4].

Molecular analysis of NF2 revealed that the mutation affects a gene that encodes a protein with 595 amino acids – the protein schwannomin/merlin. This protein is related to a family of proteins – the ezrin-radixin-moesin family – that link the actin cytoskeleton to the cell membrane molecules important for cellular remodeling and growth regulation [1, 6].

Both unilateral and bilateral VSs arise at the border between the central and peripheral segments of the VIIIth cranial nerve. Approximately

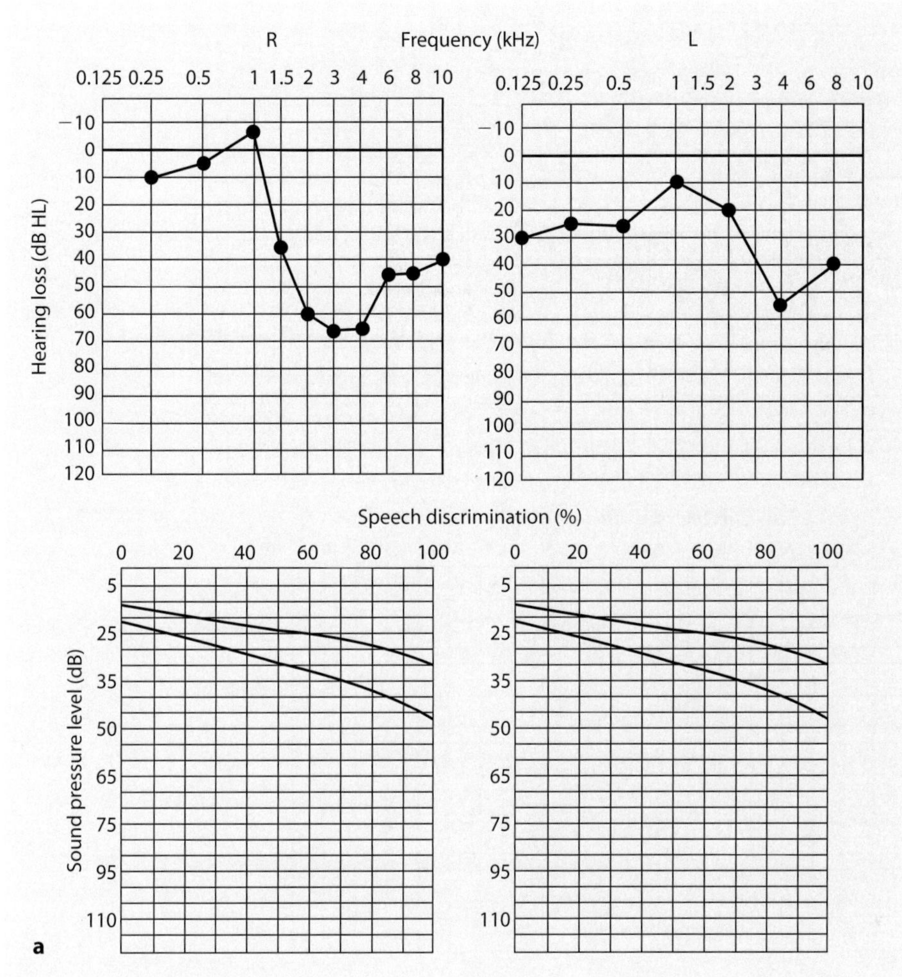

Fig. 2. a Preoperative audiogram of the same patient.

40% of the NF2-associated VS appear to have grape-like clusters. It is supposed that this multilobular structure is a consequence of the polyclonal origin of schwannomas, the latter being proved at the molecular level [7]. In some cases, nerves and vessels pass between the tumor lobules. The tumor can infiltrate the fibers of individual nerves, what is seldom found in unilateral tumors. Differences in tumor vascularity also have been reported, the NF2 tumors being highly vascularized. There might even be significant difference in both VSs in a single patient. One of the lesions could be much more adherent to the surrounding neural structures than the other [3, 4].

Although longitudinal studies of the growth rate of VS in NF2 indicate that it is generally higher in younger patients, some studies and the author's experience show that there are great variations, both between patients and over time in the same patient. No predictors for the rate of increase of the tumors have been identified. Clinical management of such patients cannot be based on the expectation of similar natural evolution [1].

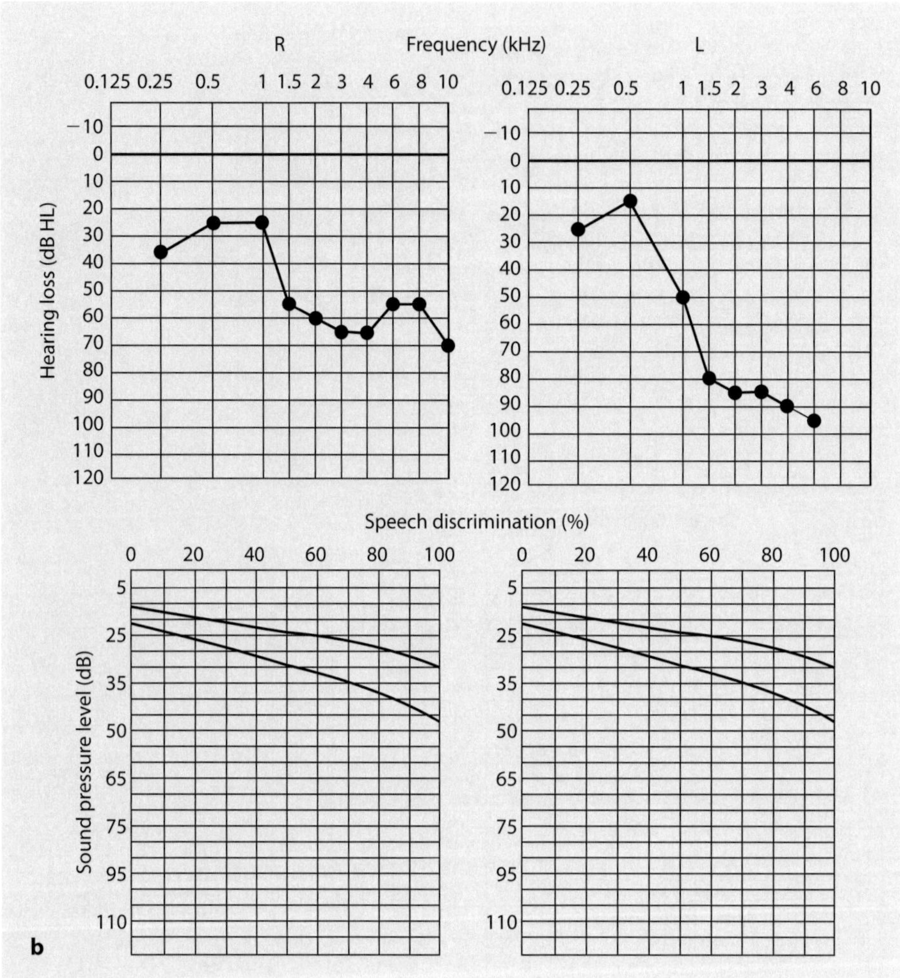

Fig. 2. b Preserved bilateral hearing is demonstrated by the postoperative audiological examination.

All these characteristics as well as the association with other central nervous system tumors determine the scope of the problems facing the neurosurgeon. Management of bilateral VS differs in a number of ways from sporadic unilateral tumors [8, 9]. The major management issue is the disabling consequences of acquired deafness.

Treatment options of patients with bilateral VS include observation, radiosurgery or surgical treatment [9]. Several surgical approaches have been put forward: partial or total tumor removal via the retrosigmoid or the middle fossa approach aiming at hearing preservation, total removal of the tumor with placement of an auditory brainstem implant (ABI), and decompression of the cochlear nerve at the IAC.

Facial Nerve Preservation

Regarding the preservation of the facial nerve, some surgeons advocate subtotal tumor removal. According to their observations, the absence of clear arachnoidal plane renders facial nerve injury unavoidable [10]. Recurrences after the subtotal removal are highly probable because most of these patients are relatively young and the VSs are typically rapidly growing. Surgeries in cases of recurrences are more difficult and more dangerous. Our treatment goal has always been total tumor removal. The only exceptions have been made in order to preserve hearing function or facial nerve integrity. Deliberate subtotal resections have been performed for brain stem decompression and for hearing preservation in the last hearing ear. Facial nerve preservation was possible in all cases except if the schwannoma (or multiple schwannomas) arose from the facial nerve or no cleavage plane between the cranial nerves and the tumor could be found. In 187 cases (89%), the facial nerve could be separated from the VS and its continuity preserved.

Hearing Preservation

Some surgeons propose a more conservative approach in order to preserve hearing – simple observation of the patient and subtotal intracapsular resection if the VS increases in size [2]. They advise that surgery should be postponed as long as possible [10]. Hearing conservation should be attempted on the side with the larger tumor and surgery on the better hearing ear is to be avoided. If this treatment strategy is followed, surgery is usually performed when the tumors have reached a considerable size, which significantly worsens the outcome. We accept an initial observational period in selected cases, such as the elderly, those with poor surgical risks, or those who refuse surgery.

Proponents of the active treatment strategy state that surgical removal of bilateral VS should occur as early as possible if the tumor is small (up to 1.5 cm), the hearing is usable and hearing preservation is possible [4, 11]. In order to maximize the chance of hearing preservation, the smallest tumor should be approached initially. If hearing is not preserved, the second tumor is followed expectantly until either hearing is lost or brainstem compression requires removal. Brackmann et al. [12] also favor an early proactive management of patients with bilateral VS. If the VSs are of equal size, they attempt hearing preservation for the ear with slightly worse hearing. If the hearing is equal in both ears, then hearing preservation is attempted on the side with the larger tumor.

Our treatment philosophy is based on the assumption that surgical removal of VS can preserve hearing. Our goal has always been preservation of functional hearing for as long as possible. If the chances of functional hearing preservation are realistic, our recommendation is to perform early surgery. Tumor extension, audiometry data, and auditory brainstem responses (ABR) determine which side should be operated on initially. The side with the best chances for hearing preservation is treated first. The main predictors of successful hearing preservation are tumor extension, preoperative hearing level and quality of ABR. We recommend initial treatment on the side with the smaller tumor or the side with a better hearing level. If the hearing and tumor size are similar on both sides, our decision is based on the preoperative ABR. The side with better quality is operated on first, because the chances of successful hearing preservation are better on that side. Thus, we achieved bilateral hearing preservation in 23% of the patients. 65% of the patients had preserved unilateral hearing after surgery with useful preoperative hearing level.

For VS on the only hearing side, osseous decompression of the cochlear nerve in the IAC, with or without partial tumor removal, has been proposed as a means of slowing the hearing loss [13]. It is presumed that reducing the pressure within the IAC will permit continued tumor growth for a time with preservation of hearing. Some surgeons state that wide bony removal and dural decompression are sufficient and the tumor should not be manipulated [12]. In order to minimize the risk of deafness in such cases, we offer IAC decompression and complete or partial tumor removal, depending on the intraoperative ABR. If slight microsurgical actions are followed by severe deterioration in ABR, only partial resection is performed. With this strategy, we succeeded in preserving hearing in 15 patients. Follow-up examinations indicated that preserved hearing remained functional for periods of up to 15 years. Tumor regrowth has been moderate and has not necessitated reoperations.

Radiosurgery is another treatment option. It provides tumor control and hearing preservation of approximately 33–43%, although some deterioration occurs during the ensuing 6 years [14, 15]. Radiation therapy is best reserved for NF2 patients who have particularly aggressive tumors, those with medical contraindications for microsurgery, patients who refuse surgery, or for the elderly [1, 12]. In our opinion, radiosurgery is not the optimal primary therapy in NF2. When offering such treatment, issues such as the long-term hearing preservation, danger of malignant transformation of the tumor, and the local effects that render later surgery more difficult, should be considered [1, 16].

Bilateral deafness of NF2 patients is often inevitable. The introduction of the ABI in the clinical practice offers hope for such patients. The ABI is designed to stimulate directly the second-order neurons [17, 18]. The main goal is to help patients to receive environmental sounds and to enhance their lip-reading ability for better communication. Clinical examinations indicate that auditory sensations appear immediately after the activation of the ABI, but a certain period is necessary for the readaptation of the central auditory system [17]. At the 6th month, over 60% of our patients with ABI achieved significant improvement of communication skills. In most patients, the performance continues to improve for up to 8 years after implantation [18].

All patients with NF2 and their families should have access to genetic testing because early, at best presymptomatic, diagnosis improves clinical outcome. Some authors even suggest that magnetic resonance tomography scanning for members of NF2 families should start at 10–12 years of age [7].

Treatment of NF2 patients should be individualized. Close collaboration with the patient and his family is essential. Patient's attitude and expectations should guide the decision making process.

Conclusion

Patients with NF2 should be referred to specialty treatment centers. The goal of VS surgery in NF2 patients should be complete tumor removal but not at the expense of functional impairment. Carefully individualized treatment strategy offers the possibility of prolongation of life and preservation of neurological functions.

References

1 Baser ME, Gareth DR, Evans DG, Gutmann DH: Neurofibromatosis 2. Curr Opin Neurol 2003;16:27–33.

2 National Institutes of Health Consensus Development Conference: Statement on Acoustic Neuroma. Arch Neurol 1994;51:201–207.

3 Samii M, Matthies C, Tatagiba M: Management of vestibular schwannomas (acoustic neuromas): auditory and facial nerve function after resection of 120 vestibular schwannomas in patients with neurofibromatosis 2. Neurosurgery 1997;40:696–706.

4 Samii M, Matthies C: Management of 1,000 vestibular schwannomas (acoustic neuromas): hearing function in 1,000 tumor resections. Neurosurgery 1997;40:248–262.

5 Bradley WD: Clinical Manifestations of Mutations in the Neurofibromatosis Type 2 Gene in Vestibular Schwannomas (Acoustic Neuromas). Laryngoscope 1998;108:178–189.

6 Meng JJ, Lowrie DJ, Sun H, Dorsey E, Pelton PD, Bashour AM, Groden J, Ratner N, Ip W: Interaction between two isoforms of the NF2 tumor suppressor protein, merlin, and between merlin and ezrin, suggests modulation of ERM proteins by merlin. J Neurosci Res 2000;62:491–502.

7 Evans DG, Baser ME, O'Reilly B, Rowe J, Gleeson M, Saeed S, King A, Huson SM, Kerr R, Thomas N, Irving R, MacFarlane R, Ferner R, McLeod R, Moffat D, Ramsden R: Management of the patient and family with neurofibromatosis 2: a consensus conference statement. Br J Neurosur 2005;19:5–12.

8 Wiegand ME, Haid T, Goertzen W, Wolf S: Preservation of hearing in bilateral acoustic neurinomas by deliberate partial resection. Acta Otolaryngol 1992;112:237–241.

9 Neff BA, Welling DB: Current concepts in the evaluation and treatment of neurofibromatosis type II. Otolaryngol Clin North Am 2005;38:671–684.

10 Blomstedt GC, Jääskeläinen JE, Pyykkö I, Ishizaki H, Troupp H, Palva T: Recovery of sutured facial nerve after removal of acoustic neuroma in patients with neurofibromatosis-2. Neurosurg 1994;35:364–369.

11 Slattery WH III, Brackmann DE, Hitselberger W: Hearing preservation in neurofibromatosis type 2. Am J Otol 1998;18:638–643.

12 Brackmann DE, Fayad JN, Slattery WH III, Friedman RA, Day JD, Hitselberger WE, Owens RM: Early proactive management of vestibular schwannomas in neurofibromatosis type 2. Neurosurg 2001;49:274–280.

13 Gadre AK, Kwartler JA, Brackmann DE, House WF, Hitselberger WE: Middle fossa decompression of the internal auditory canal in acoustic neuroma surgery: a therapeutic alternative. Laryngoscope 1990;100:948–952.

14 Prasad D, Steiner M, Steiner L: Gamma surgery for vestibular schwannoma. J Neurosurg 2000;92:745–759.

15 Subach BR, Kondziolka D, Lunsford LD, Bissonette DJ, Flickinger JC, Maitz AH: Stereotactic radiosurgery in the management of acoustic neuromas associated with neurofibromatosis type 2. J Neurosurg 1999;90:815–822.

16 Thomsen J, Mirz F, Wetke R, Astrup J, Bojsen-Moller M, Nielsen F: Intracranial sarcoma in a patient with neurofibromatosis type 2 treated with gamma knife radiosurgery for vestibular schwannoma. Am J Otol 2000;21:364–370.

17 Lenarz T, Moshrefi M, Matthies C, Frohne C, Lesinski-Schiedat A, Illg A, Rost U, Battmer RD, Samii M: Auditory brainstem implant: part I. Auditory performance and its evolution over time. Otol Neurotol 2001;22:823–833.

18 Otto SR, Brackmann DE, Hitselberger WE, Shannon RV, Kuchta J: Multichannel auditory brainstem implant: update on performance in 61 patients. J Neurosurg 2002;96:1063–1071.

Prof. M. Samii, MD, PhD
Rudolf Pichlmayrstrasse 4
DE–30625 Hannover (Germany)
Tel. +49 511 27092 700, Fax +49 511 27092 706, E-Mail samii@ini-hannover.de

Régis J, Roche P-H (eds): Modern Management of Acoustic Neuroma.
Prog Neurol Surg. Basel, Karger, 2008, vol 21, pp 176–182

Radiosurgery for Type II Neurofibromatosis

Jeremy Rowe · Matthias Radatz · Andras Kemeny

National Centre for Stereotactic Radiosurgery, Royal Hallamshire Hospital, Sheffield, UK

Abstract

A summary of our radiosurgical experience treating type II neurofibromatosis (NF2) vestibular schwannomas (VSs), based on a retrospective consecutive series of 122 tumours in 92 patients, with an extended series of a further 22 patients (906 patient-years of follow-up) to investigate the risk of malignancy after radiosurgery. With current techniques, we estimate that 8 years after radiosurgery for NF2 VS, 20% of patients will have required further treatment, 50% will be well controlled, and in 30% there will have been some concern about control, but they will have been managed conservatively. Three years after treatment, approximately 40% retain their functional hearing, 40% have some deterioration, 20% becoming deaf in that ear. The risk of facial palsy was 5%. Two malignancies were recorded after radiosurgery, in one the malignant behaviour preceded treatment. This is less than the previously reported rate of spontaneously developing malignant gliomas in NF2. Whilst the clinical results are far worse than those achieved treating sporadic tumours, this applies equally to the results of surgery or observation when treating NF2 tumours. It is important therefore that these patients are given advice specific for NF2. Considering this, we believe that radiosurgery remains a valuable minimally invasive treatment option for selected NF2 patients.

The continuing debate about the management of type II neurofibromatosis (NF2) vestibular schwannomas (VSs) reflects that there is no ideal treatment option for this condition [1]. The limitation of observation and a conservative management policy is that the natural history of NF2 is well known: these patients go deaf with tumours which present earlier and grow more rapidly than their sporadic counterparts. The limitations of surgery are reflected by the increasing emphasis placed on conservative management strategies, deferring operative interventions and the morbidity that may result [1]. In contrast, stereotactic radiosurgery is attractive in offering active management whilst being minimally invasive. That is not to say, however, that radiosurgery is without potential risks or complications. Indeed, both the Marseille radiosurgical group and our own have held the view that radiosurgery is less effective in treating NF2 VS compared with unilateral sporadic tumours [2, 3], although the same can be said for surgical excision. Furthermore, there is concern about irradiating a condition with abnormal tumour suppressor genes, and whether this can cause malignancy. In this paper, we review our experience treating NF2 and summarise how this experience influences the advice and guidance we offer these patients.

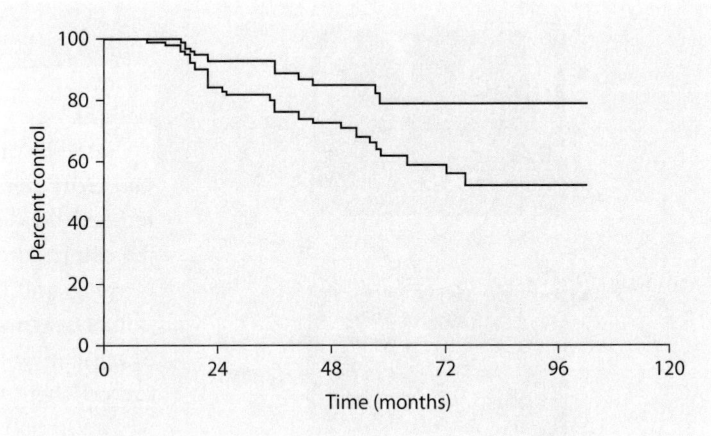

Fig. 1. Kaplan-Meier plots illustrating the rate at which salvage procedures are taken after radiosurgery (21% at 8 years, or 79% controlled) and recalculated defining a loss of control by the need for further therapy or radiological growth or any clinical concern of symptom progression (52% controlled at 8 years).

Methods

Patient Details

This review is based on two overlapping series of patients. From 1986 to December 2000, 123 radiosurgery treatments were undertaken for 122 VSs in 96 patients with an established diagnosis of NF2. The patients had an equal sex distribution, a mean age at presentation of 24.1 (11.1) years and a mean age at treatment of 28.9 (11.6) years. Twenty-seven of the 96 patients (28%) fulfilled the criteria of early presentation, multiple intracranial tumours other than VS and spinal disease for the severe Wishart phenotype of NF2. Of the 122 tumours, radiosurgery was performed as the initial treatment in 97, 20 having undergone one previous resection and five multiple operations. Ninety-two of the tumours were treated from 1993 onwards using MRI localisation, modern planning software allowing the use of multiple isocentres to generate conformal plans and prescribing a mean marginal dose of 13.4 (1.6) Gy, this effectively reflecting our current practice. Results of tumour control, hearing preservation and cranial nerve complications are based on this 'current practice' material.

In addition, we have clinical information on a further 22 patients with NF2, treated variously for an additional 24 VSs (from 2001 to 2004), for 23 meningiomas, and four trigeminal neuromas. Overall, this totals 118 patients treated with radiosurgery or a total of 906 patient-years of follow-up from first radiosurgical treatment. The mean age at first treatment for this extended series is 32.0 (14.0) years. These patients were cross-referenced against national mortality and cancer databases to investigate the long-term risk of malignant neoplasms [4].

Patient Assessment, Follow-Up and Analysis

Clinical, radiological and audiometric examinations were reviewed. Tumour control was defined both by the need for further therapeutic intervention (surgery in all but one instance), and when there was any clinical or radiological concern about symptom progression or tumour growth. Control rates were calculated from Kaplan-Meier plots. Hearing preservation was defined as a change in Gardner-Robertson hearing grade estimated on average more than 3 years after radiosurgery. In addition, pure tone audiogram thresholds were used. Adverse changes in facial and trigeminal nerve function were recorded. New intracranial malignancies reported after the radiosurgery were recorded. A regression analysis was performed investigating factors determining tumour control. Comparisons use t and χ^2 tests as appropriate. Values are expressed as mean (SD).

Results

Based on a Kaplan-Meier plot of the rate of surgical intervention after radiosurgery (fig. 1), 8 years after radiosurgery 21% of patients will have required further treatment for their VSs. If this plot is recalculated combining those patients undergoing further treatment with those whose imaging shows tumour growth, and those with increasing symptoms possibly attributed to a growing VS, the control rate falls to 52% at 8 years. These results are generated from the 92

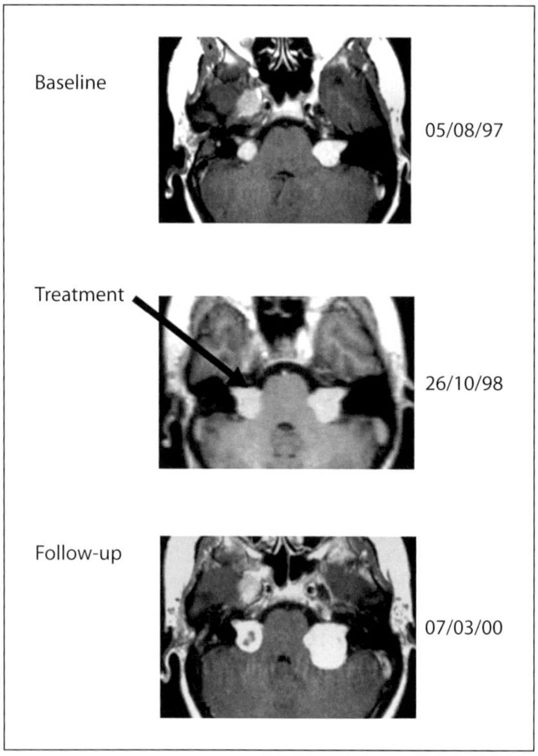

Fig. 2. An illustration of the efficacy of radiosurgery in NF2. Between diagnosis (August 1997) and treatment (October 1998) both VSs are growing. After radiosurgery to the right side, it shrinks with central signal change, whilst the opposite side continues to grow. Analysing all patients with untreated contralateral tumours, radiosurgery significantly decreases growth compared with the opposite side.

'current practice' tumours treated since 2003, but are not statistically different from the overall population. Examining individuals with an untreated contralateral VS acting as an internal control (fig. 2), radiosurgery statistically decreases growth relative to the contralateral side ($p < 0.01$) [3].

Analysing growth control in terms of patient and treatment variables, shows that tumour volume at the time of treatment is the most significant determinant of outcome ($p < 0.001$). If only tumours of 10 cm^3 volume or less were treated, this would encompass 94–96% of patients who had good clinical outcomes (defined as tumour control for at least 5 years) [5]. There is also a tendency for the more severe phenotypes to fare less well [5].

Patterns of hearing preservation or loss vary markedly between individuals. We have documented rapid and more gradual declines in hearing after radiosurgery, exceptionally recovery of hearing, and we have also documented preservation of hearing in excess of 10 years. Overall, 23 of 61 patients with hearing before radiosurgery preserved their Gardner-Robertson grades (38%), whilst 26 had some decrease in grade (42%), 12 patients becoming totally deaf. Examination of pure-tone audiograms showed hearing deterioration before radiosurgery, but this is expected as hearing loss was a factor precipitating treatment in 34% of the patients.

Persisting facial nerve weakness after radiosurgery occurred in 5% of patients and, excluding individuals with trigeminal neuromas, 2% developed trigeminal neuropathy.

In the extended series of 118 NF2 patients, comprising 906 patient-years of follow-up, two new intracranial malignancies were recorded after radiosurgery. One of these was a tumour previously described in detail, with atypical rapid growth before radiosurgery, the growth continuing after treatment and at subsequent surgery the histology was malignant [6]. The second case was a patient who developed a malignant glioma 3 years after radiosurgery for a VS.

Discussion

In advising NF2 patients, perhaps the most fundamental point to make is that whilst the histology may be the same as for unilateral sporadic VS, this is a very different disease entity. Simple comparisons and extrapolations based on experience largely with sporadic tumours should not be made. We would regard all treatment options: observation and conservative management, microsurgery, and radiation treatments as being less effective treating NF2 VS compared with sporadic tumours. Whilst surgical excision may be a major but attractive undertaking for some patients with sporadic tumours, hopefully curing the individual, NF2 is not curable: these individuals develop further tumours in time. Furthermore, with multiple tumours and multiple treatments, the morbidity faced by NF2 patients is very much greater. Additionally, past experiences with other tumours or treatments, or with other family members undergoing treatment, may influence the way that an individual with NF2 perceives the balance of risk and benefit of different treatment options. For these reasons, we believe that it is essential that patients are given advice specific for NF2, and that generalisations and results based on series and experiences treating largely sporadic tumours, are not simply applied. Indeed, given the complexity of the problems faced by these individuals, ideally they should be seen or at least have access to a specialist multi-disciplinary NF2 clinic [1].

Tumour Control

Appreciation of the complexity of this is reflected in the way that we have chosen to report tumour control rates. The simplest measure of tumour control, or the loss of it, is the rate at which salvage surgical resection is undertaken after radiosurgery. This is what patients ask: after all they undergo radiosurgery with the specific aim of avoiding surgery. As a measure, it is attractive as surgery is a discreet and definite event, and therefore it can be answered precisely: in our material 79% of patients avoided surgery for at least 8 years.

This however, is simplistic. Whilst surgery is a clear event, the decision to undergo it is anything but and, in practice, there may be significant reticence on the part of the patient and the surgeon with regard to undertaking it. An extreme example of this was afforded by one of our early patients dying of pneumonia 14 months after radiosurgery. Factors in his death included his end-stage NF2 condition, hypostasis from paraparesis and spinal disease, and concern about growing infra- and supra-tentorial tumours. With decreasing treatment options, he withdrew from radiological follow-up and neurosurgical review, there being no record of his bulbar function. In essence, it is not clear whether the radiosurgery controlled the tumour for the rest of his natural life or whether there was increasing tumour growth contributing to his deteriorating state. To express this, we recalculated the Kaplan-Meier plots, but included as uncensored observations, not only patients undergoing surgery, but in whom there was any concern about tumour control. This offers a best and worst case scenario. We would summarise this as saying that with current doses within eight years of radiosurgery we would estimate that approximately 20% of NF2 patients will have undergone surgery, 50% will have well controlled tumours and in 30% there may have been variable concerns about tumour control, but they will have continued to be managed conservatively.

Time limits are important, not only to reflect our experience with current treatment protocols, but because we have seen tumour growth 12 years after apparently successful radiosurgery. Whether this is tumour recurrence or a new lesion arising is debatable, but the implication is clearly that long-term follow-up and radiological surveillance of NF2 is required.

Hearing

The main problem in advising patients about hearing preservation is that individual responses are highly variable. We have seen long-term hearing preservation 10–12 years after radiosurgery, and exceptionally have seen hearing recovery, although our view and advice to patients is that hearing once lost is never expected to recover. Overall, we summarise our findings as estimating that approximately 40% of patients will retain their functional hearing grade, meaning that if they have speech discrimination before, they will retain it after treatment, whilst 40% of patients have some loss in hearing and 20% go completely deaf. The mean time interval after treatment for these estimations was in excess of 3 years.

Patient and Tumour Selection

The major factors in deciding to treat a VS are tumour growth and the size of the tumours and the hearing in both ears. If a tumour is not growing, there is no clear indication for radiosurgery, although in NF2 this is rare. Even with limited follow-up, 75–79% of NF2 VSs are actively growing [3]. The timing of radiosurgery is further influenced by tumour size. Given that approximately 95% of good results (defined as tumour control for 5 years or more) are achieved treating tumours of 10 cm^3 or less, we are very reluctant to consider tumours larger than this. If a patient presented with asymmetrical tumours, one larger than 10 cm^3 we might very well suggest surgery on the first side, possibly with consideration of an auditory brain stem implant.

With bilateral tumours, we would treat the larger side with generally the worst hearing first, and would consider treatment on the second side only after an interval when the results of hearing preservation or hearing loss were known on the first side. We would also actively encourage these patients to learn how to lip read whilst they still had useful hearing, before undergoing sequential treatments. Whilst previously bilateral VS treatments with radiosurgery on a single day were performed, we no longer offer this, and prefer stage treatment. This partly reflects the risk of irradiating the brainstem by treating tumours on either side of it (although no patient so treated developed a brainstem radiation reaction), and partly the uncertainty of what we are achieving with regard to hearing preservation in any individual.

Other Complications

With regard to cranial nerve palsies, 5% of the NF2 patients treated with the current dose protocol and methodology developed persisting facial nerve palsies, considerably higher than our experience with unilateral VS. Excluding patients with trigeminal neuromas, the trigeminal neuropathy rate was 2%, more in keeping with the sporadic VS experience.

The other complication of major concern is that of radiation causing further neoplastic complications. This could be by inducing a malignant transformation in a pre-existing tumour or by inducing a new tumour. Most of the literature has concerned the former, although applying a two-hit hypothesis where an individual inherits one abnormal tumour suppressor gene, but requires a mutation in a corresponding healthy allele to generate tumours, the formation of new tumours may be of concern.

In an effort to address the risk of malignancy after radiosurgery, we recently cross-referenced our UK patient database against national cancer and mortality registries [4]. Treating 118 NF2 patients with over 900 patient years of follow-up, we detected two malignant tumours. One was well known to the Department, the malignant behaviour probably pre-dating the radiosurgery [6]. The second case was of a glioma not evident on scans 3 years earlier when radiosurgery for a VS was performed. The problem with this material is the lack of an adequate control group. In an attempted review of the UK NF2 population, the risk of a malignant glioma was put at 4% with an average patient life expectancy that was less than we are achieving in the patients treated with radiosurgery [4]. Whilst we would not wish to underestimate the risks of radiosurgery, these data are reassuring in that despite the size and follow-up of this series, we are not seeing an increased risk of malignancy. In practice, patients seeking a radiosurgical opinion have their own views on the safety and acceptability not only of radiosurgery, but of the other treatment modalities, principally that of surgical resection.

Treatment Options

The principal active treatment option in the management of NF2 VS is surgical resection. Comparisons are difficult as clearly this is a very different undertaking. In its favour, surgery recreates space in the posterior fossa, hence the emphasis placed on surgery for larger tumours. Furthermore, surgery can be combined with an auditory brainstem implant to augment hearing, although such a strategy will not currently restore speech discrimination.

Against surgery is not only the morbidity associated with precipitated hearing loss or facial nerve damage, but also mortality. Even the largest series, that of Samii, described 82 patients, 2 of whom died [7]. Reviewing our own series, not only were all of the documented deaths due to the consequences of NF2, but 20% were directly related to neurosurgical complications. This is not to say that the neurosurgery was ill-considered. In the later stages of the disease, when options are limited it can be hard to deny a neurosurgical operation to a patient with benign tumours, although they may not do well as a result. Such experiences may however colour the view that NF2 patients have of neurosurgery.

The other active treatment option to consider is that of fractionated stereotactic radiotherapy. Conceptually, this may be attractive as fractionating a course of treatment might be kinder to the cochlear nerve, yielding better hearing preservation. In practice, the evidence for this in the context of unilateral sporadic VS is lacking, and there are no major series using fractionation for NF2. There is also the concern that fractionation may be less effective for benign tumours. Furthermore, a fractionated treatment may increase the likelihood of genetic mutations without cell death increasing the long-term risk of secondary neoplasms. For these reasons, we are not currently fractionating VS treatments for sporadic or NF2 tumours.

Conclusions

All treatment options are less effective in managing NF2 VS compared with unilateral sporadic tumours. This, combined with the morbidity of multiple tumours and treatments, makes it essential that patients are given advice specific for NF2. Currently, we estimate that 8 years after radiosurgery for NF2 VS, 20% of patients will have required further treatment, 50% will be well controlled, and that in 30% there will have been some concern about control but that they will have been managed conservatively. Three years after radiosurgery, we estimate that 40% of patients will retain their hearing grade, 40% have some deterioration, 20% becoming deaf in that ear. We put the risk of facial paresis at 5%. Tumour size is the most important factor in determining outcome, and we are reluctant to treat tumours larger than 10 cm^3. The risk of malignancy remains a concern, although with 900 patient-years of follow-up, we are not identifying an increased risk. We continue to offer radiosurgery to selected NF2 patients because, considering the therapeutic options and the dilemmas faced by these individuals, we believe it a valuable, minimally invasive, alternative management strategy.

References

1 Evans DGR, Baser ME, O'Reilly B, et al: Management of the patient and family with neurofibromatosis 2: a consensus conference statement. Br J Neurosurg 2005;19:5–12.

2 Roche PH, Regis J, Pellet W, et al: Neurofibromatosis type 2. Preliminary results of gamma knife radiosurgery of vestibular schwannomas. Neurochirugie 2000;46:339–353.

3 Rowe JG, Radatz MWR, Walton L, Soanes T, Rodgers J, Kemeny AA: Clinical experience with Gamma Knife stereotactic radiosurgery in the management of vestibular schwannomas secondary to type 2 neurofibromatosis. JNNP 2003;74:1288–1293.

4 Rowe J, Grainger A, Walton L, et al: Safety of radiosurgery applied to conditions with abnormal tumor suppressor genes. Neurosurgery 2007;60:860–864.

5 Rowe JG, Radatz MWR, Walton L, Kemeny AA: Stereotactic radiosurgery for type 2 neurofibromatosis acoustic neuromas: patient selection and tumour size. J Funct Stereotact Neurosurg 2002;79:107–116.

6 Bari M, Forster D, Kemeny A, Walton L, Hardy D, Anderson J: Malignancy in a vestibular schwannoma. Report of a case with central neurofibromatosis treated by stereotactic radiosurgery and surgical excision with a review of the literature. Br J Neurosurg 2002;16:284–289.

7 Samii M, Matthies C, Tatagiba M: Management of vestibular schwannomas (acoustic neuromas): auditory and facial nerve function after resection of 120 vestibular schwannomas in patients with neurofibromatosis 2. Neurosurgery 1997;40:696–706.

Jeremy Rowe
National Centre for Stereotactic Radiosurgery, Royal Hallamshire Hospital
Glossop Road
Sheffield S10 2JF (UK)
Tel. +44 114 271 3572, Fax +44 114 275 4930, E-Mail Jeremy.Rowe@sth.nhs.uk

Régis J, Roche P-H (eds): Modern Management of Acoustic Neuroma.
Prog Neurol Surg. Basel, Karger, 2008, vol 21, pp 183–191

Microsurgical Treatment of Intracanalicular Vestibular Schwannomas

R. Noudel[a] · T. Ribeiro[b] · P.-H. Roche[b]

[a]Department of Neurosurgery, Maison Blanche Hospital, University of Reims, Reims,
[b]Department of Neurosurgery, Sainte Marguerite Hospital, University of Marseille, Marseille, France

Abstract

Early treatment of intracanalicular vestibular schwannomas (IVSs) may be advisable because their spontaneous course will show hearing loss in most cases. Advanced microsurgical techniques and continuous intraoperative monitoring of cranial nerves may allow hearing preservation (HP) without facial nerve damage. However, there are still controversies about the definition of HP and the best surgical approach that should be used. In this study, we reviewed the main data from the recent literature on IVS surgery and compared hearing, facial function and complication rates after the retrosigmoid and middle fossa approaches, respectively. The results showed that the average HP rate is approximately 45% after IVS surgery whatever the surgical route. HP varied widely depending on the audiometric criteria that were used for definition of serviceable hearing. There was a trend to show that middle fossa approach offered a better quality of postoperative hearing (not statistically significant), whereas the retrosigmoid approach offered a better facial nerve preservation and fewer complications (not statistically significant). We believe that the timing of treatment in the course of the disease and selection between radiosurgical versus microsurgical procedure are key issues in the management of IVS. Once open surgery has been decided, selection of the approach mainly depends on individual anatomical considerations and experience of the surgeon.

Incidence of vestibular schwannomas (VSs) in the general population was estimated at 9 per million and per year and intracanalicular VSs (IVSs) had been reported with a 0.32% rate in a total of 615 consecutively diagnosed VSs [1]. Routine use of gadolinium-enhanced MRI for the evaluation of patients with asymmetric hearing loss has led to an increasing tendency to diagnose small VSs that are amenable to hearing preservation (HP) surgery [2, 3]. Samii et al. [4] have reported 16 IVSs (2.7%) among 600 patients with VS consecutively operated on. Early detection of IVS raises the issue of whether or not treatment is required and, if so, whether surgical removal is the most appropriate treatment [3, 5]. IVS is not a life-threatening disease. The rationale for treatment is the likelihood of hearing loss and the potential growth to a high surgical risk size: therefore, to be justified, any treatment should provide better results than the expected risks of a conservative attitude [6].

In recent years, great advances in neuroimaging, intraoperative cranial nerve monitoring and microsurgical techniques have shifted the focus of VS surgery from prolonging life to preserving cranial nerve function [7], especially for small tumors. If preservation of serviceable binaural hearing is an objective in the management of IVS, early surgery should be considered to prevent progressive or sudden hearing loss and tumor progression to a size that would increase risks

Table 1. Review of the literature on HP or serviceable HP (SHP), facial nerve function preservation rates (FP; H-B grades 1 and 2) and postoperative complications via the RS approach for IVS removal

First author	Cases	HP and SHP rates, %	FP rates, %	Complications
Samii, 1991	14	57, HP 40, SHP	100	CSF leak (NR) 14% residual tinnitus
Cohen, 1993	21	33, SHP	100	
Samii, 1997	37	51, HP	94	
Rowed, 1997	26	50, SHP	96	
Irving, 1998	17	12, SHP	88	
Staecker, 2000	15	47, SHP	93	CSF leak, 27% headaches, 46%
Coletti, 2005	35	57, SHP	91	CSF leak, 9% brain edema, 17% headache, 9%
Samii, 2006	22	57, SHP	90	

NR = Not reported

related to surgical removal, particularly with respect to facial nerve function. Surgical approaches that permit HP include the retrosigmoid (RS) and the middle fossa (MF) approaches [3, 5]. The selection of the optimal surgical approach for the treatment and the indications for performing HP surgery still remain a matter of debate. The goal of the present study was to compare the results obtained after microsurgical removal of IVS within the medical literature in terms of quality of resection, HP, facial nerve function outcome and postoperative complications according to surgical routes.

Materials and Methods

The published data about the functional results and postoperative complications after microsurgical removal of IVS were reviewed. We selected the main series that were reported in the last 20 years. We eliminated the series recording the data from less than 10 patients. Audiologic measurements included pure tone average (PTA) and word recognition score (WRS) determined pre- and postoperatively. Criteria used for definition of serviceable or useful hearing which are in agreement with most large series included a PTA of less than 50 dB and a WRS greater than 50% [8, 9]. Facial nerve outcome was determined by the House and Brackmann (H-B) grading system [10]. Normal or near-normal function corresponded to grades 1 and 2. Additional outcome measures included postoperative cerebrospinal fluid (CSF) leaks, postoperative headaches, epileptic seizures and persistent otological signs.

Results

The results obtained after RS and MF approaches are summarized in tables 1 and 2, respectively. The main parameters of interest were the rates of functional HP and good facial function. HP rates for the MF and RS approaches range from 38 to 66% and 12 to 57%, respectively, but analysis of the results does not show a statistically significant difference in favor of either approach. Good

Table 2. Review of the literature on SHP, FP (normal or near normal function) and postoperative complications via the MF approach for IVS removal

First author	Cases	SHP rates, %	FP rates, %	Complications
Brackmann, 1979	11	45	73	gait disturbances, 36%
Gantz, 1986	16	38	82	
Cannoni, 1989	13	46	NR	
Brackmann, 1994	19	63	92	
Irving, 1998	25	44	72	
Staecker, 2000	15	57	93	CSF leak, 20% headaches, 16%
Satar, 2003 (meta-analysis)	209	60	98.9 (for 189 cases)	
Coletti, 2005	35	66	77	brain edema, 14% headache, 3% extradural hematoma, 6%

NR = Not reported

facial nerve function (grades 1 and 2) at late evaluation (1 year postoperatively) is reported in 88–100% of patients operated on via the RS route and in 72–98.9% in cases of MF approach and does not show any statistical advantage in favor of either surgical route.

Discussion

Diagnostic Considerations

VSs are mainly revealed by gradual increasing symptoms with insidious asymmetrical hearing loss followed by tinnitus and vertigo (+/– severe vertiginous ataxia) or one or several incidences of acute hearing loss, with or without remission [3, 4]. In cases of IVS, clinical presentation is markedly different from other VSs. In the series of Samii et al. [4] the diagnostic delay is shorter and the severity of hearing loss is considerable, given the tiny size of the tumor (2 patients deaf and 7 patients with bad hearing among 16 patients with IVS). In the affected side of 156 patients with IVS, Caye-Thomasen et al. [3] reported at diagnosis a hearing loss significantly higher than in the contralateral ear, with a mean PTA of 51dB and a mean WRS of 60%. However, 45% of those patients had AAO-HNS class A or B at the time of diagnosis. Vestibular signs appear early and as frequently as cochlear signs, in contrast to larger VSs where incidence of vestibular signs is 40–60%.

Radiologically, on the bone window CT scans, different stages of internal auditory canal (IAC) enlargement can be described: initially, a bulb-like deformation appears in the middle of the canal because the nidus of the tumor starts growing at the neuroglia-Schwann cells interface that is located further distal in the IAC for the vestibular nerve than for the cochlear portion. Then, the enlargement of the mid-portion and the fundus of the IAC lead to a bud type feature. Later in the evolution, if silent, further enlargement of the canal develops at the porus and forms the funnel type [4, 11].

Natural History of Intracanalicular Vestibular Schwannomas

Most VSs show growth during long-term follow-up review: variable growth rates have been reported with a mean of 0.1–0.2 cm per year [12]. The very limited available information about the natural history of untreated IVSs suggests that about 50% of patients with serviceable hearing at the time of diagnosis of an IVS will show progressive hearing deterioration and will loose serviceable hearing over the next 2 years [3, 13]. Caye-Thomasen et al. [3] who examined prospectively the spontaneous course of 156 patients with IVS found that 43% of the tumors had increased at a mean follow-up of 4.6 years, with a relative growth rate of 46% per year. In their study, the PTA deterioration rate correlated positively with the mean absolute growth rate, but the risk of hearing loss was not related either to diagnostic sublocalization (fundus, central, porus), size of the tumor at diagnosis, or the tumor-induced expansion of the IAC. These findings suggest that tumor pressure on the cochlear nerve induces the hearing loss but other mechanisms such vascular compromise, abnormal inner ear fluid composition and cochlear hair cell loss may also be implicated [14]. Since tumor growth and initial hearing level are the only predictive factors of hearing loss, clinical and radiological observation is the only way to decide whether to treat or not.

General Considerations about Treatment

Goals of Surgery

Hearing loss in a typical middle-aged VS patient can lead to significant physical and psychosocial dysfunction. The goals of VS surgery should be total tumor removal and preservation of neuro-otological functions, especially facial nerve function and hearing level, which are both the most important predictors of quality of life [15]. In cases of VS confined to the IAC, these goals are more likely to be achieved, thanks to technical refinements in the operative evoked potential recording and in microsurgical procedure [4].

Considering that it is of benefit to preserve serviceable binaural hearing, early treatment may be advisable since hearing loss may frequently occur in the 5 years after diagnosis of IVS [3, 5, 16]. In addition, some authors have suggested that surgeons should try to save hearing in any patient who displays some degree of measurable hearing before surgery regardless of tumor size [17, 18] but this recommendation remains controversial. Supporters of the early proactive treatment of VS consider that the smaller the VS is, the easier and safer will be its surgery as well its postoperative course. Caye-Thomasen et al. [3] suggest that HP treatment should be applied to patients with good hearing in the nontumor ear and a speech discrimination score (SDS) in the tumor ear >70%, or in case of poor hearing in the nontumor ear, patients with an SDS >50%; based on these criteria, 33% of the patients were eligible for HP treatment at diagnosis in their study.

Hearing Preservation in Intracanalicular Vestibular Schwannoma Surgery. The initial cases of HP after surgical removal of VS were reported by Elliot and McKissock [19]. During the 1960s, House [20] developed the MF approach to the IAC and was able to preserve hearing in a few intracanalicular tumors. In the mid- to late 1970s, a new interest in HP was raised by neurosurgeons employing the RS transmeatal route [17, 21]. Since 1985, overall results have improved steadily and HP in unilateral VS has increasingly been documented [9, 22, 23]. Global HP in operated VS varies from 12 to 66% [24–28].

There is some flow remaining in the analysis of HP since there is no agreement about what constitutes serviceable or useful hearing. Some authors consider preservation of any hearing a success, whereas others used different audiometric parameters to define serviceable hearing: in most studies, the threshold for serviceable hearing is a PTA <50 dB and an SDS >50% [8, 9] but Samii and Matthies [4] define useful hearing as a PTA

<40 dB and an SDS >70%. There is no consensus about the selection criteria for a patient to undergo HP, grading and postoperative hearing results as well as what defines preserved hearing [15]. The most helpful criteria are given by Gardner and Robertson [8] because both PTA and SDS are considered and the classification used is that indicated by the worst of these 2 measurements. Preserved hearing is achieved when the patient keeps 'serviceable' (Gardner and Robertson 1 or 2, class A or B AAO-HNS) hearing postoperatively [6].

The MF approach has been thought to provide better results of HP than the RS approach but analysis of the results previously reported shows that outcome with respect to preservation of serviceable hearing does not statistically differ as a result of using either the posterior or the MF surgical approaches (tables 1 and 2). More than the selected approach, tumor size and preoperative hearing status are the main predictors of success rate in preserving VIIIth cranial nerve function [29, 30].

The potential for HP is inversely related to the size of the tumor. Haines and Levine [6] reported an HP rate of 82% among 11 patients operated on for IVS, compared to 33–50% HP rates regardless of the tumor size. In another study [15], patients with intracanalicular or 11- to 25-mm tumor had better results with a 33% rate of serviceable HP than larger tumors that were associated with a 12.5% rate of serviceable HP. Therefore, some authors have suggested that attempts to preserve hearing should only be done in VSs less than 20 mm in maximal diameter [31, 32]. According to Mohr et al. [11], the critical 'cut-off' size for serviceable HP treatment is an extrameatal diameter of 15 mm. Cohen et al. [33] found that a maximum IVS diameter of 7 mm was associated with significantly greater likelihood of serviceable postoperative HP. The strong correlation between the tumor size and the immediate postoperative hearing was also confirmed by Post et al. [26]: the HP rate decreased from 83% with small tumors of less than 1 cm to 52% with tumors of less than 2 cm. In the meta-analysis conducted by Satar et al. [28], HP rate for 209 IVSs operated on via an MF route reached 56.5% and was significantly higher than for larger tumors with more than 1 mm of extracanalicular extension. Paradoxically, in several series of Samii et al. [4, 34, 35] the HP associated with IVSs (51 to 57%) operated on via the RS approach were not better and even less favorable than those associated with small VSs (grade 2) that displayed both intra- and extracanalicular portions (56–58%).

Therefore, in some cases of IVS, the HP rate also depends on the level of preoperative hearing. In cases of a good preoperative hearing, HP rates may reach an average of 60% while the chances of saving or improving hearing are poor if only measurable hearing is present preoperatively [4, 26–28, 36, 37]. In addition, short duration of hearing loss preoperatively might signify slight alterations of the cochlear nerve and better postoperative results. Samii [34] found that a <1.5 years' duration of hypoacousia was a good predictor of HP.

Tumor size and preoperative hearing level, however, are not the only predictors of HP. Individual surgical experience plays a significant role in the postoperative HP rate, as commented by authors that compared their results in two consecutive groups of patients [35].

The influence of monitoring cochlear nerve auditory evoked potentials (CNAP) or brain stem auditory evoked potentials (BAEPs) on HP is controversial. Continuous intraoperative monitoring of the CNAP, with or without BAEPs, did not prevent loss of serviceable hearing in half of the patients with intracanalicular tumors either in the series of Rowed [5], or Cohen et al. [33]. Conversely, other authors reported a better outcome for patients with preserved intraoperative CNAPs [4, 15, 26] or suggested that BAEPs would be helpful if surgery was momentarily stopped at the time where intraoperative changes of either latency or amplitude were noted [26]. Therefore, delayed hearing loss despite preserved BAEPs and maintenance of anatomical continuity of the VIIIth nerve probably occurs as a result of traction of the myelin sheath or ischemia affecting the cochlea or cochlear nerve by injury to the labyrinthine artery [38].

The rate of HP also varies according to the length of the postoperative follow-up [29]. Patients with intact postoperative hearing may subsequently experience hearing decline. In the series of Shelton et al. [32], as many as 56% of patients were found to experience a decline in hearing quality with a follow-up of 8–20 years. Such valuable long-term data are usually not given in the surgical series.

Anatomical considerations brought by radiological analysis and operative findings have been reported as predictive factors of HP. Superior vestibular nerve tumors may be associated with a better outcome probably because they invade the cochlear nerve at a later stage than inferior vestibular nerve tumors [27]. Involvement of the fundus of the IAC is considered as an unfavorable feature [11]. Elevation of pressure within the IAC due to intracanalicular extension may increase the vulnerability of the already compromised nerve and its tiny vasculature within the IAC during drilling and dissection, decreasing the likelihood of HP [39]. In addition, the lack of CSF space between the tumor and the fundus constitutes a surgical challenge: exposure of the entire fundus may violate the labyrinth in the absence of exact anatomical landmarks to identify the posterior semicircular canal and the crus commune, but overheating and vibration damage contributes to hearing loss. Consistency of the tumor is not an important factor [4, 26]. Moriyama et al. [40] have shown that adhesion between the tumor and cochlear nerve may influence the functional results.

Hearing results should not only consider the postoperative hearing levels in the operated ear but should also take into account the hearing levels in the opposite ear. According to Jaisinghani [15], cases of preserved hearing are patients who have measurable hearing in the operated ear postoperatively, which can be improved with a hearing aid and with contralateral good function. In small tumors, there is little difference in the outcome of HP attempts between familial and sporadic tumors, though it has been generally believed that HP is more difficult in patients with NF2 [41].

Facial Nerve Function Preservation. Pre- and postoperative facial nerve function is normal or almost normal (H-B grades 1 and 2) in most cases of the surgically treated IVS [4–6, 18, 26, 27, 36]. A recent meta-analysis of surgical series suggested a statistical significant advantage for the RS approach in regard to facial nerve outcome ($p = 0.05$) [5]. Irving et al. [27] showed that there was an increased incidence of transient facial palsy in patients who underwent surgery via the MF route, but the results at 1 year were equal between the 2 surgical approaches. Coletti and Fiorino [30] also demonstrated better results of facial nerve function with the RS approach, with a statistical significant difference ($p < 0.05$) only in the immediate postoperative period; at 1 year, the rate of patients with good facial function (grades 1 and 2) was still superior in the RS group (91%) than in the MF group (77%) but the difference was not statistically significant. The MF approach requires greater manipulation of the nerve for tumor access and removal. Thereby, a neuropraxic injury is possible and may explain more transient deficits.

A very tight relationship was reported between the VIIth cranial nerve preoperative condition and the clinical result as reflected by facial function [39]. Such statistically significant correlation was also found to exist between the postoperative facial function and the tumor size that is the main predictor of facial nerve preservation [35, 38].

Extent of Resection. One of the major arguments against HP attempts is that they will lead to limited resection and increase the rate of recurrences. Actually, most series report a complete surgical removal of IVS whatever the surgical approach with no recurrences at long-term follow-up [4, 26, 35].

Results According to Surgical Approach

As the translabyrinthine and transotic approaches destroy hearing, only the middle and posterior fossa approaches must be compared because only these offer the opportunity of preserving both facial and cochlear functions that are the main goals of IVS surgery [4, 28, 30, 42]. In selecting an approach for IVS, tumor size plays an important role, in association with factors such as preoperative hearing level and facial function, extension of the tumor toward the porus or the fundus. However, in most cases, the choice is based on the surgeon's experience and preferences [30, 35]. Otologists prefer the MF approach [8, 20, 28, 31, 42–44] whereas neurosurgeons generally perform the RS approach [4, 11, 24, 34, 35].

The MF approach has been described as the best technique in terms of auditory results [4, 15, 20, 42], probably because the cochlear nerve is more remote and therefore protected from inadvertent manipulation when the IAC is approached from above rather than from behind [6]. However, few retrospective studies [5, 27, 38, 45] have directly compared hearing results with the MF and RS approach and suggested a better chance of HP or improving slightly using the MF approach than the RS route, but the differences were not statistically significant. The prospective and randomized study conducted by Coletti and Fiorino [30] also failed to show any significant difference in auditory results between the 2 techniques, except for tumors reaching the fundus: when the distance from the IAC fundus was 3 mm or less, the MF approach afforded a significantly higher HP rate (60%) than the RS route (44%). Indeed, the RS approach is associated with greater risk of injury to the cochlear nerve, because exposure of the lateral end (the last 4 mm) of the IAC is limited by potential damage of the posterior semicircular canal [5], leading to cerebellar retraction that may cause traction of the nerve, especially at the level of the mechanically weak Obersteiner-Redlich zone [46]. These difficulties may also result in an incomplete tumor resection. However, visual access to the inside of the IAC via the RS approach can be gained by using an endoscope. The MF approach affords easy access and better exposure to the fundus of the IAC and avoidance of cerebellar retraction. In the MF operation, a direct approach to the IAC allows exposure of the medial portion first reducing the risk to the inner ear: this results in less traction on the distal end of the VIIIth nerve at its weak point and on the distal labyrinthine artery at its foraminal end. In this approach, drilling of the IAC is conducted via an epidural way with no bone dust in direct contact with the nerves and vessels. In the series of Staecker et al. [38] the cochlear nerve was anatomically preserved at similar rates in the MF and RS groups but HP was better in the MF group (not statistically significant; tables 1 and 2): this would support the hypothesis that either vascular damage or mechanical intraneural disruption is the cause of poor hearing outcome.

On the other hand, supporters of the RS approach advocate better visualization of the brain stem structures and ability to remove tumors of all sizes with greater ease of medial to lateral dissection [4, 35, 39]: in the study of Coletti and Fiorino [30], HP was significantly better with the RS approach when the IAC enlargement was greater than 7 mm. In addition, vestibular and facial functions are thought to be more vulnerable with the MF approach, especially in the early postoperative period [4, 5, 30, 40, 43, 44, 47–49]: transient facial palsy is significantly higher with the MF route [27, 30]. In addition, temporal lobe retraction, even staying epidural in the MF approach is at risk of neurological deficits and seizures. The incidence of postoperative headaches is higher with the RS approach, while CSF leak and persistent otological signs are reported with variable rates in the literature [4, 15, 27, 35, 38, 44].

Schematically, it has been suggested that the MF approach should be reserved for tumors that reach the fundus of the IAC with good preoperative levels, whereas the RS approach is more suitable for medially based tumors extending to the cerebellopontine angle with poor preoperative hearing levels [3, 15, 38].

Conclusion

In selected cases of intracanalicular VS, microsurgical treatment may remain an option where the goals are tumor resection, hearing and facial nerve preservation with no complications. By following operative guidelines of microsurgical techniques with intraoperative monitoring of the cochlear and facial nerves, HP can be achieved in a high percentage of patients, whatever the surgical route. Taking into account the respective advantages of the MF and the RS approach, there is no prospective randomized study that indicates better results with one of them. However, in tumors reaching the IAC fundus the MF approach may provide better HP. This surgery should be discussed in a case by case manner by a multidisciplinary team who can propose all therapeutic options, including radiosurgery. Taken collectively, the following parameters: young age, small tumor size, lack of extension to the fundus, normal shape of the IAC, excellent preoperative hearing with good ABR, are good predictors of a successful microsurgical treatment but also of radiosurgery, which is a less invasive option.

References

1 Tos M, Thomsen J, Charabi S: Epidemiology of acoustic neuromas: has the incidence increased during the last years? in Tos M, Thomsen J (eds): Acoustic Neuroma. Proceedings of the First International Conference on Acoustic Neuroma. Copenhagen, Denmark, August 25–29, 1991. Amsterdam, Kugler, 1992, pp 3–6.
2 Strangerup SE, Tos M, Caye-Thomasen P, Tos T, Klokker M, Thomsen J: Increasing annual incidence of vestibular schwannoma and age at diagnosis. J Laryngol Otol 2004;118:622–627.
3 Caye-Thomasen P, Dethloff T, Hansen S, Stangerup SE, Thomsen J: Hearing in patients with intracanalicular vestibular schwannomas. Audiol Neurootol 2007;12:1–12.
4 Samii M, Matthies C, Tatagiba M: Intracanalicular acoustic neurinomas. Neurosurgery 1991;29:189–199.
5 Rowed DW, Nedzelski JM: Hearing preservation in the removal of intracanalicular acoustic neuromas via the retrosigmoid approach. J Neurosurg 1997;86:456–461.
6 Haines SJ, Levine SC: Intracanalicular acoustic neuroma: early surgery for preservation of hearing. J Neurosurg 1993;79:515–520.
7 Sampath P, Rini D, Long DM: Microanatomical variations in the cerebellopontine angle associated with vestibular schwannomas (acoustic neuromas): a retrospective study of 1006 consecutive cases. J Neurosurg 2000;92:70–78.
8 Gardner G, Robertson JH: Hearing preservation in unilateral acoustic neuroma surgery. Ann Otol Rhinol Laryngol 1988;97:55–66.
9 Committee on Hearing and Equilibrium Guidelines for the evaluation of hearing preservation in acoustic neuroma (vestibular schwannoma). American Academy of Otolaryngology-Head and Neck Surgery foundation, Inc. Otolaryngol Head Neck Surg 1995;113:179–180.
10 House JW, Brackmann DE: Facial nerve grading system. Otolaryngol Head Neck Surg 1985;93:146–147.
11 Mohr G, Sade B, Dufour JJ, Rappaport JM: Preservation of hearing in patients undergoing microsurgery for vestibular schwannoma: degree of meatal filling. J Neurosurg 2005;102:1–5.
12 Strasnick B, Glasscock ME III, Haynes D, Mc menomey SO, Minor LB: The natural history of untreated acoustic neuromas. Laryngoscope 1994;104:1115–1119.
13 Gardner G, Moretz WH Jr, Robertson JH, Clark C, Shea JJ Jr: Non surgical management of small and intracanalicular acoustic tumors. Otolaryngol Head Neck Surg 1986;94:328–333.
14 Kobayashi T, Aslan A, Chiba T, Takasaka T, Sanna M: Measurement of endocochlear DC potentials in ears with acoustic neuromas: a preliminary report. Acta Otolaryngol 1996;116: 791–795.
15 Jaisinghani VJ, Levine SC, Nussbaum E, Haines S, Lindgren B: Hearing preservation after acoustic neuromas surgery. Skull Base Surgery 2000;10:141–147.
16 Wazen J, Silverstein H, Norrell H, Besse B: Preoperative and postoperative growth rates in acoustic neuromas documented with CT scanning. Otolaryngol Head Neck Surgery 1985;93:151–155.
17 Janetta PJ, Moller AR, Moller MB: Technique of hearing preservation in small acoustic neuromas. Ann Surg 1984;200:513–523.
18 Samii M, Turel KE, Penkert G: Management of seventh and eighth nerve involvement of cerebellopontine angle tumors. Clin Neurosurg 1985;32: 242–272.
19 Elliot FA, McKissock W: Acoustic Neuroma: Early diagnosis. Lancet 1954;2:1189–1191.
20 House WF: Surgical exposure of the internal auditory canal and its contents through middle cranial fossa. Laryngoscope 1961;71:1363.
21 Ojemann RG, Levine RA, Montgomery WW, McGaffigan P: Use of intraoperative evoked potentials to preserve hearing in unilateral acoustic neuroma removal. J Neurosurg 1984;61: 938–948.
22 Frerebeau P, Benezech J, Uziel A, Coubes P, Segnarbieux F, Malonga M: Hearing preservation after acoustic neurinoma operation. Neurosurgery 1987;21:197–200.

23 Glasscock ME III, Hays WJ, Minor ZB, Haynes DS, Carrasco VN: Preservation of hearing in surgery for acoustic neuromas. J Neurosurg 1993;78:864–870.
24 Fischer G, Fischer C, Rémond J: Hearing preservation in acoustic neurinoma surgery. J Neurosurg 1992;76: 910–917.
25 Maw AR, Coakham HB, Ayoub O, Butler SR: Hearing preservation and facial nerve function in vestibular schwannoma surgery. Clin Otolaryngol 2003;28:252–256.
26 Post KD, Eisenberg MB, Catalano PJ: Hearing preservation in vestibular schwannoma surgery: what factors influence outcome ? J Neurosurg 1995;83:191–196.
27 Irving R, Jackler R, Pitts LH: Hearing preservation in patients undergoing vestibular schwannoma surgery: comparison of middle fossa and retrosigmoid approaches. J Neurosurg 1998;88: 840–845.
28 Satar B, Yetiser S, Ozkaptan Y: Impact of tumor size on hearing outcome and facial function with the middle fossa approach for acoustic neuroma: a meta-analytic study. Acta Otolaryngol 2003;123(4):499–505.
29 Betchen SA, Walsh J, Post KD: Long-term hearing preservation after surgery for vestibular schwannoma. J Neurosurg 2005;102:6–9.
30 Coletti V, Fiorino F: Is the middle fossa approach the treatment of choice for intracanalicular vestibular schwannoma? Otolaryngol Head Neck Surg 2005 123:459–466.
31 Harner SG, Laws ER Jr, Onofrio BM: Hearing preservation after removal of acoustic neruomas. Laryngoscope 1984;94:1431–1434.
32 Shelton C, Brackmann DE, House WF, Hitselberger WE: Acoustic tumor surgery. Prognostic factors in hearing conservation. Arch Otolaryngol Head Neck Surg 1989;115:1213–1216.
33 Cohen NL, Lewis WS, Ransohoff J: Hearing preservation in cerebellopontine angle tumor surgery: the NYU experience 1974–1991. Am J Otol 1993;14:423–433.
34 Samii M, Matthies C: Management of 1000 vestibular schwannomas (acoustic neuromas): hearing function in 1000 tumor resection. Neurosurgery 1997;40:248–262.
35 Samii M, Gerganov V, Samii A: Improved preservation of hearing and facial nerve function in vestibular schwannoma surgery via the retrosigmoid approach in a series of 200 patients. J Neurosurg 2006;105:527–535.
36 Brookes GB, Woo J: Hearing preservation in acoustic neuroma surgery. Clin Otolaryngol 1994;19:204–214.
37 Kansaki J, Ogawa K, Inoue Y, Shiobara R, Toya S: Quality of hearing preservation in acoustic neuroma surgery. Am J Otol 1998;19:644–648.
38 Staecker H, Nadol Joseph B Jr, Ojeman R, Ronner S, McKenna MJ: Hearing preservation in acoustic neuroma surgery: middle fossa versus retrosigmoid approach. Am J Otol 2000;21:399–404.
39 Koos WT, Diaz Day J, Matula C, Levy DI: Neurotopographic considerations in the microsurgical treatment of small acoustic neurinomas. J Neurosurg 1998;88:506–512.
40 Moriyama T, Fukushima T, Asaoka K, Roche PH, Barrs DM, McElveen JT Jr. Hearing preservation in acoustic neuroma surgery: importance of adhesion between the cochlear nerve and the tumor. J Neurosurg 2002;97:337–40.
41 Miyamoto RT, Campbell RL, Fritsch M, Lochmueller G: Preservation of hearing in neurofibromatosis 2. Otolaryngol Head Neck Surg 1990;103:619–624.
42 Brackmann DE, House JR III, Hitselbeger WE: Technical modifications to the middle fossa craniotomy approach in removal of acoustic neuromas. Am J Otol 1994;15:614–619.
43 Gantz BJ, Parnes LS, Harker LA, McCabe BF: Middle cranial fossa acoustic neuroma excision: results and complications. Ann Otol Rhinol Laryngol 1986;95:454–459.
44 House WF, Hitselberger WE: The middle fossa approach for removal of small acoustic tumors. Acta Otolaryngol (Stockh) 1969;67:413–427.
45 Holsinger FC, Coker N, Jenkins HA: Hearing preservation in conservation surgery for vestibular schwannoma. Am J Otol 2000;21:695–700.
46 Sekiya T, Moller AR, Janetta PJ: Pathophysiological mechanisms of intraoperative and postoperative hearing deficits in cerebellopontine angle surgery: an experimental study. Acta Neurochir 1986;81:142–152.
47 Dugar J, Nikolopoulos TP, O'Donoghue GM: Hearing preservation in acoustic neuroma surgery: the impact of different patient selection criteria. Laryngoscope 2002;112:2051–2053
48 Cannoni M, Pech A, Pellet W: Experiences at the Timone Hospital, Marseille in acoustic neuroma surgery. Arch Otorhinolaryngol 1989;246: 297–298.
49 Brackmann DE: Middle cranial fossa approach; in House WF, Luetje CM (eds): Acoustic tumors. Baltimore, University Park Press, 1979 Volume 2, Management.

Dr. Rémy Noudel
Department of Neurosurgery, Maison Blanche Hospital, University of Reims
FR–51100 Reims (France)
Tel. +33 661 127 429, Fax +33 326 784 097, E-Mail remynoudel@yahoo.fr

Régis J, Roche P-H (eds): Modern Management of Acoustic Neuroma.
Prog Neurol Surg. Basel, Karger, 2008, vol 21, pp 192–199

Radiosurgery for Intracanalicular Vestibular Schwannomas

Ajay Niranjan · David Mathieu · Douglas Kondziolka · John C. Flickinger · L. Dade Lunsford

Departments of Neurological Surgery, Radiology and Radiation Oncology, University of Pittsburgh, and Center for Image-Guided Neurosurgery, University of Pittsburgh Medical Center-Presbyterian, Pittsburgh, Pa., USA

Abstract

Advances in central nervous system imaging have resulted in early detection of a greater number of intracanalicular vestibular schwannomas. Early detection of intracanalicular vestibular schwannomas raises the issue of whether or not treatment is required and, if so, whether radiosurgery is the most appropriate option. Available evidence indicates that a majority of intracanalicular lesions are observed to grow and most will be associated with progressive hearing loss or, less frequently, sudden persistent hearing loss. If the objective of treatment is to preserve serviceable binaural hearing, early intervention is advisable. Early intervention is advantageous only if serviceable hearing can be maintained in the majority of patients along with low perioperative morbidity. Radiosurgery seems to achieve these goals ideally. Radiosurgery is a minimally invasive management option for patients with intracanalicular tumors. Radiosurgery provides high rate of long-term hearing preservation with minimal morbidity.

In the past, the diagnosis of vestibular schwannoma (VS) was often made at an advanced growth stage and surgical removal was the only reasonable choice because these tumors often caused symptoms of mass effect. Nowadays, increasing numbers of patients are diagnosed when their tumors are still intracanalicular or small. Several factors are responsible for this change. These include availability of improved imaging modalities such as contrast-enhanced computed tomography and magnetic resonance (MR) scanning with paramagnetic contrast agents, and a better-informed population. These advances have led to increasing numbers of newly diagnosed, smaller volume tumors [1–3]. Although the majority of intracanalicular contrast-enhancing lesions are presumed to be VSs, in rare instances other lesions may present with similar clinical and radiological behavior. These rare lesions include mycotic aneurysm of the AICA [4], cavernous hemangioma [5, 6] meningioma [7–9], lipomas [10], hemangioblastoma [11] and chronic inflammation [12, 13].

There is no consensus on the management of minimally symptomatic intracanalicular VS with regard to selection of therapeutic modality and the timing of intervention. Some physicians recommend 'wait and scan' as the nonsurgical option, arguing that tumor growth is extremely slow [14, 15]. Others advocate early intervention in the form of surgery or radiosurgery shortly after imaging diagnosis. Proponents of surgery report favorable results when surgery is performed at this early growth stage [16–18]. Radiosurgery has emerged as a minimally invasive therapeutic option for most patients with VS, especially intracanalicular tumors [19–24]. High rates of long-term tumor growth control have been reported subsequent to intracanalicular VS radiosurgery.

Preservation of hearing is now the most important criterion for successful management of intracanalicular VSs, whether observation, microsurgery or radiosurgery is chosen. The facial nerve function is almost always preserved after radiosurgery. The selection of a management option is related to the factors such as the patient's age, tumor size, hearing status, occupation, the patient's desire for hearing preservation versus tumor removal and patient's preference for a particular option after honest and accurate informed consent.

Observation

The rationale for recommending observation is that some tumors have a very slow growth rate so that few symptoms may affect an individual's quality of life. Not surprisingly, no consensus exists on the growth rate of acoustic tumors. Charabi et al. [25] followed 123 patients with 127 tumors with a wait and scan policy in the period from 1973 to 1999. Three sets of growth results were obtained. The results at 1993 revealed tumor growth in 74%, no growth in 18% and shrinkage in 8%. By 1996, the results changed to: tumor growth in 82%, no growth in 12% and shrinkage in 6%. By 1999, tumor growth was detected in 85%, no growth in 9% and shrinkage in eight tumors (6%). This study showed that tumor growth is time dependent and most tumors ultimately grow over 10–20 years.

To compare conservative management with surgery Bozorg Grayeli et al. [26] followed 693 patients with small VS between 1991 and 2002. One hundred and fourteen (16%) had intracanalicular tumors. Conservative management was chosen in patients aged >60 years and in those who refused surgery. In this subgroup, the mean follow-up period was 33 months. In the conservative management group, 47% of tumors showed significant growth, 47% were stable and 6% showed regression. Deterioration of hearing function by one or more class was observed in 56% of cases. In the conservative management group, 17% were lost during follow-up. These authors concluded that a high rate of deterioration in hearing function and the loss of patient compliance during conservative management should be taken into account when considering hearing preservation strategies for patients with VS [26]. Observation may be appropriate initial strategy for selected elderly patients or those with major medical comorbidity.

Microsurgery

Proponents of early surgery recommend excision of intracanalicular VS because the results are better when tumor is small. However, there is no consensus on which microsurgical approach is better. The quality of life after VS surgery was investigated in a series of 227 patients [27]. In this study, patients with poor functional outcomes were evenly distributed over the medium and large tumor size groups, and patients with small tumors (diameter <15 mm) had significantly better outcomes. Normal or nearly normal function of the facial nerve had always been considered an important criterion in the evaluation of the surgical outcome of VS surgery. Intrameatal VSs show excellent functional facial nerve results in all large series reported, regardless of the applied surgical approach.

Two institutions, the University of California at San Francisco (UCSF) [28] and Harvard [29], published their results for hearing preservation for both the middle fossa and retrosigmoid approaches matching patients for tumor size and preoperative hearing level. For both institutions, the best match for tumor size between groups occurred for intracanalicular tumors. When success was defined as hearing preserved in the same or better class for patients with intracanalicular tumors and class A, B, or C hearing preoperatively, the UCSF middle fossa patients had better hearing preservation [retrosigmoid success was 0 of 16 (0%); middle fossa success was 10 of 25 (40%)] [28]. However, the Harvard patients had comparable hearing results between their groups [retrosigmoid success was 6 of 15 (40%); middle fossa success was 6 of 13 (46%)] [29]. When success was defined as maintaining serviceable hearing in patients with preoperative class A hearing, the difference in success between the two approaches was not statistically significant at either institution. Hearing preservation when compared across-institution for middle fossa patients ranged from 33 to 57%, with a median rate of 48% (preserved in the same class). Hearing preservation in the same class for retrosigmoid patients ranged from 0 to 68%, with a median rate of 39%. The difference between the median results for each group was not significant. Preservation of serviceable hearing in middle fossa patients with preoperative class A hearing ranged from 50 to 71%, with a median rate of 69%. Serviceable hearing preservation in retrosigmoid patients with preoperative class A hearing ranged from 17 to 88% with a median rate of 54% [30]. Delayed hearing deterioration after microsurgical removal of acoustic neuromas is known to occur, although most surgical series do not report long-term data [31, 32]. Goel et al. [31] reported delayed hearing deterioration in 3 (20%) of 15 patients in whom hearing preservation had been successful. Shelton et al. [32] evaluated the durability of preserved postoperative hearing in 25 middle fossa acoustic tumor patients over time. The mean follow-up time for this group was more than 8 years. They noted a significant loss of the preserved hearing in 56% of patients. The mean loss of speech discrimination was 25%, and the mean loss of speech reception threshold was 12 dB.

Facial nerve outcome was significantly better for retrosigmoid patients in both the within-institution and across-institution comparisons (81% median success rate for middle fossa vs. 95% for retrosigmoid) [30]. In middle fossa surgery the individual surgeon's experience may play a significant role in the patient's final facial nerve outcome. Other surgical complication such as headache and CSF leak may be significant factors that impact on the quality of life of patients. The Harvard series, demonstrated a trend toward a greater number of headaches in the retrosigmoid group (3 of 15 in the middle fossa group vs. 7 of 15 in the retrosigmoid group) [29]. Eleven of the 73 patients (15%) in the Seattle series had postoperative headache [30]. Seattle series also reported 4% incidence of a cerebrospinal fluid leak that required treatment. Tumor recurrence was noted in 3% of patients who had complete tumor removal [30].

Radiosurgery

The goal of microsurgery in VS is radical tumor removal with preservation of neurological function, while the goal of radiosurgery is control of tumor growth (defined as the absence of tumor growth or a reduction in tumor volume) with preservation of neurological function. A very important aspect to consider in comparing the results of microsurgery and radiosurgery is the patient selection for hearing preservation surgery. The technique of VS with stereotactic radiosurgery has improved since the initial reports by Leksell. Advances in MRI, computers and robotics have improved functional outcome of acoustic tumor radiosurgery. No mortality associated with this treatment modality has been reported.

University of Pittsburgh Experience

Preradiosurgery Evaluations

At the University of Pittsburgh between 1987 and 2003, 161 patients (105 men, 57 women) underwent Gamma Knife radiosurgery (GKR) for intracanalicular tumor. The median patient age was 56 years (range: 22–89). Tinnitus was a presenting symptom in 108 (67%) patients. All were evaluated with high-resolution MRI and underwent clinical evaluation as well as audiological tests which included pure tone average (PTA) and speech discrimination score (SDS) measurements. Hearing was graded using the Gardner-Robertson's modification (GR) of the Silverstein and Norell classification [33] and facial nerve function was assessed according to the House-Brackmann (H-B) grading system [34]. 'Serviceable' hearing (GR class I and II) was defined as a PTA or speech reception threshold lower than 50 dB and SDS better than 50%. Hearing was also graded using the guidelines suggested by the Committee on Hearing and Equilibrium of the American Academy of Otolaryngology-Head and Neck surgery (AAO-HNS) [35]. In this classification, hearing loss at higher frequency (3,000 Hz) is also included in calculating the PTA. 'Serviceable' hearing (class A and B) is similar to class I and II of Gardner-Robertson's hearing classes.

Radiosurgery Technique

The procedure began with rigid fixation of an MRI-compatible Leksell stereotactic frame (model G, Elekta Instruments, Atlanta, Ga., USA) to the patient's head. Local anesthetic scalp infiltration (5% marcaine and 1% xylocaine) was used, occasionally supplemented by mild intravenous sedation. At present, titanium pins with plastic inserts are used to avoid any chance of heating of pins due to radiofrequency currents that may form during MRI. High-resolution images were acquired with a fiducial system attached to the stereotactic frame. For radiosurgery of intracanalicular lesions, a 3-D volume acquisition MRI using a spoiled-gradient recalled acquisition in steady state (SPGR) pulse sequence (divided into 1-mm-thick 28 axial slices) was performed in order to cover the entire lesion and surrounding critical structures. In addition, a 3-D T_2-weighted volume sequence was also performed to delineate tumor as well as inner ear structures (cochlea and semicircular canals).

The tumor volume was determined first by outlining the tumor using contrast-enhanced SPGR images. The tumor volume was further modified using T_2 volume images. The cochlea was also outlined using T_2 images. Planning was performed on narrow slice thickness axial MR images with coronal and sagittal reconstructions. A highly conformal dose plan using only 4-mm collimators covering the entire lesion was created. Preservation of cochlear and facial nerve function was the aim during planning. Our prior analysis indicated that hearing preservation rates were enhanced when a combination of only 4-mm collimators were used to irradiate intracanalicular portions of acoustic tumors [36]. Because the facial nerve and the acoustic nerve complex generally course along the anterior margin of the tumor, the dose plan should by highly conformal in this region. The treatment isodose, maximum dose, and dose to the margin were jointly decided by a neurosurgeon and radiation oncologist. For the past 10 years, we selected 12–13 Gy as the usual tumor margin dose.

Highlights of our current dose planning technique for intracanalicular lesions include use of 3-D SPGR as well as 3-D T_2-weighted MRI, multiple 4-mm isocenters, and beam weighting (fig. 1). For intracanalicular lesions, 100% of the tumor is covered by prescribed dose level. Currently, we prescribe a margin dose of 12.5 Gy to the isodose line covering the lesion. Dose volume histograms on tumor, cochlea and brainstem are evaluated. The treatment is accomplished in a single session by positioning the head serially for each subsequent isocenter with the robotic APS (automated positioning system) until a fully conformal field encompasses the tumor volume (like a glove fitting the hand).

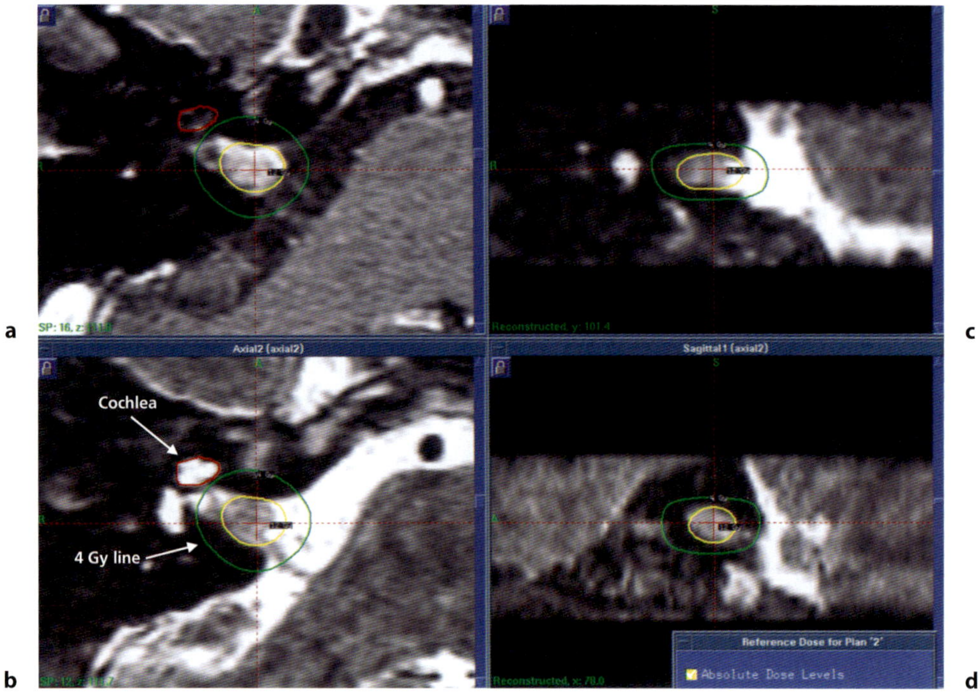

Fig. 1. Radiosurgery dose plan showing axial contrast-enhanced gradient-recalled MR image (**a**) with 3-D T_2 weighted axial (**b**), coronal (**c**) and sagittal (**d**) MR images. Dose plan shows 50% isodose line (12 Gy line) covering the tumor. The cochlea (outlined in red) receives less than 4 Gy.

Postoperative Care and Evaluations

All patients received an intravenous dose of 40 mg of methylprednisolone at the conclusion of the procedure. The stereotactic frame was removed, immediately after radiosurgery. Patients were observed for few hours in the same day surgery unit and were discharged within 24 h. After radiosurgery, all patients were followed up with serial gadolinium-enhanced MRI scans, which were requested at 6 months, 12 months, 2, 4, 8, and 16 years. All patients who had any preserved hearing were advised to obtain audiological tests (PTA and SDS) near the time of their MRI follow-up.

Outcome of Intracanalicular Lesion Radiosurgery

Tumor Control

Post-SRS imaging was available in 145 patients. At a median follow-up of 24 months (range: 12–144) tumors regressed in 56 (35%), remained unchanged in 82 (51%) patients. Slight initial tumor enlargement (1–3 mm) followed by stabilization was noted in 6 patients. None of theses patients required any further intervention. One additional patient who had noted tumor growth at 1 year and was eligible for repeat SRS instead underwent elective surgical excision 18 months after radiosurgery. Thus, tumors were controlled in 144 of 145 evaluable patients after single SRS procedure. The tumor control rate (freedom from additional intervention) was 99.3% in this series.

Hearing Preservation

Serviceable hearing is classified as AAO-HNS class A and B or GR class I and II. Differences between preoperative and postoperative hearing class were reported in most surgical series in two ways. One method was to report patients with preoperative hearing in class A, B, or C as unchanged, improved, or worse. The other method was to evaluate patients with preoperative class A hearing in order to determine the rate of retaining serviceable hearing (class A or B) after surgery. The serviceable hearing part of the evaluation was limited to preoperative class A patients to eliminate a potential selection bias introduced by including patients with poorer preoperative hearing who would be expected to have a lower likelihood of preservation of serviceable hearing. Most radiosurgical series report preservation of GR class I and II (or AAO-HNS grade A and B) as serviceable hearing. In the present series, there were 73 evaluable patients with GR grade I, II, or III hearing prior to SRS. At a median follow-up of 24 months (range: 12–144), 62 (85%) of these patients maintained GR grade I, II or III hearing after SRS. There were 29 evaluable patients with initial AAO-HNS class A hearing. Serviceable hearing (AAO-HNS class A or B) was preserved in 21 (72.5%) patients. Of 35 patients who had pre-SRS GR grade I hearing, serviceable hearing (grade I or II) was preserved in 26 (74.3%) patients. There were 61 evaluable patients with Gardner-Robertson grade I or II hearing prior to radiosurgery. Serviceable gearing (GR grade I or II) was preserved in 35 (61%) of these patients. Trigeminal nerve function was preserved in all patients. No patient developed a permanent facial paresis. Two patients noticed temporary facial spasms and facial nerve paresis (H-B grade 2) which improved on a short course of corticosteroids.

Clinical results after VS radiosurgery have been extensively documented in the published literature. In most series, the subset of intracanalicular lesions is included with medium and large tumors in the data analysis. However, there are few reports that only studied the subset of intracanalicular tumor radiosurgery [36–38]. Flickinger et al. [20] recently studied Pittsburgh data for long-term hearing preservation after VS radiosurgery using 12–13 Gy as tumor margin dose. Twenty-five patients in this series had intracanalicular tumors. The crude hearing preservation rate in this subset was 84% for preservation of the same Gardner-Robertson hearing level and 92% for preservation of serviceable hearing in patients with preoperative class 1 and 2 hearing. Massager et al. [39] analyzed the relationship between hearing preservation after GKR and volumetric and dosimetric parameters of the intracanalicular components of VS. These authors noted that hearing preservation after GKR was significantly correlated with the intracanalicular tumor volume, as well as with the integrated dose delivered to the intracanalicular tumor volume. Sixteen patients in this series (19.5%) had a purely intracanalicular VS. Of this group, the audiologic status of 9 patients (56%) remained at the same Gardner-Robertson class, whereas 7 patients (44%) had worsened hearing after GKR. Regis et al. [40] analyzed their VS series and concluded that the hearing preservation depended on numerous factors related to the patient and to the 'operative technique'. The main parameters of predictability in this series were limited preoperative pure tone loss, Gardner and Robertson class 1 (vs. 2), multi-isocentric dose planning, and margin lower than 13 Gy. They reported a greater than 95% functional hearing preservation rate at 2 years for patients with intracanalicular tumor with a Gardner and Robertson class 1 hearing that were treated with a 'state of the art' Gamma Knife using a marginal dose of less than 13 Gy [40].

Acute complications following intracanalicular radiosurgery are rare. Transient complications of intracanalicular lesion radiosurgery include headache, vomiting, dizziness, hemifacial spasm and facial and acoustic neuropathy [38, 41, 42]. Long-term facial nerve function preservation (H-B grade 1) using current technique is approximately 99%.

Conclusions

Attempts to predict the lesion growth rate on the basis of patient age and sex and the histological or immunohistochemical characteristics of the lesion have thus far yielded disappointing results. Progressive hearing loss probably occurs in most intracanalicular tumors. It therefore appears that if preservation of serviceable hearing is an objective in the management of intracanalicular tumors, early intervention should be considered to prevent progressive or sudden hearing loss and lesion progression to a size that would increase risks related to preservation of cochlear and facial function if intervention is ultimately needed. The success rates for serviceable hearing preservation by radiosurgery are superior to microsurgery using either the retrosigmoid or middle fossa approach. There is sufficient long-term outcome data on preservation of serviceable hearing after GKR of intracanalicular tumors. Smaller intracanalicular tumors are associated with a significantly greater likelihood of serviceable hearing preservation after radiosurgery. The complications associated with open surgical approaches are also eliminated by radiosurgery with comparable tumor growth control rates.

Considering that a reliable means of predicting growth of intracanalicular lesions is not available, the preservation of serviceable hearing and normal facial nerve function is best served by early intervention. Radiosurgery is now considered as management of first choice for intracanalicular acoustic tumors.

References

1 Tos M, Charabi S, Thomsen J: Clinical experience with vestibular schwannomas: epidemiology, symptomatology, diagnosis, and surgical results. Eur Arch Otorhinolaryngol 1998;255:1–6.

2 Tos M, Charabi S, Thomsen J: Incidence of vestibular schwannomas. Laryngoscope 1999;109:736–740.

3 Tos M, Charabi S, Thomsen J: Increase of diagnosed vestibular schwannoma in Denmark. Acta Otolaryngol Suppl 1997;529:53–55.

4 DiMaio S, Mohr G, Dufour JJ, et al: Distal mycotic aneurysm of the AICA mimicking intracanalicular acoustic neuroma. Can J Neurol Sci 2003;30:388–392.

5 Petit-Lacour MC, Marsot-Dupuch K, Hadj-Rabia M, et al: Hemangioma of the porus acusticus. Impact of imaging studies: case reports. Neuroradiology 2001;43:1102–1107.

6 Sepehrnia A, Rebolledo Godoy AP, Reusche E: A cavernous hemangioma simulating an intracanalicular acoustic neurinoma–a case report. Zentralbl Neurochir 2000;61:194–197.

7 Asaoka K, Barrs DM, Sampson JH, et al: Intracanalicular meningioma mimicking vestibular schwannoma. AJNR Am J Neuroradiol 2002;23:1493–1496.

8 Dinh DH, Clark SB, Whitehead M, et al: Intracanalicular meningioma. South Med J 2000;93:618–621.

9 Haught K, Hogg JP, Killeffer JA, et al: Entirely intracanalicular meningioma: contrast-enhanced MR findings in a rare entity. AJNR Am J Neuroradiol 1998;19:1831–1833.

10 Braun V, Kretschmer T, Sommer C, et al: Lipomas of the internal auditory canal–report of two cases and review of the literature. Zentralbl Neurochir 2004;65:88–94.

11 Resto VA, Lustig LR: Hemangioblastoma of the internal acoustic canal in a patient with von Hippel-Lindau disease: a case report and review of the literature. Arch Otolaryngol Head Neck Surg 2000;126:85–88.

12 Charabi S, Thomsen JC, Tos M: False-positive diagnostic findings in acoustic neurinomas. Ugeskr Laeger 1991;154:19–22.

13 Maeta M, Saito R, Nameki H: False-positive magnetic resonance image in the diagnosis of small acoustic neuroma. J Laryngol Otol 2001;115: 842–844.

14 Jorgensen BG, Pedersen CB: Acoustic neuroma. Follow-up of 78 patients. Clin Otolaryngol Allied Sci 1994;19:478–484.

15 Nedzelski JM, Canter RJ, Kassel EE, et al: Is no treatment good treatment in the management of acoustic neuromas in the elderly? Laryngoscope 1986;96:825–829.

16 Charabi S, Thomsen J, Mantoni M, et al: Acoustic neuroma (vestibular schwannoma): growth and surgical and nonsurgical consequences of the wait-and-see policy. Otolaryngol Head Neck Surg 1995;113:5–14.

17 Charabi S, Thomsen J, Tos M, et al: Acoustic neuroma/vestibular schwannoma growth: past, present and future. Acta Otolaryngol 1998;118:327–332.

18 Samii M, Matthies C, Tatagiba M: Intracanalicular acoustic neurinomas. Neurosurgery 1991;29:189–198; discussion 198–189.

19 Chung WY, Liu KD, Shiau CY, et al: Gamma knife surgery for vestibular schwannoma: 10-year experience of 195 cases. J Neurosurg 2005;102 (Suppl):87–96.

20 Flickinger JC, Kondziolka D, Niranjan A, et al: Acoustic neuroma radiosurgery with marginal tumor doses of 12 to 13 Gy. Int J Radiat Oncol Biol Phys 2004;60:225–230.

21 Hasegawa T, Kida Y, Kobayashi T, et al: Long-term outcomes in patients with vestibular schwannomas treated using gamma knife surgery: 10-year follow up. J Neurosurg 2005;102:10–16.

22 Kondziolka D, Lunsford LD, Flickinger JC: Acoustic neuroma radiosurgery. Origins, contemporary use and future expectations. Neuro-Chirurgie 2004;50:427–435.

23 Noren G: Gamma knife radiosurgery of acoustic neurinomas. A historic perspective. Neurochirurgie 2004;50:253–256.

24 Wackym PA, Runge-Samuelson CL, Poetker DM, et al: Gamma knife radiosurgery for acoustic neuromas performed by a neurotologist: early experiences and outcomes. Otol Neurotol 2004;25:752–761.

25 Charabi S, Tos M, Thomsen JC, et al: Vestibular schwannoma. A new interpretation of tumor growth. Ugeskr Laeger 2000;162:5497–5500.

26 Bozorg Grayeli A, Kalamarides M, Ferrary E, et al: Conservative management versus surgery for small vestibular schwannomas. Acta Otolaryngol 2005;125:1063–1068.

27 Irving RM, Beynon GJ, Viani L, et al: The patient's perspective after vestibular schwannoma removal: quality of life and implications for management. Am J Otol 1995;16:331–337.

28 Irving RM, Jackler RK, Pitts LH: Hearing preservation in patients undergoing vestibular schwannoma surgery: comparison of middle fossa and retrosigmoid approaches. J Neurosurg 1998;88:840–845.

29 Staecker H, Nadol JB Jr, Ojeman R, et al: Hearing preservation in acoustic neuroma surgery: middle fossa versus retrosigmoid approach. Am J Otol 2000;21:399–404.

30 Mangham CA Jr: Retrosigmoid versus middle fossa surgery for small vestibular schwannomas. Laryngoscope 2004;114:1455–1461.

31 Goel A, Sekhar LN, Langheinrich W, et al: Late course of preserved hearing and tinnitus after acoustic neurilemoma surgery. J Neurosurg 1992;77:685–689.

32 Shelton C, Hitselberger WE, House WF, et al: Hearing preservation after acoustic tumor removal: long-term results. Laryngoscope 1990;100: 115–119.

33 Gardner G, Robertson JH: Hearing preservation in unilateral acoustic neuroma surgery. Ann Otol Rhinol Laryngol 1988;97:55–66.

34 House JW, Brackmann DE: Facial nerve grading system. Otolaryngol Head Neck Surg 1985;93:146–147.

35 Anonymous: Committee on Hearing and Equilibrium guidelines for the evaluation of hearing preservation in acoustic neuroma (vestibular schwannoma). American Academy of Otolaryngology-Head and Neck Surgery Foundation, INC. Otolaryngol Head Neck Surg 1995;113:179–180.

36 Niranjan A, Lunsford LD, Flickinger JC, et al: Dose reduction improves hearing preservation rates after intracanalicular acoustic tumor radiosurgery. Neurosurgery 1999;45:753–762; discussion 762–755.

37 Ogunrinde OK, Lunsford DL, Kondziolka DS, et al: Cranial nerve preservation after stereotactic radiosurgery of intracanalicular acoustic tumors. Stereotact Funct Neurosurg 1995;64(Suppl 1):87–97.

38 Vermeulen S, Young R, Posewitz A, et al: Stereotactic radiosurgery toxicity in the treatment of intracanalicular acoustic neuromas: the Seattle Northwest gamma knife experience. Stereotact Funct Neurosurg 1998;70(Suppl 1):80–87.

39 Massager N, Nissim O, Delbrouck C, et al: Role of intracanalicular volumetric and dosimetric parameters on hearing preservation after vestibular schwannoma radiosurgery. Int J Radiat Oncol Biol Phys 2006.

40 Regis J, Delsanti C, Roche P, et al: Preservation of hearing function in the radiosurgical treatment of unilateral vestibular schwannomas. Preliminary results. Neurochirurgie 2002;48:471–478.

41 Pollack AG, Marymont MH, Kalapurakal JA, et al: Acute neurological complications following gamma knife surgery for vestibular schwannoma. Case report. J Neurosurg 2005;103:546–551.

42 Stieglitz LH, Samii A, Kaminsky J, et al: Nausea and dizziness after vestibular schwannoma surgery: a multivariate analysis of preoperative symptoms. Neurosurgery 2005;57: 887–890; discussion 887–890.

Ajay Niranjan, MBBS, MCh
Department of Neurological Surgery, University of Pittsburgh, Suite B-400
200 Lothrop St.
Pittsburgh, PA 15213 (USA)
Tel. +1 412 647 9699, Fax +1 412 647 6483, E-Mail niranjana@upmc.edu

Régis J, Roche P-H (eds): Modern Management of Acoustic Neuroma.
Prog Neurol Surg. Basel, Karger, 2008, vol 21, pp 200–206

Hydrocephalus and Vestibular Schwannomas: Considerations about the Impact of Gamma Knife Radiosurgery

Pierre-Hugues Roche[a] · Muhamad Khalil[a] · Outouma Soumare[a] · Jean Régis[b]

[a]Service de Neurochirurgie, Hôpital Sainte-Marguerite, et [b]Service de Neurochirurgie Stéréotaxique et Fonctionnelle, Hôpital de la Timone, Assistance Publique-Hôpitaux de Marseille, Marseille, France

Abstract

Hydrocephalus may occur at various stages of the natural course of vestibular schwannoma and can also be diagnosed after the therapeutic procedure. The aim of the present study was to analyze the impact of Gamma Knife radiosurgery (GKR) on previously diagnosed hydrocephalus (group A patients) and to evaluate the incidence of de novo hydrocephalus after GKR (group B patients). We reviewed retrospectively our case material and the data from the literature. Among the first 1,000 vestibular schwannoma patients treated by GKR in our institution, 30 patients (3%) belonged to group A and 1% to group B. In both groups, hydrocephalus was more often associated with the following data: Elderly, large tumor, previous MS, NF2 disease and bilateral tumors. Cerebrospinal fluid (CSF) shunting system was needed in 25% of the group A and in all of the group B patients. In this latter group, CSF shunting was justified by poor clinical tolerance, and the mean interval between GKR and CSF shunting was 14.8 months (range: 4–31 months). These data suggest that GKR does not decompensate the majority of preexisting radiological hydrocephalus. De novo post-GKR hydrocephalus is of low incidence, comparable to the postoperative rate. Generally, it comes early after GKR and justifies CSF shunting. Thus, it may be postulated that in a small subgroup of patients, GKR may disturb the normal hydrodynamic pathway. Mechanisms of such event remain controversial.

The occurrence of hydrocephalus is a well-known situation in the course of vestibular schwannoma (VS), particularly in cases of large tumors. Mechanisms and management remain controversial except if symptoms are obviously linked to an active hydrocephalus due to the obstruction of the cerebrospinal fluid (CSF). Hydrocephalus may also complicate the outcome of operated cases. Some cases may also occur after radiosurgical treatment and the implication of radiation is unclear. In order to verify this latter assertion, we reviewed our own experience of patients who underwent radiosurgical treatment in our institution and analyzed the data from previous studies of the microsurgical and radiosurgical literature.

Patients and Methods

Study Design

The 1,000 consecutive first VS patients who underwent Gamma Knife radiosurgery (GKR) in our institution from July 1992 to January 2002 were retrospectively investigated for evidence of hydrocephalus diagnosed before the procedure (group A) and were also checked for the occurrence of hydrocephalus after the GKR (group B). Both groups were studied, and search was made to find any correlation of hydrocephalus with clinical, radiological and treatment protocol parameters (this latter parameter only for group B). Statistical comparison of patients from group A and group B was done using the Mann-Whitney U test and the Fisher exact test for quantitative parameters and for qualitative parameters, respectively. Parts of this study have been published in a previous paper [1].

We also conducted a PubMed search with a crossed selection of the following key words: acoustic neuroma, hydrocephalus, gammaknife, radiosurgery, VS.

Population and Methods

Enlargement of the ventricles was defined as hydrocephalus in the present study regardless of symptomatology. The bicaudate CVI was used to describe the ventricle size. In case of hydrocephalus, systematic search for clinical manifestations of communicating hydrocephalus including short memory disturbance, ataxia and loss of sphincter control was conducted. Signs of obstructive hydrocephalus including headaches, nausea, vomiting, and altered levels of consciousness were also searched. For the group A patients, the Gamma Knife treatment protocol was not influenced in any parameter by the evidence of hydrocephalus. Modalities of follow-up were done as usual, including clinical examination and MR study at 6 months, 1 year, 2, 3, 5, 7, 9 years after the treatment. Patients were aware that in case of special clinical event, it was recommended to check their status by their referring physician.

The CSF shunting procedure was decided based on the association of clinical symptoms and contemporary enlargement of ventricular size.

Results

Patient Characteristics

Among the 1,000 consecutive VS patients who underwent GKR in our institution, 32 displayed a hydrocephalus before treatment (group A) while 11 cases of de novo hydrocephalus were identified in the follow-up (group B). The main characteristics of both groups are shown in table 1. In both groups, patient age and tumor size were significantly higher than in the global population of treated cases. In group A, previous microsurgery was observed in 6 cases (20%) and NF2 disease was noted in 4 cases (13%), which is also significantly higher than for the whole population.

Patients from group A displayed mainly isolated radiological hydrocephalus. In group B, the majority of patients had altogether radiological and clinical signs of hydrocephalus. Comparison of both groups in respect of patient age, tumor size, and treatment parameters did not show statistical difference (table 2).

Patient Management

In group A, it was possible to obtain enough follow-up information duration in only 20 patients (table 3). Median follow-up of these patients was 39.5 months. Five (25%) of them underwent a CSF shunting procedure. Shunting was motivated by clinical deterioration caused by active hydrocephalus associated with increasing ventricular size. In all cases, shunting was efficient to improve the symptoms. In this group, 2 patients (10%) underwent additional therapeutic procedure on their VS because of failed GKR, which means that there is a correlation between hydrocephalus decompensation and GKR failure in some cases.

All the 11 patients from group B required a shunt that was motivated by clinical worsening contemporary of ventricular enlargement. The interval between GKR and ventriculoperitoneal (VP) shunt ranged between 4 and 31 months with a mean interval of 14.8 months. The patient who underwent shunting at 4 months was a neurofibromatosis type 2 (NF2) patient treated simultaneously for both large VSs. She needed to be operated on facing a severe ataxia and intracranial hypertension signs due to enlargement of tumors and ventricular signs. VP shunting and removal of the largest tumor where done in the same procedure. Whatever the studied group, clinical manifestations were those of communicating hydrocephalus in the majority of patients. In group A, a history of NF2 was noted in 4 patients before treatment and none of these patients required CSF shunting.

Table 1. Main characteristics of the patients regarding epidemiology, radiological aspects, dosimetry and evolution

	Group A (n = 32)	Group B (n = 11)
Age, years		
Mean (range)	62.7 (25–81)	62.9 (21–80)
Median	70	68
Previous MS/NF2 patient	6/4	0/1
Koos grading of the tumor sizew		
Stage II	13	3
Stage III	13	7
Stage IV	6	1
Tumor volume, mm^3		
Median	2,412	2,160
Mean	2,707	3,172
Isocenters		
Mean	9.1	5
GP	11/32	1/11
Outcome of patients with enough informative follow-up		
Patients	20	11
Follow-up, months		
Mean (range)	43.4 (12–86)	50.5 (14–102)
Median	39.5	50
Tumor control	18 controlled, 2 failed	8 controlled, 3 failed
VP shunt after GKR	5	11
Interval GKR to VP shunt, months		
Median		14
Mean (range)		14.8 (4–31)

GP = Gamma plan; MS = microsurgery.

Discussion

Incidence
Incidence of hydrocephalus associated with VS is difficult to determine because of heterogeneity of case selection with respect to the patient age, tumor size, radiological definition. Nevertheless, this incidence ranges from 3.7 [2] to 15% [3] of cases. Early experience with CT mentioned a clear correlation between hydrocephalus and tumor size, particularly for tumors exceeding 3 cm [4]. In the study [5] about 236 VS patients, age

Table 2. Statistical comparison of groups A and B

Assessed variables in groups A and B	Statistical significance
Quantitative variables	
Age	0.63
Volume	0.85
Maximum tumor diameter	0.41
Peripheral dose	0.41
Number of isocenters	0.85
Qualitative variables	
NF2	1
Previous microsurgery	0.31
Koos grading (1, 2 or 3 versus 4)	0.65

Statistical significance was set at $p < 0.05$.

was statistically correlated to hydrocephalus ($p = 0.015$). Tumor size was also a significant influencing factor ($p < 0.0001$). In this study, these factors appeared to be statistically independent. In several other studies, tumor size also appeared as a determinant factor [3, 6, 7]. More recently, Rogg et al. [8] observed that in the subgroup of non-communicating type of hydrocephalus (NCTH) that constituted 30% of their cases, there was a positive correlation between the grade of NCTH and tumor volume. This correlation was also found between the severity of fourth ventricle compression and the extent of hydrocephalus.

Clinical Manifestations

The complete or incomplete Hakim triad is the usual presentation, while intracranial hypertension manifestations are found in a few cases (15% of the largest published series [6]). It should be noted that it is sometimes difficult to attribute the ataxia to the tumor mass or to the hydrocephalus.

Patients from group A displayed mainly isolated radiological hydrocephalus, which explains that none of them required CSF shunting before GKR. In group B, the majority of patients had altogether radiological and clinical signs of hydrocephalus and required CSF shunting. Signs where mainly comparable to what is described in the case of chronic idiopathic hydrocephalus of the adult.

Mechanism of Hydrocephalus

Obstruction is rarely observed even if correlation with size is well recognized. Actually, tumor removal does not always resolve the hydrocephalus. Obstruction mechanism is encountered in cases of extra-large VS where V4 is distorted, in young patients with papillary edema and ICH symptoms. As a rule, slow growth of tumors allows gradual remodeling and adaptation of the CSF way of drainage. In the study of Rogg et al. [8], about 157 VS patients, 28 of them (18%) presented a hydrocephalus before any treatment. Thirty-nine percent of them displayed NCTH, while 61% had a communicating type (CTH). In this latter group, there was a poor correlation between the tumor volume and the severity of hydrocephalus. CTH may have several explanations. It has been suggested that resorption was impaired because of an accumulation of proteinaceous material into the CSF. Although not tested in ordinary practice, excessive level of proteins is usually observed in cases of VS, usually exceeding 1 g/l. Blood-brain barrier disruption and inflammatory processes inside the tumor may allow diffusion of proteins in the CSF, thereby blocking the action of arachnoid villi. Gardner et al. [9] postulated that this phenomenon was equivalent to the mechanism of hydrocephalus that occurs in the context of intramedullary tumors. Other authors have suggested [10, 11] that an excessive rate of proteins and microhemorrhagic events around the tumor may be responsible for fibrosis and cohesion of the arachnoid membranes. It may also

Table 3. Comparison of management and follow-up of patients from groups A and B

	Group A (n = 20)	Group B (n = 11)
Follow-up, months		
Mean (range)	43.4 (12–86)	50.5 (14–102)
Median	39.5	50
Tumor control at last follow-up	18 control, 2 failure	8 control, 3 failure
CSF shunting after GKR	5	11
GKR to shunt interval, months		
Mean (range)		14.8 (4–31)
Median		14

be possible to consider complex mechanisms associating both etiologies.

It is also of interest to understand the mechanism of hydrocephalus while the treatment has been given. After microsurgical treatment, local inflammatory processes are naturally suspected of causing the circulation trouble. Direct manipulation of the tumor capsule, delivery of intracisternal hemoglobin and of proteinaceous material are always observed. Understanding the hydrocephalus mechanism after radiosurgery is far more unclear due to the rarity of this situation. Obstructive mechanism is exceptional if care is taken to avoid the treatment of large tumors with a significant mass effect. As mentioned above, it has been observed in one of our patients from group B. Sawamura et al. [12] have studied a group of patients who underwent stereotactic radiation therapy. They suggested that radio-induced modifications of the tumor biology entailed accumulation of cellular and proteinaceous material from the degradation and necrosis of the tumor. Our personal surgical observations after failed GKR showed that in most cases, scarring and thickening of the arachnoid membranes were common findings. However, these modifications were located around the tumor and did not affect remote spaces.

What Is the Fate of Preexisting Hydrocephalus before Treatment of VS?

In the microsurgical series, several authors adopted a wait and see policy and focused only on the surgery of the tumor. In most cases, resolution of hydrocephalus was observed and there was no need for additional shunting. Atlas et al. [3] reported 14 patients with hydrocephalus in a series of 104 consecutive cases of VS. In 9 cases, treatment was tumor removal only, and there were no cases that required ventricular drainage or shunting following surgery. In the large series of about 1,000 VS from Samii and Matthies [11], a preexisting hydrocephalus required CSF shunt insertion in 9 cases (1%) before tumor removal. In our own practice, we try to adopt a conservative policy and avoid shunting whenever possible in respect of the clinical tolerance. In other cases, where ataxia or intracranial hypertension is significant, we may prefer to put a shunt before surgical removal of the VS.

Considering that only 20% of the patients who harbored hydrocephalus before treatment (group A) required additional shunting after radiosurgery, it can be postulated that radiosurgery does not significantly influence the process of hydrocephalus, when excluding the cases for failure with continuous tumor growth (fig. 1).

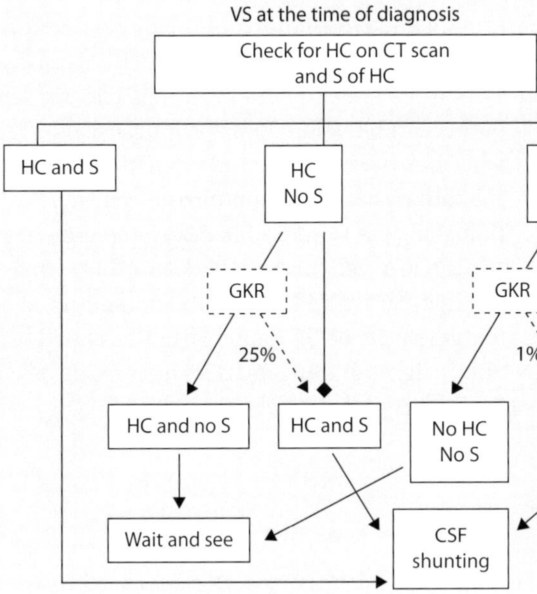

Fig. 1. Possible changes of ventricular size in a newly diagnosed VS after spontaneous evolution or after a GKR. The way to manage the ventricular enlargement is also shown. Dotted arrows indicate the potential implication of the GKR in hydrocephalus (HC) decompensation (25% of cases that came to GKR with previous HC) or in de novo hydrocephalus (1% of the whole VS patients who underwent GK). These data are extracted from our personal experience. Diamond arrows show the natural history of VS without direct implication of GKR in HC decompensation or in de novo HC. S = Signs and/or symptoms of hydrocephalus.

Actually, comparison of both groups (A versus B) of patients in our own series did not show any difference in respect of clinical and radiological parameters (table 2).

Does Treatment of a VS Patient without Previous Hydrocephalus Directly Impact on the Occurrence of Ventricle Enlargement?

Brow [13] did not mention hydrocephalus as a possible surgical complication. In the series reported by Pirouzmand et al. [6] about 173 patients who were followed after surgery for a cerebellopontine angle tumor, 2 patients experienced de novo hydrocephalus (1.2%). Even if not exactly provided by Samii and Matthies [11], it can be extracted from their data that approximately 1% of their patients experienced this event.

Little is known about the consequences of radiosurgery on CSF pathway. Noren [14] stated that treatment-related peritumoral reaction was sufficient to block the CSF circulation and required shunt insertion in 1.4% of the VS he managed with GKR, which is quite similar to the 1% we report in the present series. From other series of GKR, we learn that there was a need for shunting in 0 [15] to 3% [16], but we do not know precisely from these studies if hydrocephalus was already present before treatment. Unger et al. [17] described the outcome study of 56 VS patients treated with GKR with a median follow-up of 62 months. Little information is given but 2 patients displayed a transient enlargement of the ventricular system and 1 required a shunting procedure (2%) contemporary of a tumor increasing volume. In the Linac literature we have very scanty data with a 0% rate of hydrocephalus observed in Spiegelman's team [18], while Sawamura et al. [12] reported a 11% rate using fractionation.

In the cases of de novo hydrocephalus, it remains difficult to know if patients were already predisposed to experience hydrocephalus or if GKR induced by itself the CSF pathway disturbance. When looking at conservatively treated VS patients, the incidence of hydrocephalus is not reported but may be very low. Thus, we may assume that GKR directly affects the CSF pathway in a subgroup of patients by an unknown mechanism (fig. 1). The fact that several patients from group B experienced hydrocephalus in the early follow-up after GKR supports this assertion.

Conclusions

The data from the current series suggest that whether occurring before or after radiosurgery in the history of a VS patient, hydrocephalus is more frequent in larger-sized tumors and elderly patients. It can be assumed that in some patients, GKR plays a direct role in the occurrence of hydrocephalus without any relation to tumor growth and GKR failure. In these rare cases, ventricle enlargement is associated with significant symptoms and requires shunting. The incidence of this complication does not appear greater than what has been reported after microsurgery. On the other hand, asymptomatic ventricle dilation that was observed in 3% of patients before treatment rarely necessitated shunting. Analysis of larger series and better understanding of potential effects of GKR on CSF pathway will bring new insights into this matter and provide new information to the patients.

References

1 Roche PH, Ribeiro T, Soumare O, Robitail S, Pellet W, Régis J: Hydrocéphalie et radiochirurgie gamma knife des schwannomes vestibulaires. Neurochirurgie 2004;50:345–349.
2 Briggs RJ, Shelton C, Kwartler JA, Hitselberger W: Management of hydrocephalus resulting from acoustic neuromas. Otolaryngol Head Neck Surg 1993;109:1020–1024.
3 Atlas MD, Perez de Tagle JR, Cook JA, Sheehy JP, Fagan PA: Evolution of the management of hydrocephalus associated with acoustic neuroma. Laryngoscope 1996;106:204–206.
4 Witten RM, Wade CT: Computed tomography in acoustic tumor diagnosis; in House WF, Luetje CM: Acoustic Tumors (Vol I Diagnosis). Baltimore University Park Press, 1979, p 266.
5 Tanaka Y, Kobayashi S, Hongo K, Tada T, Sato A, Takasuna H: Clinical and neuroimaging characteristics of hydrocephalus associated with vestibular schwannoma. J Neurosurg 2003;98: 1118–1193.
6 Pirouzmand F, Tator CH, Rutka J: Management of hydrocephalus associated with vestibular schwannoma and other cerebellopontine angle tumors. Neurosurgery 2001;48:1246–1254.
7 Steenerson RL, Payne N: Hydrocephalus in the patient with acoustic acoustic neuroma. Otolaryngol Head Neck Surg 1992;107:35–39.
8 Rogg JM, Ahn SH, Tung GA, Reinert SE, Noren G: Prevalence of hydrocephalus in 157 patients with vestibular schwannoma. Neuroradiology 2005;47:344–351.
9 Gardner WJ, Spitler DK, Whitten C: Increased intracranial pressure caused by increased protein content in cerebrospinal fluid. N Engl J Med 1954;250:932–936.
10 Nassar SI, Correll JW: Subarachnoid hemorrhage due to spinal cord tumors. Neurology 1968;18:87–94.
11 Samii M, Matthies C: Management of 1,000 vestibular schwannomas (acoustic neuromas): Surgical management and results with an emphasis on complications and how to avoid them. Neurosurgery 1997;40:11–23.
12 Sawamura Y, Shirato H, Sakamoto T, Aoyama H, Suzuki K, Onimaru R, Isu T, Fukuda S, Miyasaka K: Management of vestibular schwannoma by fractionated stereotactic radiotherapy and associated cerebrospinal fluid malapsorption. J Neurosurg 2003;99: 685–692.
13 Brow RE. Pre-and Postoperative Management of the acoustic tumor patient, in: House WF, Luetje CM: Acoustic tumors (Vol II management) Baltimore University Park Press, 1979, pp 153–173.
14 Noren G: Long-term complications following gamma knife radiosurgery of vestibular schwannomas. Stereotact Funct Neurosurg 1998;70(suppl 1):65–73.
15 Prasad D, Steiner M, Steiner L: Gamma surgery for vestibular schwannoma. J Neurosurg 2000;92:745–759.
16 Kondziolka D, Lunsford D, McLaughlin MR, Flickinger JC: Long-term outcomes after radiosurgery for acoustic neuromas. N Engl J Med 1998;339: 1426–1433.
17 Unger F, Walch C, Hasselsberger K, Papaefthymiou G, Trummer M, Eustacchio S, Pendl G: Radiosurgery of vestibular schwannomas: a minimally invasive alternative to microsurgery. Acta Neurochir 1999;141:1281–1286.
18 Spiegelmann R, Lidar Z, Gofman J, Alezra D, Hadani M, Pfeffer R: Linear accelerator radiosurgery for vestibular schwannoma. J Neurosurg 2001;94: 7–13.

Prof. Pierre-Hugues Roche
Service de Neurochirurgie de l'Hôpital Nord, Assistance Publique-Hôpitaux de Marseille
Chemin des Bourrelly, FR–13915 Marseille Cedex 20 (France)
Tel. +33 4 91 96 86 20, Fax +33 4 91 96 89 15, E-Mail proche@mail.ap-hm.fr

Régis J, Roche P-H (eds): Modern Management of Acoustic Neuroma.
Prog Neurol Surg. Basel, Karger, 2008, vol 21, pp 207–213

Radiosurgery and Carcinogenesis Risk

Xavier Muracciole · Jean Régis

Service de Neurochirurgie Fonctionnelle et Stéréotaxique, Hôpital d'Adulte de la Timone, Marseille, France

Abstract

The definition of radiation-induced tumors is based on indirect criteria. They were defined initially by Cahan: the tumors must occur at the irradiated site after a time of latency longer than 5 years and be of a different pathological type from the initially irradiated tumor. The central nervous system belongs to sensitive tissue and it seems that a threshold dose does not exist. Thus, the relative risk varies from 1.57 to 8.75 for a dose of 1 Gy. It increases with the time of observation with a maximum of 18.4 between 20 and 25 years. Thus the cerebral radiation-induced tumors would be dependent on low dose for large volumes of healthy cerebral tissue (tineas, acute leukemia), and high dose for small volumes as irradiated benign lesions (pituitary tumors, meningiomas). Several factors influence the incidence of these radiation-induced tumors, of which the age at exposure and individual susceptibility are related to heredity. To date, 3 cases of radio-associated glioblastoma and 5 cases of transformed vestibular schwannoma related to radiosurgery were reported in the literature. They do not present all the traditional criteria. Thus, we reported through our experience 2 cases illustrating these problems to confront them with the published data. The long-term risk of radiation-induced tumor requires a time of observation between 5 and 30 years. This risk is estimated at less than 1 per 1,000. It must be communicated to each patient and counterbalanced with the operational risk of a benign tumor (1 per 100 of perioperative mortality) or the hemorrhagic risk of an untreated arteriovenous malformation (1 per 100 per year).

The use of ionizing radiation for benign diseases of the nervous system poses an increasing risk of primary nervous system tumors. The radiation-induced tumors vary substantially and do not have a specific pathological characteristics. The absence of a clear definition underlines the difficulty in distinguishing a radiation-induced tumor from a second spontaneous tumor. The role of radiotherapy in the development of a second tumor could perhaps be suspected by the increase in the incidence and specific mortality associated with each tumor compared to a control population. Thus, the solid tumors induced by the therapeutic medical use of the ionizing radiations were the subject of relatively recent epidemiologic studies. This is related to the time of appearance and the difficulty in isolating them from the spontaneous secondary tumors. Cahan et al. [1] defined indirect criteria to define radiation-induced sarcomas and other radiation-induced tumors. Those tumors must occur at the irradiated site after a time of latency higher than 5 years, and the pathological type must be different from the initially irradiated tumor. It is necessary to verify the absence of a second tumor at the time of radiotherapy and the absence of a pathology associated with a high susceptibility to develop tumor: Recklinghausen's disease, Li-Fraumeni syndrome, tuberosis sclerosis, xeroderma pigmentosum, retinoblastoma or genetic predisposition. Several epidemiologic studies have reported radiation-induced tumors following radiotherapy, but this risk after radiosurgery is unknown.

Factors Associated with Radiation-Induced Tumors

Several factors related to the host (age at exposition, irradiated tissue) or the methods of irradiation (dose level, irradiated volume) can influence the incidence of these tumors. The age at exposure is the major factor related to the carcinogenesis. The active periods of growth represent the most radiosensitive periods with high proliferative activity of the cells. The estimated cumulated risk at 30 years was 20% in a cohort of children who survived acute lymphoblastic leukemia after prophylactic whole brain irradiation [2]. The tissue type influences significantly the sensitivity to irradiation. Tissues are classified as: very sensitive (thyroid), sensitive (central nervous system – CNS) and moderately sensitive (mesenchymal tissue). In the same way, individual susceptibility related to heredity can significantly influence this risk. Among the parameters related to the irradiation, there is a close relationship between the dose level and the volume of irradiated healthy tissue. The cerebral radiation-induced tumors are dependent either on low dose for high volumes of healthy cerebral tissues (capitis tineas, acute leukemia) or on higher dose for benign lesions with a longer follow-up (pituitary tumors, meningioma, and pediatric glioma). Moreover, the dose-effect relation varies with age, delivered dose, dose rate, type of irradiation and healthy tissue concerned. Thus, total dose and the dose-effect relation could be illustrated with radiation thyroid pathology as low as a dose of 0.05 Gy [3] and radiation mammary malignant pathology with a linear relationship up to 5 Gy [4]. The tumors occur most frequently 15–20 years after radiotherapy, implying a long follow-up period. Radiation-induced cancers represent a frequent cause of death.

Specificities of the Central Nervous System and Radiation-Induced Tumor

The CNS belongs to sensitive tissue as well as the lung, pleura and mammary tissue. To date, no dose threshold for the CNS has been described. However the relative risk (RR) seems to lie between 1.57 and 8.75 for a dose of 1 Gy [5]. Thus, the RR according to time increases by 3.9 (between 15 and 20 years of observation) at 18.4 (between 20 and 25 years) to decrease to 3.2 (between 35 and 40 years) [6].

Radiation Dose

It seems that no threshold of exposed radiation dose exists, and each dose level could potentially cause a radiation-induced tumor. Historically, the first reported study concerned a cohort of children irradiated for tinea. An average dose to the brain was estimated at 1.5 Gy (from 1 to 6 Gy). The radiation-associated cerebral tumors were 8.4 times more frequent in the irradiated group (RR = 8.4, CI = 4.8–14.8) in comparison with the control group (5,392 not exposed children). A correlation could be highlighted with the dose of exposure. Thus, if the RR lies between 1.6 and 8.7 for a dose of 1 Gy, it increases to 20 for a dose from 2 to 3 Gy [5, 6]. Among 80,160 atomic bomb survivors, a statistically significant dose response was observed for all brain tumors and also specifically for schwannoma with a dose as low as 1 Sievert. Pui et al. [7] reported increased risk of developing of a second tumor by a factor of 3 for children who received prophylactic whole brain irradiation with a moderate dose level of 18–24 Gy for acute lymphoblastic leukemia. However, most of these second tumors were benign (schwannoma, meningioma) or with a low malignant potential [2].

Age at Exposure

Pediatric patients present higher risk than adults because the long latency of second tumors could be as long as 20–30 years [8]. A long life expectancy induces a long-term follow-up of young patients treated by radiotherapy. The age plays a major part in cerebral carcinogenesis. In the same way, the incidence of meningioma induced in the Japanese population irradiated in 1945 increased only for individuals younger than 20 years [9].

Hereditary Predisposition

Hereditary predisposition plays part in this risk. The risk of death from a second tumor at 40 years is 1.5% for patients with a unilateral not irradiated retinoblastoma, 6.4% for a bilateral not irradiated retinoblastoma and 30.3% for the bilateral retinoblastoma exposed to atomic radiation [10]. In the same way, patients with neurofibromatosis type 2 are at a higher risk for radiation-associated tumors. The pathology of these tumors was meningiomas, gliomas and sarcomas by order of decreasing frequency. The RR at 30 years increased to 9 for a benign tumor and 2.6 for a malignant tumor.

Time of Latency

The median time of diagnosis was fixed at 9 years and 14 years for the radiation-induced gliomas and meningiomas, respectively [11]. Among 253 patients with a radiation-associated meningioma after irradiation for tinea at a median age of 7 years, the median time was 36 years (from 12 to 49 years). It underlines the need of long follow-up to evaluate this risk [12].

Relative Risk and Brain Irradiation

The cumulated risk to develop a second tumor seems to vary from 1.3% at 10 years, to 2% at 20 years and 2.7% at 30 years [13]. The results of a meta-analysis werc in favor of an increased risk of secondary cerebral tumors of 6.1 (CI 3.1–10.7) [14].

Characteristics of Radiation-Induced Cerebral Tumor

The mechanisms of the carcinogenesis of these tumors are complex and unknown. It seems that a threshold dose does not exist. The severity of second tumor is not related to the total dose either. The radiation-induced tumor occurs in the areas receiving a relatively low dose (not inducing cellular death) in a large brain volume. Thus, the high dose of irradiation could destroy the cells of exposed tissue at this risk of carcinogenesis. Only the cells integrating errors of DNA repair would presented successive changes being able to lead to the malignant transformation. From cytogenetic studies of 23 radiation-associated tumors, 2 cerebral tumors presented changes of tumor suppressor genes, accumulation of genomic abnormalities (deletion) leading to the loss of the function of some genes and to the initiation of the tumoral process [15]. The time of latency could be long before the first clinical signs appear. There is no pathological difference permitting the dissociation between spontaneous glioma and radiation-associated glioma [16]. No change of the tumor suppressor PTEN gene was demonstrated for the latter. The description of a change on the P53 gene and its overexpression at the level of the transformed schwannoma were reported by Shin et al. [17]. They suggested a molecular mechanism associated with the malignant part or the malignant transformation with the tumor triton. The radiation-associated carcinogenesis suggests a relationship between low dose (calculated median dose of 1.4 Gy) and large irradiated brain volume (900 cm^3 of the healthy cerebral tissue) for taenia irradiation [14]. By comparison with radiosurgery for a schwannoma 15 mm in diameter, the same calculated volume is about 120 cm^3.

Radiosurgery and Radiation-Associated Tumor

Radiosurgery is used increasingly to treat intracranial benign tumors (meningioma, schwannoma, pituitary adenoma), vascular malformation and functional diseases. To date, a very low number of radiation-induced tumor was reported in

Table 1. Malignant, radiosurgery-associated tumors

Series	Sex/age	Initial diagnosis	Marginal dose, Gy	Free interval, years	Pathology of 2nd tumor
Shamiza [26]	F/57	VS	11	7.5	GBM
Kaido [27]	M/14	AVM	20	6.5	GBM
Yu [28]	F/57	meningioma	20	7	GBM
Salvati [29]	F/66	cavernoma	25	13	GBM
Sanno [30]	F/53	meningioma	30	4.5	osteosarcoma
Muracciole [31]	F/64	VS	13	8.4	GBM
Rowe [18]	–	cavernoma	–	8	astrocytoma

VS = Vestibular schwannoma; GBM = glioblastoma multiform.

the literature. They do not present all traditional criteria of Cahan. We report 2 cases occurring in our clinical practice. We would be emphasizing the nosologic problems inherent to the definition of the radiation-induced tumors or radiation associated in the field of radiosurgery.

Case 1

A 64-year-old woman consulted for an important decrease in hearing in October 1991. Examination revealed a vestibular schwannoma of the right acoustic nerve. After a follow-up period, a significant increase in size (15 × 18 × 10 mm) was observed on MRIin January 1993 with a major auditory degradation. This patient underwent radiosurgery in March 1993, receiving a dose of 13 Gy to the periphery by four isocenters (maximal dose of 26 Gy). In the follow-up, the lesion size increased on successive MRI and the diagnosis of recurrence was made (22 × 21 × 20 mm). The patient underwent subtotal resection with preservation of the facial nerve in March 1996. The pathological report revealed the persistence of a schwannoma type A of the Antoni classification. In July 2001, 8 years and 4 months after radiosurgery, the patient had headaches with an anxious agitation and a left hemiparesis. A cerebral MRI scan highlighted a right temporal lesion highly suggestive of high-grade glioma. The patient underwent right temporal craniotomy and total resection of the enhancing lesion. Pathological analysis revealed presence of a glioblastoma. The patient received a postoperative radiotherapy of the tumoral bed and unfortunately died 1 year after the diagnosis of glioblastoma.

The latent period and the nature of the secondary tumor strongly suspect the radiation nature of the glioblastoma. In the literature, 7 second malignant tumors (3 glioblastomas, 1 osteosarcoma and 1 astrocytoma) were reported with all Cahan' criteria (table 1). All cases must be considered as radiosurgery-induced tumors. However, it is interesting to note that in 3 cases of secondary glioblastoma, a neurosurgical procedure was taken. This surgery could contribute to local inflammatory phenomena participating potentially in tumoral promotion and proliferation. Also these 4 cases together with the number of lesions treated by radiosurgery until today (80,000 patients) could be integrated in the natural incidence of glioma in terms of coexistence without specific responsibility [19].

Case 2

A 61-year-old woman presented a tumoral lesion of the left pontocerebellar angle manifested by hypoacousia, acouphens and instability. Radiological data strongly suggested a schwannoma with a large diameter of 25 mm. The patient was then treated by Gamma Knife radiosurgery in June 1999 with a prescription dose of 10 Gy with 19 isocenters. In the follow-up, the lesion continued to increase and required neurosurgical intervention by a translabyrinthine approach 3 years and 4 months after the radiosurgery. The postoperative pathological report revealed the presence of a tumor triton, considered as a sarcomatous tumor. During the follow-up, reappearance of headaches highlighted a second

Table 2. Malignant schwannoma and radiosurgery

Series	Sex/age	Initial diagnosis	NF2	Treatment	Free interval, years	Pathology of 2nd tumor
Kurita[1]	F/26	VS	no	STR – RS	5	MS
Noren [32]	F/18	VS	yes	STR – RS	5	MS
Comey [20]	M/50	VS	no	RS – STR	5	MS
Shin [17]	F/26	VS	no	RS	5	MS
Muracciole [31]	F/63	VS	no	RS	4	MS

STR = Subtotal resection; RS = radiosurgery; MS = malignant schwannoma; NF2 = neurofibromatosis type 2.
[1]Personal communication.

important recurrence. The patient underwent a second subtotal resection 13 months after the first neurosurgical procedure and 4 years and 5 months after the radiosurgery. A conformal external radiotherapy completed the local treatment.

Four other identical cases of a tumor triton were reported after a radiosurgical treatment for vestibular schwannoma [19–21; Kurita, pers. commun.]. A malignant schwannoma named 'tumor triton' represents a specific nosologic entity which should be separated from radiation-associated tumor. This tumor derives from the nervous sheaths combining a spiculated malignant cellular quota (spindle) and a little differentiated part with immunostaining of the rhabdoid subtype. This 'tumor triton' denomination is related to the capacity of the neural tissue to stimulate an exophytic growth from mesenchymal tissue [22]. Its malignant nature tends frequently to recur locally and to disseminate in the CNS. This type of lesion does not enter stricto sensus within the framework of the radiosurgery-associated tumors. It occurs after radiosurgery for a histologically standard schwannoma. The malignant transformation of a schwannoma or a schwannoma with benign and malignant parts is extremely rare except in a context of neurofibromatosis. Thus, 3 cases were reported only in the series of neurosurgery of acoustic schwannomas [20]. It is thus difficult to evaluate the potential role of radiosurgery in the emergence of a malignant part within a schwannoma. It is possible, as Comey suggested, that the malignant part is initially present and temporarily controlled by radiosurgery. Table 2 summarizes 5 cases which were reported as radiation-associated tumors. These lesions did not present the full criteria of Cahan's definition.

Incidence of Radiation-Induced Tumor

Whole brain volume is exposed to low doses of radiation (1 Gy) by the radiosurgery procedure. This low dose is associated with an RR of radiation-induced tumor ranging from 1.57 to 18.4 for a latency period of 20–25 years. Ganz [23] reported an incidence of radiosurgery-induced tumor ranging from 0 to 3 per 200,000 patients. However, the latent period and follow-up methods of his cohort (not systematically MRI procedures) minimized the true incidence. Rowe et al. [18] reported a retrospective cohort study comparing the Sheffield England radiosurgery patient database with national mortality and cancer registries. No excess incidence of cerebral malignancy was detected among 4,877 patients treated by Sheffield Gamma Knife Unit, with a total of 29,916 patient-years of follow-up and a mean of 6.1 years per patient. Only a single new primary intracranial tumor (astrocytoma) was observed after radiosurgery when one would expect 2.47 cases of CNS malignant tumor in a cohort of more than 1,200 patients followed for 10–19 years [20]. Radiation-induced meningioma was excluded from this analysis. These benign tumors represent the majority of radiation-induced tumors [6]. Sheehan et al. [24] also reported a long follow-up of 1,333 patients treated for arteriovenous malformation (AVM) and at least 10 years of 288 patients. The risk to develop a radiosurgery-induced tumor was estimated at 0.7% with an incidence of 69 per 100,000 person-years (2 meningiomas). These data must reflect the annual incidence of primary brain tumors ranging from 10.97 to 15.5 per 100,000 person-years [25]. However, there are nearly 500,000 radiosurgery treatments at this time and probably the risk of delayed oncogenesis varies from 1 per 1,000 patients to 1–20,000 patients.

Conclusion

Radiation-associated tumors present no specific clinical, pathological, or molecular parameters. The criteria of Cahan represent highly evocative arguments of this nature without representing strict rules. The search for molecular markers associated with a genetic predisposition to develop this type of tumor will prevent exposing such patients to the risk of radiation carcinogenesis in the future. However, this risk of tumor associated with radiosurgery is significantly lower compared to conventional irradiation. This risk can be estimated at less than 1 per 1,000 patients treated by radiosurgery with a range from 0.01 to 2% in comparison to the 10% risk associated with a traditional external radiotherapy at 20 years. This partly depends on the target volume to treat much smaller, less exposed healthy tissue and a higher cytotoxicity related to the high dose of the single and mutagen treatment. However, within the field of vestibular schwannoma, this risk seems to be related to the low dose concerning surrounding healthy tissue. Two cases of radiation-induced (radiation-associated) tumor were reported and discussed. The long-term risk of radiation-associated tumor requires a long time of observation between 5 and 30 years. Thus during the first consultation for radiosurgery of a benign lesion, this risk, although extremely low (less than 1 per 1,000), must be presented to each patient and be counterbalanced with the operative risk for a benign tumoral lesion (1 per 100 of perioperative mortality) or the hemorrhagic risk of an untreated AVM (1 per 100 per year). The risk of radiosurgery-induced tumor must be weighted in the treatment of pediatric patients and patients with benign tumors and with long life expectancy.

References

1 Cahan WG, Woodard HQ, Higinbotham NL, Stewart FW, Coley BL: Sarcoma arising in irradiated bone: report of eleven cases. 1948. Cancer 1998;82:8–34.

2 Pui CH, Cheng C, Leung W, Rai SN, Rivera GK, Sandlund JT, Ribeiro RC, Relling MV, Kun LE, Evans WE: Extended follow-up of long-term survivors of childhood acute lymphoblastic leukaemia. N Engl J Med 2003;349:640–649.

3 Ron E, Lubin JH, Shore RE, Mabuchi K, Modan B, Pottern LM, Schneider AB, Tucker MA, Boice JD Jr: Thyroid cancer after exposure to external radiation: a pooled analysis of seven studies. Radiat Res 1995;141:259–277.

4 Mattsson A, Ruden BI, Palmgren J, Rutqvist LE: Dose- and time-response for breast cancer risk after radiation therapy for benign breast disease. Br J Cancer 1995;72:1054–1061.

5 Hubert D, Bertin M: Radiation-induced tumours of the nervous system in man. Bull Cancer 1993;80:971–983.

6 Ron E, Modan B, Boice JD Jr, Alfandary E, Stovall M, Chetrit A, Katz L: Tumours of the brain and nervous system after radiotherapy in childhood. N Engl J Med 1988;319:1033–1039.

7 Pui CH, Pei D, Sandlund JT, Campana D, Ribeiro RC, Razzouk BI, Rubmitz JE, Howard SC, Hijiya N, Jeha S, Cheng C, Downing JR, Evans WE, Relling MV, Hudson M: Risk of adverse events after completion of therapy for childhood acute lymphoblastic leukaemia. J Clin Oncol 2005;23:7936–7941.

8 Sznajder L, Abrahams C, Party DM, Gierlowski TC, Shore-Freedman E, Schneider AB: Multiple schwannomas and meningiomas associated with irradiation in childhood. Arch Intern Med 1996;156:1873–1878.

9 Shibata S, Sadamori N, Mine M, Sekine I: Intracranial meningiomas among Nagasaki atomic bomb survivors. Lancet 1994;344:1770.
10 Eng C, Li FP, Abramson DH, Ellsworth RM, Wong FL, Goldman MB, Seddon J, Tarbell N, Boice JD Jr: Mortality from second tumours among long-term survivors of retinoblastoma. J Natl Cancer Inst 1993;85:1121–1128.
11 Dalton VMK, Gelber RD, Li F, Donnelly MJ, Tarbell NJ, Sallan SE: Second malignancies in patients treated for childhood acute lymphoblastic leukemia. J Clin Oncol 1998;16:2848–2853.
12 Sadetzki S, Flint-Richter P, Ben-Tal T, Nass D: Radiation-induced meningioma: a descriptive study of 253 cases. J Neurosurg 2002;97:1078–1082.
13 Breen P, Flickinger JC, Kondziolka D, Martinez AJ: Radiotherapy for nonfunctional pituitary adenoma: analysis of long-term tumour control. J Neurosurg 1998;89:933–938.
14 Erfurth EM, Bulow B, Mikoczy Z, Svahn-Tapper G, Hagmar L: Is there an increase in second brain tumours after surgery and irradiation for a pituitary tumour. Clin Endocrinol 2001;55:613–616.
15 Chauveinc L, Dutrillaux AM, Validire P, Padoy E, Sabatier L, Couturier J, Dutrillaux B: Cytogenetic study of eight new cases of radiation-induced solid tumours. Cancer Genet Cytogenet 1999;114:1–8.
16 Brat DJ, James CD, Jedlicka AE, Connolly DC, Chang E, Castellani RJ, Schmid M, Schiller M, Carson DA, Burger PC: Molecular genetic alterations in radiation-induced astrocytomas: Am J Pathol 1999;154: 1431–1438.
17 Shin M, Ueki K, Kurita H, Kirino T: Malignant transformation of a vestibular schwannoma after gamma knife radiosurgery. Lancet 2002;360:309–310.
18 Rowe J, Grainger A, Walton L, Silcocks P, Radatz M, Kemeny A: Risk of malignancy after gamma knife stereotactic radiosurgery. Neurosurgery 2007;60:60–65.
19 McLean CA, Laidlaw JD, Brownbill DS, Gonzales MF: Recurrence of acoustic neurilemoma as a malignant spindle-cell neoplasm. Case report. J Neurosurg 1990;73:946–950.
20 Comey CH, McLaughlin MR, Jho HD, Martinez AJ, Lunsford LD: Death from a malignant cerebellopontine angle triton tumour despite stereotactic radiosurgery. Case report. J Neurosurg 1998;89:653–658.
21 Hanabusa K, Morikawa A, Murata T, Taki W: Acoustic neuroma with malignant transformation. Case report. J Neurosurg 2001;95:518–521.
22 Brooks JS, Freeman M, Enterline HT: Malignant 'Triton' tumours. Natural history and immunohistochemistry of nine new cases with literature review. Cancer 1985;55:2543–2549.
23 Ganz JC: Gamma knife radiosurgery and its possible relationship to malignancy: a review. J Neurosurg 2002;9:644–652.
24 Sheehan J, Yen CP, Steiner L: Gamma knife surgery-induced meningioma. Report of two cases and review of the literature. J Neurosurg 2006;105: 325–329.
25 Christensen HC, Kosteljanetz M, Johansen C: Incidences of gliomas and meningiomas in Denmark 1943–1997. Neurosurgery 2003;52: 1327–1334.
26 Shamisa A, Bance M, Nag S, Tator C, Wong S, Noren G, Guha A: Glioblastoma multiforme occurring in a patient treated with gamma knife surgery. Case report and review of the literature. J Neurosurg 2001;94: 816–821.
27 Kaido T, Hoshida T, Uranishi R, Akita N, Kotani A, Nishi N, Sakaki T: Radiosurgery-induced brain tumour. Case report. J Neurosurg 2001;95:710–713.
28 Yu JS, Yong WH, Wilson D, Black KL: Glioblastoma induction after radiosurgery for meningioma. Lancet 2000;356:1576–1577.
29 Salvati M, Frati A, Russo N, Caroli E, Polli FM, Minniti G, Delfini R: Radiation-induced gliomas: report of 10 cases and review of the literature. Surg Neurol 2003;60:60–67.
30 Sanno N, Hayashi S, Shimura T, Maeda S, Teramoto A: Intracranial osteosarcoma after radiosurgery : case report. Neurol Med Chir 2004;44:29–32.
31 Muracciole X, Cowen D, Regis J: Radiosurgery and brain radio-induced carcinogenesis : update. Neurochirurgie 2004;50:414–420.
32 Noren G: Long-term complications following gamma knife radiosurgery of vestibular schwannomas. Stereotact Funct Neurosurg 1998;70:65–73.

Dr. Xavier Muracciole
Service de Neurochirurgie Fonctionnelle et Stéréotaxique
Hôpital d'Adulte de la Timone, 264 bvd Saint Pierre
FR–13385 Marseille Cedex 05 (France)
E-Mail xavier.muracciole@ap-hm.fr

Régis J, Roche P-H (eds): Modern Management of Acoustic Neuroma.
Prog Neurol Surg. Basel, Karger, 2008, vol 21, pp 214–221

Vestibular Schwannomas: Complications of Microsurgery

Pierre-Hugues Roche[a] · Telmo Ribeiro[a] · Henri-Dominique Fournier[c] · Jean-Marc Thomassin[b]

[a]Service de Neurochirurgie, Hôpital Sainte-Marguerite, [b]Fédération d'Oto-Rhino-Laryngologie, Hôpital la Timone, Assistance Publique-Hôpitaux de Marseille, Marseille, [c]Service de Neurochirurgie, Hôpital Larrey, Centre Hospitalier Universitaire d'Angers, Angers, France

Abstract

Current microsurgical treatment of vestibular schwannomas usually brings satisfactory results for the patients. However, transient or permanent complications may occur, especially when treating large tumors. Precise information about these potential complications has to be given to the patient at the time of the surgical decision. Based on their personal experience of large operated vestibular schwannomas and analyzing a review of the international literature, the authors detail these complications and the way to prevent and manage them. The problems that are linked to the variety of surgical approaches are also commented. The most frequent complication is cerebrospinal fluid leak that requires medical management and in less than one third of cases, surgical exploration. Vascular problems including ischemia or hemorrhage inside the posterior fossa represent the main source of permanent morbidity. Lower cranial nerve deficits are unusual but may expose to early and delayed aspiration pneumonias. The authors conclude that careful selection of cases, meticulous operative management and intensive postoperative care are essential steps to prevent and to treat these complications.

Despite significant development of radiosurgical techniques, microsurgical resection remains the first intention treatment of large vestibular schwannomas (VSs). The goal of this treatment is to obtain maximal resection with functional preservation. However, complications may occur once the patient's skin is opened under general anesthesia.

The aim of this chapter is to detail these complications and their mechanisms, to indicate the way to avoid them and to explain how to manage them when they occur.

Design of the Study

This study incorporated data from our previously published experience of large VSs [1] and reviewed the recent series from the international literature. To select these series, we used a Medline and Pubmed search using the following key words: 'complication', 'mortality', 'middle fossa approach', 'retrosigmoid approach', 'translabyrinthine approach', 'vestibular schwannoma' covering the period from 1985 to present in English. We excluded small series (less than 90 operated cases).

We excluded from the scope of this chapter problems that are linked to facial nerve injury and evaluation of the cochleovestibular function after surgery. Both aspects are detailed in separate chapters. The issue of recurrence is also debated elsewhere.

Results

Mortality

The current mortality rate is approximately 1–2% in main series dealing with large VS. Main causes of death are aspiration pneumonia, cerebellopontine angle (CPA) hemorrhage, and myocardial infarction.

Samii and Matthies [2] reported a 1% rate of mortality among 1,000 operated cases, and distinguished three groups of patients who were considered to be at major risk: (1) premorbid patients with previous surgery or with severe brain stem compression, (2) tumors with caudal cranial nerve involvement and complete palsy after surgery, (3) possible postoperative hemorrhage (cystic or nonencapsulated tumors).

Better selection of cases for surgery and orientation toward conservative treatment are strongly recommended for high-risk patients. In cases of large tumors with significant brain shift and premorbid state, a quick procedure of internal debulking using a retrosigmoid (RS) approach can be advised.

Cranial Nerve Deficits

Some of these deficits are routinely discussed with the patient during the preoperative step. Facial palsy and cochleovestibular dysfunction may be expected and are well known issues that are discussed in different chapters.

Other cranial nerve deficits are usually not expected. Trigeminal nerve injury may lead to facial numbness and more rarely to anesthesia dolorosa. Trigeminal injury may occur in the case of large tumors extending cranially. It is not unusual to observe operatively that the tumor distorts the trigeminal root that courses in the same cisternal space. However, by comparison with the acousticofacial bundle, the nerve seems resistant to a considerable shifting, surgical manipulation and devascularization. Combined deficit of facial and trigeminal nerve is usually responsible for serious eye trophic problems (corneal ulceration). Such situation may be more frequently observed in giant tumors and in neurofibromatosis type 2 patients, where previous surgery of the CPA has been done for another tumor or recurrent schwannoma.

Lower cranial nerve (LCN) dysfunction is rarely reported. Among 707 operated cases, Sanna et al. [3] described 1 case (0.14%), while we described a 4.2% incidence of deficits, mainly transient [1]. Caudal extension of large VSs is routinely observed but LCNs are protected by the arachnoid sheath of the cerebellomedullary cistern. However, once this cistern has been opened, the LCNs must be considered as very fragile. In cases of operative doubt about potential damage of these nerves, it is advised to examine the pharyngeal motility and vocal cord motion before feeding the patient. True adhesion is encountered in some giant tumors; in these cases, it may be preferable to leave some of the tumor capsule along the nerve course.

Oculomotor deficits are exceptional. The 1.68% rate of deficit that has been reported by Sanna et al. [3] and the 7% reported by Kanzaki et al. [4] has not been confirmed by other series. This rarity is probably due to distinct cisternal course of these nerves that are usually not exposed in the operative field. In giant tumors only, the upper pole reaches the free edge of the tentorium and puts the IVth nerve at jeopardy while the ventral part of the tumor may push the cisternal portion of the VIth nerve.

Vascular Complications

Vascular complications have been reported in up to 7% of patients and can have devastating consequences with significant risks of morbidity and death. In a recent study conducted by Sade et al. [5], vascular complications were detected in 11 patients (2.7%) among a series of 413 operated VS. Eight of them were hemorrhagic complications (2 CPA, 1 intracerebellar, and 5 epidural hematomas) while 3 patients experienced ischemic problems (1 venous thrombosis, 2 arterial infarct due to perioperative inappropriate coagulations).

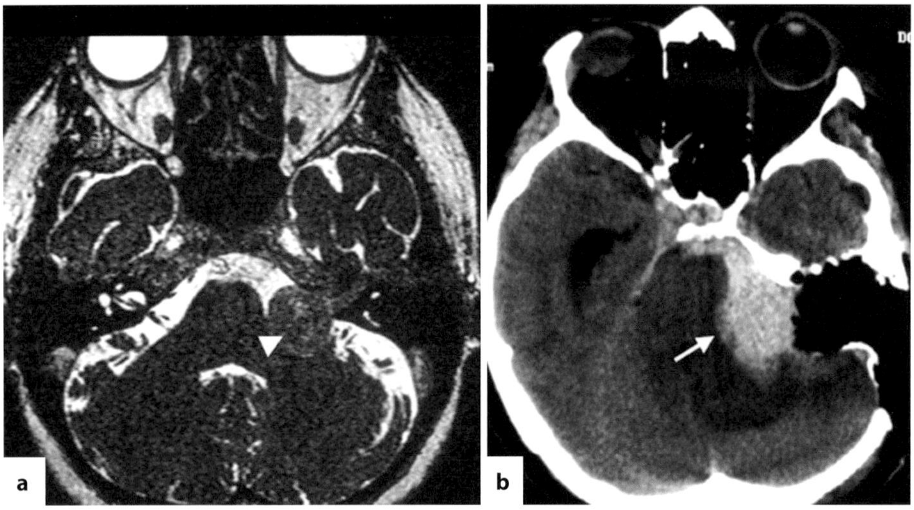

Fig. 1. a This T_2-weighted axial MRI shows a left schwannoma (white arrowhead) in the CPA and in the internal auditory meatus in a 63-year-old woman presenting with tinnitus and imbalance. **b** This axial CT can that was performed in the early postoperative course shows a large CPA hematoma with brain shift that required emergency evacuation.

Hemorrhagic Complications

The incidence of posterior fossa hematomas is around 1% of operated cases, ranging from 0.8 [6] to 2.4% of cases [7]. The most common type of postoperative bleeding is an intracisternal CPA hemorrhage, as illustrated by one of our observation in figure 1. In most cases, bleeding is detected within the first 24 h after surgery. Cystic and/or unencapsulated tumors have been reported to increase the risk of postoperative hematoma [2]. Injury to the venous structures (bridging veins, sinuses, jugular bulb) may be responsible for insidious postoperative bleeding. Yamakami et al. [8] suggested that the semi-sitting position, in reducing the venous pressure, might contribute to overlook a bleeding vein until a postoperative hematoma develops. In order to reduce the risk of hematoma, careful inspection of the operative field under saline irrigation is recommended at the completion of surgery. Hematoma is depicted because of neurological worsening and comatous state and confirmed by emergency computed tomography (CT) scan. It requires an emergency microsurgical re-exploration where suction irrigation of the clots, identification of the source of bleeding and hemostasis are performed. The origin of the bleeding is not always found at the time of surgery and this second exploration of the operative field puts the cranial nerves at jeopardy. In cases of acute hydrocephalus, an external ventricular drainage is required.

Ischemic Complications

This problem may be of arterial or venous origin and may affect the brain stem or the cerebellar hemisphere. Adhesion of the tumor with the lateral aspect of the brainstem and middle cerebellar peduncle is responsible of microtraumatisms of the small vessels that course at the interface of both structures. In cases of large tumors, it remains possible to preserve the arachnoid plane over the cerebellar hemisphere, but this plane is usually disrupted deeper at the level of the brain stem and subpial vessels may be damaged there. Coagulation of small arterial perforators must be avoided to prevent brainstem infarction. Major injury of cerebellar arteries (AICA or PICA) is exceptional because these vessels are usually well identified and can be dissected and preserved. Kania et al. [9] reported 3 cases of partial AICA syndrome among 6 vascular complications in a series of 432 operated cases. Vasospasm has been a described mechanism of ischemic complications during cranial base surgery [9]. Usually, tears from the small subpial veins can be coagulated with no consequences but care should be taken to preserve large veins.

Sinus thrombosis is an underestimated complication: Keiper et al. [10] reported a 4.7% incidence of sinus thrombosis after the RS and TL procedures. Venous infarction with acute symptoms of headache and visual deterioration is the consequence of sudden raised intracranial pressure. Tolerance to the thrombosis depends on preoperative individual caliber of the involved sinus and of drainage pattern of the whole brain. A late presentation is possible (as late as 4 weeks after surgery). Keiper et al. [10] described 5 cases of pseudotumor cerebri responsible for visual obscuration, papilledema and headaches in the days (ranging from J1 to J35) following the thrombosis of a transverse sinus after suboccipital or translabyrinthine (TL) removal of a CPA tumor. In 2 cases, medical treatment was given while a lumboperitoneal shunt allowed recovery of all symptoms in 3 cases. In order to avoid such complication, the same authors advised to (1) maintain an adequate hydration during and after surgery, (2) limit the bony exposure to what is necessary, (3) minimize the retraction against venous structures. In one of our operated cases, aphasia followed by a decreased level of consciousness and left hemiparesis occurred at 3 days after the uneventful TL removal of a left-sided VS (fig. 2). Despite the normality of a venous angiogram, the ischemia that was observed at the level of the left temporal lobe and in the basal ganglia could be attributed to venous thrombosis. Under anticoagulation treatment, the patient improved in a few days but some of his language difficulties pertained.

Meningitis

Postoperative meningitis is a rare but not exceptional event that has been reported in 1.3 [2] to 9.2% [6] of large series. It may be associated with cerebrospinal fluid (CSF) leak or not. In the study from the House Ear Clinic about 723 operated cases, incidence of CSF leaks and meningitis was 6.8 and 2.9%, respectively. Meningitis occurred more frequently in larger tumors, but the occurrence of a CSF leak did not predispose to meningitis [11].

Clinical inflammatory syndrome and headaches may be attenuated by the systematic use of paracetamol in the postoperative course. Persistent lethargic status and signs of meningeal irritation with a normal CT scan should lead to perform a lumbar puncture. Hypoglycorrachia is the most important stigma of bacterial meningitis because the level of albumin and count of polynuclear cells is usually seriously modified by the previous intracisternal surgery. Direct examination of the CSF, Gram staining and culture will be able to confirm the pathogenic agent and provide an adapted antibiogram. Intravenous administration of high doses of antibiotics that are able to cross the blood-brain barrier are started once the CSF has been withdrawn and analyzed. In a second step, the treatment is adapted to the identification of the pathogenic agent.

Cerebrospinal Fluid Leak

CSF leak is defined as a persistent communication between the cisternal space and the external environment. It is the most frequent complication. Its incidence ranges between 0 and 30%, with the average around 10%: 8.4% in our own series [1], 9.2% in the 1,000 cases managed by Samii and Matties [2] and 10.7% in the 624 cases reported by Brennann et al. [12]. Although usually benign and easy to cure, the CSF leak may expose to meningitis or tension pneumocephalus if not identified and treated early. It is necessary

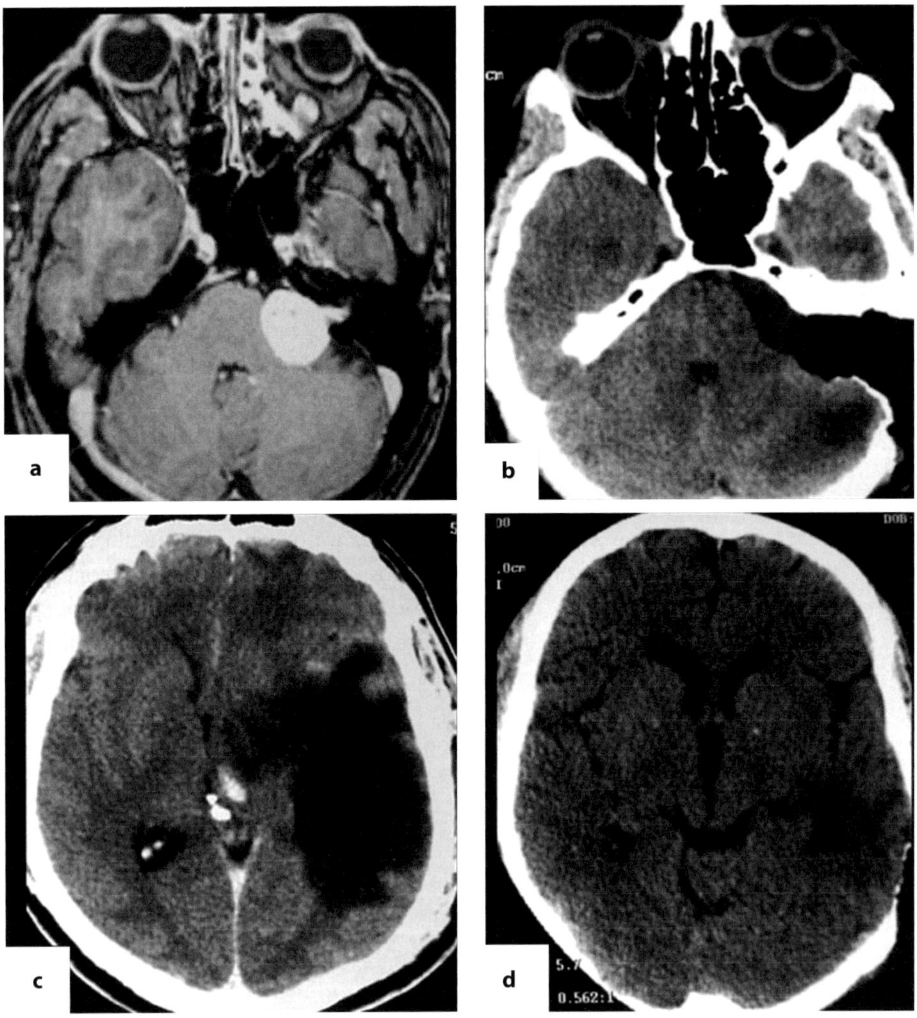

Fig. 2. a Axial T_1-weighted MRI study showing a left CPA schwannoma that was still growing at 2 years after radiosurgery. **b** This axial CT scan was done on the day that followed the left widened TL approach of the tumor. **c** This axial CT scan was performed at 3 days after surgery because of clinical worsening and showed a deep and superficial hypodensity in the posterior region of the left temporal lobe, with brain shift. **d** This axial CT scan showed a near-total resolution of the ischemic feature at 1 month following this venous complication.

to distinguish the leaks through the incision from rhinorrhea or otorrhea. In a recent study, the most frequent site of CSF leak was the skin incision (45% of cases) with rhinorrhea and otorrhea accounting for 38 and 16%, respectively [12]. Otorrhea was explained by the positioning of transtympanic promontory electrodes.

Variables that may influence this complication are debatable. Influence of tumor size is not clearly recognized in all studies. The same conclusion is brought for the influence of the surgical approach. Brennan et al. [12] reported that there were no significant differences in the incidence of leak between the RS and the TL approach (7.9

compared with 10%), but the RS approach was significantly more associated with rhinorrhea and otorrhea while TL approach was mainly responsible for leaks through the wound. This information may reflect a more watertight closure in the RS approach. Becker et al. [13] concluded that neither surgical approach nor tumor size affected the rate of CSF leakage. They also observed that the rate of leaks remained stable in recent decades despite numerous refinements of closure technique. Taken collectively, these data suggested that transient or permanent postoperative rises in the CSF pressure may explain this complication [13]. Preoperative hydrocephalus may influence the rate of CSF leakage. In the study from Tanaka et al. [14], CSF leakage was encountered in 12 (5.1%) out of 236 patients. In the group of 24 patients with hydrocephalus who did not have a shunt at the time of tumor resection, the incidence of postoperative CSF leakage was 29.2%, while it was 0% in the group of 9 patients with hydrocephalus who had a previous shunting.

There is a general agreement to manage CSF leaks in a stepwise way. The majority of leaks resolve with medical treatment that comprises head elevation, compression bandage, administration of acetazolamide and a 3-day protocol of lumbar drainage or lumbar punctures. Failed cases that require surgical revision represent less than one third of the total number of leaks [2, 12]. In the TL approach, because of the use of duraplasty and not watertight closure, because of the wide area of air cell opening, the leak has less chance to seal with simple CSF diversion when compared with the use of the RS approach [12]. Even sealed with medical treatment, late recurrence is an indication for repair and necessitates a preoperative high-resolution cisternography with CT scan.

Complications following the Approach

Surgical removal of VS may be conducted through several surgical corridors. Each of them offers specific advantages that may be used for selected cases. However, the main criterion of choice is usually the surgeon's experience in a single approach. Each approach may also expose to specific complications that deserve several comments.

Retrosigmoid Approach

When used during this approach, the semisitting position risks air embolism irrespective of anesthetic monitoring to prevent this complication [15]. Drilling of the internal auditory meatus may expose to venous injury and bleeding in case of high jugular bulb position [16].

Excessive retraction of the cerebellum under a spatula may also induce a parenchymal traumatism where multiple mechanisms (contusion, vascular problem, ...) are implicated. This retraction may be responsible for persistent deficit in the case of severe damage. However, a recent case-controlled study analyzed the cerebellar function in matched groups operated via the TL and the RS approach, and was able to show a significant difference of incidence in both groups [17]. It has also been shown that the incidence of long-lasting headaches after surgery was more frequent than after using the TL route.

Translabyrinthine Approach

This approach needs a special expertise of the petrous anatomy and is usually conducted by a neuro-otologist. The facial nerve may be injured during the approach in case of inappropriate drilling around the Fallopian canal.

The issue of direct venous injury has never been specifically addressed for the TL approach but was analyzed for the presigmoidal-transpetrosal procedure [18]. This report indicated that 7 out of 143 patients (5%) developed a sigmoid sinus occlusion within 40 days after surgery (5 cases) or in the long-term (2 cases). Possible causes of occlusion were sinus injury in 5 cases and compression by bone chip in 2 cases. Various treatments including immediate removal of the bone fragment, anticoagulation therapies, and sinojugular bypass were used depending on individual circumstances. In the absence of sinus injury, the role played by the retraction of the sigmoid sinus during a lengthy procedure is probably significant in the mechanism of occlusion.

In the series from Sluyter et al. [6] about the TL removal of large VSs, an aphasia occurred in 12 of the 58 patients (21%) who where operated on the left side. Note that in this series, division of the tentorium was systematically performed, which is not common during the standard approach. In the same series, 3.3% of 120 patients had persistent epileptic seizures requiring drug treatment while we personally reported an incidence of seizure in 1% of cases [1]. Both manifestations may be attributed to the damage of the temporal lobe venous drainage.

The skin incision that is needed at the site of the harvested fat may sometimes be responsible for subcutaneous hematoma: 3.2% in one study [3] and 4% in our experience [1].

Middle Fossa Approach

During the middle fossa approach, the neuro-otologist pays special attention to separate the great superficial petrosal nerve from the temporal dura in order to preserve lacrimation. So far, the issue of eye dryness has never been addressed in the literature but we have personally observed several cases of permanent dryness when using properly this approach for petrous apex tumors while the acousticofacial bundle was preserved. Care is also taken not to open the bone shell over the superior semicircular canal or around the cochlea. One of the major issues is the consequence of the temporal lobe retraction, particularly on the left side. A study conducted in 160 patients described an incidence of 15.3% of transient temporal lobe symptoms (language disturbances or epilepsia) that were mainly associated with large tumors [4]. Another difficulty of the middle fossa approach is to manage the facial nerve inside the internal auditory canal since it is permanently interposed between the surgeon and the tumor. This position puts the nerve at risk, particularly when the internal auditory canal is widened and entirely filled by a large tumor.

Conclusions

Even drastically reduced to a small amount of cases, operative complications still exist. Problems are of various degrees, concern various mechanisms, and sometimes lead to permanent deficits. This information should be clearly given to the patient when the benefit/risk ratio is to be evaluated at the time of the treatment decision. Microsurgical removal of VS is a stepwise procedure where it is usually possible to plan each difficulty. Most complications are due to inadequate operative maneuvers. Vascular complications carry the most significant rate of severe morbidity, regardless of the surgical approach. Appropriate selection of cases, meticulous surgical technique and careful postoperative care are crucial to lower the rate of complications. Since tumor size is an important influencing parameter, combined micro-and radiosurgical strategies may be an alternative option to minimize nerve and vessel manipulation and shorten the operative time. These new strategies deserve special consideration and evaluation.

References

1 Deveze A, Roche PH, Facon F, Gabert K, Pellet W, Thomassin JMT: Résultats de l'exérèse par voie translabyrinthique élargie des schwannomes vestibulaires. Neurochirurgie 2004;50:244–252.

2 Samii M, Matthies C: Management of 1,000 vestibular schwannomas (acoustic neuromas): Surgical management and results with an emphasis on complications and how to avoid them. Neurosurgery 1997;40:11–23.

3 Sanna M, Taibah A, Russo A, Falcioni M, Agarwal M: Perioperative complications (vestibula r schwannoma) surgery. Otol Neurotol 2004;25:379–386.

4 Kanzaki J, Ogawa K, Tsuchihashi N, Inoue Y, Yamamoto M, Ikeda S: Perioperative complications in acoustic neuroma surgery by the extended middle cranial fossa approach. Acta Otolaryngol Suppl 1991;487:75–79.
5 Sade B, Mohr G, Dufour JJ: Vascular complications of vestibular schwannoma surgery: a comparison of the suboccipital retrosigmoid and translabyrinthine approaches. J Neurosurg 2006;105:200–204.
6 Sluyter S, Graamans K, Tulleken CAF, Van Veelen WM: Analysis of the results obtained in 120 patients with large acoustic neuromas surgically treated via the translabyrinthine-transtentorial approach. J Neurosurg 2001;94:61–66.
7 Briggs RJS, Luxford WM, Atkins JS, Hitselberger WE: Translabyrinthine removal of large acoustic neuromas. Neurosurgery 1994;34:785–792.
8 Yamakami I, Uchino Y, Kobayashi E, Yamaura A, Oka N: Removal of large acoustic neurinomas (vestibular schwannomas) by the retrosigmoid approach with no mortality and minimal morbidity. J Neural Neurosurg Psychiatry 2004;75:433–458.
9 Kania R, Lot G, Herman P, Tran Ba Huy P: Vascular complications after acoustic neurinoma surgery. Ann Otolaryngol Chir Cervicofac 2003;120:94–102.
10 Keiper GL, Sherman JD, Tomsick TA, Tew JM: Dural sinus thrombosis and psudotumor cerebri: unexpected complications of suboccipital craniotomy and translabyrinthine craniectomy. J Neurosurg 1999;91:192–197.
11 Rodgers GK, Luxford WM: Factors affecting the development of cerebrospinal fluid leak and meningitis after translabyrinthine acoustic tumor surgery. Laryngoscope 1993;103:959–962.
12 Brennan JW, Rowed DW, Nedzelski JM, Chen JM: Cerebrospinal fluid leak after acoustic neuroma surgery: Influence of tumor size and surgical approach on incidence and response to treatment. J Neurosurg 2001;94:217–223.
13 Becker SS, Jackler RK, Pitts LH: Cerebrospinal fluid leak after acoustic neuroma surgery: a comparison of the translabyrinthine, middle fossa, and retrosigmoid approaches. Otol Neurotol 2003;24:107–112.
14 Tanaka Y, Kobayashi S, Hongo K, Tada T, Sato A, Takasuna H: Clinical and neuroimaging characteristics of hydrocephalus associated with vestibular schwannoma. J Neurosurg 2003;98:1118–1193.
15 Duke DA, Lynch JJ, Harner SG, Faust RJ, Ebersold MJ: Venous air embolism in sitting and supine patients undergoing vestibular schwannoma resection. Neurosurgery 1998;42: 1282–1286.
16 Shao KN, Tatagiba M, Samii M: Surgical management of high jugular bulb in acoustic neurinoma via retrosigmoid approach. Neurosurgery 1993;32:32–37.
17 Kim HH, Johnston R, Wiet RJ, Kumar A: Long-term effects of cerebellar retraction in the microsurgical resection of vestibular schwannomas. Laryngoscope 2004;114:323–326.
18 Ohata K, Haque M, Morino M, Nagai K, Nishio A, Nishijima Y, Hakuba A: Occlusion of the sigmoid sinus after surgery via the presigmoidal-transpetrosal approach. J Neurosurg 1998;89:575–584.

Prof. Pierre-Hugues Roche
Service de Neurochirurgie de l'Hôpital Nord
Assistance Publique-Hôpitaux de Marseille
Chemin des Bourrelly
FR–13915 Marseille Cedex 20 (France)
Tel. +33 4 91 96 86 20, Fax +33 4 91 96 89 15, E-Mail proche@mail.ap-hm.fr

Régis J, Roche P-H (eds): Modern Management of Acoustic Neuroma.
Prog Neurol Surg. Basel, Karger, 2008, vol 21, pp 222–227

Vestibular Schwannoma Management: An Evidence-Based Comparison of Stereotactic Radiosurgery and Microsurgical Resection

Bruce E. Pollock

Departments of Neurological Surgery and Radiation Oncology, Mayo Clinic College of Medicine, Rochester, Minn., USA

Abstract

Background: The best management of vestibular schwannoma (VS) patients is controversial. **Methods:** A comparison of surgical resection and stereotactic radiosurgery based on recent studies using evidence-based medicine standards. Level 1 evidence is derived from randomized clinical trials, whereas levels 2, 3, 4, and 5 refer to prospective cohort studies, case-control series, case series, and expert opinions, respectively. **Results:** The vast majority of studies on VS management are either retrospective case-series or opinions (level 4 and 5 evidence). Five retrospective case-control series (level 3 evidence) have shown improved cranial nerve outcomes, better cost effectiveness, and less impact on patients' activities of daily living for patients having radiosurgery. One prospective cohort study (level 2 evidence) found outcomes were superior for patients having radiosurgery compared to surgical resection with regard to facial movement, hearing preservation and quality of life measures. No randomized clinical trial has been performed to compare these two techniques. **Conclusion:** The best quality of evidence (levels 2 and 3) show superior outcomes for VS patients having stereotactic radiosurgery compared to surgical resection allowing a grade B recommendation for this approach. Unless long-term follow-up shows frequent tumor progression at currently used radiation doses, radiosurgery should be considered the best management strategy for the majority of VS patients.

Evidence-based medicine (EBM) is the conscientious, explicit and judicious use of the current best evidence in making decisions about the care of individual patients [1]. In the late 1970s, Suzanne Fletcher and Dave Sackett generated the idea of 'levels of evidence' to rank the validity of evidence of preventive healthcare measures and linked them to 'grades of recommendations' for different interventions [2]. Briefly, the most valid information (level 1) is obtained when a particular therapy has been studied with multiple randomized clinical trials (RCTs) with little variation in the direction or magnitude of the results. In situations where consistent level 1 studies exist, a grade A recommendation can be made for that particular therapy. Levels 2, 3, 4, and 5 refer to cohort studies, case-control series, case series, and expert opinions, respectively. Grade B recommendation can be made with consistent level 2 or 3 studies, grade C recommendations can be made from level 4 studies, and grade D recommendations can be made from level 5 studies (or inconsistent or inconclusive studies of any level). By incorporating the best available external evidence together with our clinical expertise and consideration of an individual's life situation and preferences, a physician is able to employ an EBM practice.

A variety of reasons exist that limit the practical ability of physicians to perform RCTs for each situation. First, the condition of interest may be rare. Even in settings where the magnitude of effectiveness between different treatments is large, a sufficient number of patients must be enrolled to show this difference in a statistically meaningful way. Second, for benign tumors such as vestibular schwannomas (VSs), the success of an operation in preventing tumor recurrence or progression may not be evident for 10 or more years after surgery. Thus, the information derived from case series (level 4 evidence) may be the best available data to base clinical decision making for patients with benign tumors and extended life expectancies. Third, and particularly relevant to radiosurgery, is the fact that few patients are willing to participate in randomized trials in which one group has open surgery whereas the other undergoes radiosurgery. So although an RCT comparing outcomes after surgical resection and radiosurgery for VS would likely yield critical information, the 'trial ability' of such proposed studies is low. For these and many other reasons, clinicians most often have to base their decision making on rather poor quality evidence.

This chapter will compare recent studies on VS resection and radiosurgery according to EBM guidelines. Specifically, radiosurgery is defined as single-session procedures as opposed to image-guided, multiple session radiation delivery (stereotactic radiation therapy) [3].

Materials and Methods

This is a limited review of recently published, commonly referred to studies on VS resection and radiosurgery. The studies were grouped according to the quality of the information provided (level 1–5), and the conclusions summarized (table 1).

Table 1. Comparison of surgical resection and radiosurgery by EBM standards

Level of evidence	Preferred treatment
1 – RCT	no studies available
2 – prospective cohort study	radiosurgery[1]
3 – case-control series	radiosurgery[2]
4 – case series	conflicting conclusions
5 – expert opinion	conflicting opinions

[1]One study available [21].
[2]Five studies available [16–20].

Results

Level 5 Evidence

Literature reviews have been published that promote both surgical resection [4, 5] and radiosurgery [6] as the best treatment for VS patients. Ironically, the diametrically opposed opinions expressed in these different papers were derived from the same body of information (papers on VS resection of radiosurgery from the 1980s until the late 1990s).

Level 4 Evidence

Large case series are available for surgical resection from the retrosigmoid [7, 8], translabyrinthine [9], and middle fossa approaches [10]. Likewise, large case series are available after radiosurgery performed with the Gamma Knife [11–14] and modified linear accelerators [15]. Similar to expert opinions on this topic, advocates of surgical resection and radiosurgery typically argue that the published results favor their particular method of treatment.

Level 3 Evidence

Five retrospective case-control series have been performed comparing surgical resection and radiosurgery [16–20]. These studies found

Table 2. Case-control series (level 3 evidence) comparing surgical resection and radiosurgery for patients with VSs

Study	Treatment with better outcome				
	trigeminal	facial	hearing	ADL	cost/charges
Pollock, 1995	ND	RS	RS	NT	RS
Roijen, 1997	ND	ND	NT	RS	RS
Karpinos, 2002	RS	RS	RS	ND	NT
Regis, 2002	RS	RS	RS	RS	NT
Myrseth, 2005	NT	RS	RS	RS	NT

ND = No difference; NT = not tested; RS = radiosurgery.

radiosurgery had improved facial nerve outcomes and hearing preservation rates. Patients returned to work faster after radiosurgery, and the costs associated with radiosurgical management were less than open surgery. Table 2 outlines the major findings of these studies.

Level 2 Evidence

We recently completed a prospective cohort study of adult patients with unilateral, unoperated VS less than 3 cm in average diameter [21]. Eighty-two patients had either surgical resection (n = 36) or radiosurgery (n = 46). The groups were similar with regard to hearing loss, associated symptoms, and tumor size. Patients having resection were younger (48.2 vs. 53.9 years, $p = 0.03$). The mean follow-up was 42 months (range, 12–62). Importantly, blinded observers determined tumor size, facial weakness, and hearing preservation.

Normal facial movement and preservation of serviceable hearing was more frequent in the radiosurgical group at 3 months ($p < 0.001$), 1 year ($p < 0.001$), and at last follow-up ($p < 0.01$) compared to the surgical resection group. Patients having surgical resection had a significant decline in the following subscales of the Health Status Questionnaire (HSQ) 3 months after surgery: physical functioning ($p = 0.006$), role-physical ($p < 0.001$), energy/fatigue ($p = 0.02$), and overall physical component ($p = 0.004$). Patients in the surgical resection group continued to have a significant decline in the physical functioning ($p = 0.04$) and bodily pain ($p = 0.04$) subscales at 1 year, and in bodily pain ($p = 0.02$) at last follow-up. The radiosurgical group had no decline on any component of the HSQ after the procedure. The radiosurgical group had lower mean Dizziness Handicap Inventory scores (16.5 vs. 8.4, $p = 0.02$) at last follow-up. There was no difference in tumor control (100 vs. 96%, $p = 0.50$).

Level 1 Evidence

No RCTs are available to compare VS resection with radiosurgery.

Discussion

In 2002, Nikolopoulos and O'Donoghue [22] reviewed the English literature published over the past 23 years (111 papers) and found no level 1 or 2 evidence to support either surgical resection or radiosurgery as the preferred management for VS patients. They concluded that the quality of the evidence on this topic was poor, and emphasized the need for better studies in the future. Ideally an RCT could be performed to compare outcomes for VS patients having surgical resection or stereotactic radiosurgery. However, such a study would be difficult to perform because patients may be reluctant to undergo randomization between open brain surgery or an outpatient-based procedure done under local anesthesia. Also, many physicians who regularly manage VS patients are polarized in their thinking on this topic and would be unwilling to participate in an RCT. Recognizing these limitations, we performed a prospective observational study of VS patients managed at our center over a 2-year interval. The preoperative patient characteristics of the two treatment groups were similar with regard to presenting symptoms, neurologic deficits, and tumor size. Patients in the radiosurgical group were slightly older, but this small difference in age should have little bearing on the results of this study. Blinded, independent observers graded facial nerve outcomes, determined hearing preservation, and measured the tumors. So although our study is not an RCT, it does provide solid level 2 evidence comparing cranial nerve outcomes for VS patients having either surgical resection or radiosurgery.

At every time point examined, patients having radiosurgery more frequently had normal facial movement and retained serviceable hearing compared to the microsurgical group. Despite the importance typically placed on cranial nerve function after VS management, more important is the effect of treatment on VS patients' quality of life (QOL). Studies have shown that more than half of patients undergoing surgical resection felt their QOL was worse after surgery [23], and only one third of patients resumed their normal activities of daily living within 1 month of their operation [18, 20]. Betchan et al. [24] and Martin et al. [25] both found a significant decline in the physical functioning, role-physical, and social functioning components of the HSQ after VS resection when compared to published normal controls. Conversely, the effect of radiosurgery on QOL for VS patients in retrospective studies has been less significant than surgical resection [17–20]. Myrseth et al. [17] used the SF-36 to compare the QOL in 140 VS patients having microsurgery or radiosurgery at a mean of 5.9 years after treatment. They noted significant deviations from age-adjusted values in the microsurgical group for physical functioning, role-physical, and role-emotional when compared to the radiosurgical patients. Our prospective data also showed the surgical resection group suffered a significant decline in several components of the HSQ at 3 months, 1 year, and at last follow-up compared to their preoperative level of functioning. The radiosurgical group showed no decline in any subset of the HSQ at any point during the follow-up interval.

The effect of surgical resection and radiosurgery were quite similar for the symptoms associated with VS. The only significant difference noted for the associated symptoms was that the radiosurgical group had a lower mean Dizziness Handicap Inventory score at last follow-up, suggesting fewer problems with imbalance.

A number of factors need to be remembered when comparing the different treatments for VS patients. (1) Not every VS patient is appropriate for radiosurgery. Observation with serial imaging can be used to effectively manage many elderly patients with small or minimally symptomatic VSs [26]. In addition, patients with large tumors are poor candidates for radiosurgery and should undergo surgical resection. (2) Comparison studies to date provide no meaningful information regarding tumor control rates after surgical resection or radiosurgery of VSs. It is generally accepted that VS recurrence after total excision is approximately 3%, whereas numerous radiosurgical series have been published demonstrating a similar failure rate after VS radiosurgery. The primary complaint is that earlier studies have reported patients treated with higher radiation doses than commonly used today [27]. Hasegawa et al.

[12] recently reported outcomes for 317 VS patients undergoing radiosurgery between 1991 and 1998. The average tumor margin dose was 13.2 Gy. At a mean follow-up of 7.8 years, the 10-year progression-free survival for patients with tumors less than 15 cm^3 was 97%. Nonetheless, more data are needed on the long-term tumor control at the lower doses to conclude that tumor control rates between the two techniques are similar. (3) If radiosurgery does fail and the tumor continues to enlarge, the published results suggest that tumor removal is more difficult and patient outcomes are poor compared to patients never undergoing radiosurgery [28, 29]. Last, it is now recognized that patients having radiosurgery are at some risk for developing radiation-induced neoplasms [30]. The best estimate of this complication at this time is approximately 0.1–0.01%, although this number may increase as more patients are followed for longer intervals after radiosurgery. By comparison, a recent series of 707 patients operated between 1987 and 2001 found the risk of death after VS resection to be 0.1% [9].

Conclusions

The best quality of evidence (levels 2 and 3) shows superior outcomes for VS patients having stereotactic radiosurgery compared to surgical resection, allowing a grade B recommendation for this approach. Unless long-term follow-up shows frequent tumor progression at currently used radiation doses, radiosurgery should be considered the best management strategy for the majority of VS patients.

References

1 Sackett DL, Rosenberg WM, Gray JA, Haynes RB, Richardson WS: Evidence based medicine: what it is and what it isn't. BMJ 1996;312:71–72.
2 Canadian Task Force on the Periodic Health Examination: the periodic health examination. CMAJ 1979;121:1193–1254.
3 Pollock BE, Lunsford LD: A call to define stereotactic radiosurgery. Neurosurgery 2004;55:1371–1373.
4 Kaylie DM, McMenomey SO: Microsurgery vs gamma knife radiosurgery for the treatment of vestibular schwannomas. Arch Otolaryngol Head Neck Surg 2003;129:903–906.
5 Sekhar LN, Gormley WB, Wright DC: The best treatment for vestibular schwannoma (acoustic neuroma): microsurgery or radiosurgery? Am J Otol 1996;17:676–682.
6 Pollock BE, Lunsford LD, Noren G: Vestibular schwannoma management in the next century: a radiosurgical perspective. Neurosurgery 1998;43:475–483.
7 Samii M, Matthies C: Management of 1000 vestibular schwannomas (acoustic neuromas): hearing function in 1000 tumor resections. Neurosurgery 1997;40:248–260.
8 Sampath P, Holliday MJ, Brem H, Niparko JK, Long DM: Facial nerve injury in acoustic neuroma (vestibular schwannoma) surgery: etiology and prevention. Neurosurgery 1997;87:60–66.
9 Sanna M, Taibah A, Russo A, Falcioni M, Agarwal M: Perioperative complications in acoustic neuroma (vestibular schwannoma) surgery. Otol Neurotol 2004;25:379–386.
10 Brackmann DE, Owens RM, Friedman RA, Hitselberger WE, De la Cruz A, House JW, Nelson RA, Luxford WM, Slattery WH III, Fayad JN: Prognostic factors for hearing preservation in vestibular schwannoma surgery. Am J Otol 2000;21:417–424.
11 Flickinger JC, Kondziolka D, Niranjan A, Maitz A, Voynov G, Lunsford LD: Acoustic neuroma radiosurgery with marginal tumor doses of 12 to 13 Gy. Int J Radiat Oncol Biol Phys 2004;60:225–230.
12 Hasegawa T, Fujitani S, Katsumata S, Kida Y, Yoshimoto M, Koike J: Stereotactic radiosurgery for vestibular schwannomas: analysis of 317 patients followed more than 5 years. Neurosurgery 2005;57:257–264.
13 Iwai Y, Yamanaka K, Shiotani M, Uyama T: Radiosurgery for acoustic neuromas: results of low-dose treatment. Neurosurgery 2003;53:282–287.
14 Petit JH, Hudes RS, Chen TT, Eisenberg HM, Simard JM, Chin LS: Reduced-dose radiosurgery for vestibular schwannomas. Neurosurgery 2001;49:1299–1306.
15 Foote KD, Freidman WA, Buatti JM, Meeks SL, Bova FJ, Kubilis PS: Analysis of risk factors associated with radiosurgery for vestibular schwannoma. J Neurosurg 2001;95:440–449.
16 Karpinos M, The BS, Zeck O, Carpenter LS, Phan C, Mai W, Lu H, Chiu JK, Butler EB, Gormley WB, Woo SY: Treatment of acoustic neuroma: stereotactic radiosurgery vs. microsurgery. Int J Radiat Oncol Biol Phys 2002;54:1410–1421.
17 Myrseth E, Moller P, Pedersen P, Vassbotn FS, Wentzel-Larsen T, Lund-Johansen M: Vestibular schwannomas: clinical results and quality of life after microsurgery or gamma knife radiosurgery. Neurosurgery 2005;56: 927–935.

18 Pollock BE, Lunsford LD, Kondziolka D, Flickinger JC, Bissonette DJ, Kelsey SF, Jannetta PJ: Outcome analysis of acoustic neuroma management: a comparison of microsurgery and stereotactic radiosurgery. Neurosurgery 1995;36:215–223.
19 Regis J, Pellet W, Delsanti C, Dufour H, Roche PH, Thomassin JM, Zanaret M, Peragut JC: Functional outcome after gamma knife surgery or microsurgery for vestibular schwannomas. J Neurosurg 2002;97:1091–1100.
20 Van Roijen L, Nijs HGT, Avezaat CJJ, Karlsson G, Linquist C, Pauw KH, Rutten FFH: Costs and effects of microsurgery versus radiosurgery in treating acoustic neuromas. Acta Neurochir (Wein) 1997;139:942–948.
21 Pollock BE, Driscoll CLW, Foote RL, Link MJ, Bauch CD, Mandrekar JN, Krecke KN, Johnson CH: Patient outcomes after vestibular schwannoma management: a prospective comparison of microsurgical resection and stereotactic radiosurgery. Neurosurgery (submitted).
22 Nikolopoulos TP, O'Donoghue GM: Acoustic neuroma management: an evidence-based medicine approach. Otol Neurotol 2002;23:534–541.
23 Da Cruz MJ, Moffat DA, Hardy DG: Postoperative quality of life in vestibular schwannoma patients measured by the SF-36 Health Questionnaire. Laryngoscope 2000;110:151–155.
24 Betchan SA, Walsh J, Post KD: Self assessed quality of life after acoustic neuroma surgery. J Neurosurg 2003;99:818–823.
25 Martin HC, Sethi J, Lang DL, Neil-Dwyer G, Lutman ME, Yardley L: Patient-assessed outcomes after excision of acoustic neuroma: postoperative symptoms and quality of life. J Neurosurg 2001;94:211–216.
26 Raut VV, Walsh RM, Bath AP, Bance ML, Guha A, Tator CH, Rutka JA: Conservative management of vestibular schwannomas-second review of a prospective longitudinal study. Clin Otolaryngol 2004;29:505–514.
27 Kondziolka D, Lunsford LD, McLaughlin MR, Flickinger JC: Long-term outcomes after radiosurgery for acoustic neuromas. N Engl J Med 1998;339: 1426–1433.
28 Friedman RA, Brackmann DE, Hitselberger WE, Schwartz MS, Iqbal Z, Berliner KI: Surgical salvage after failed irradiation for vestibular schwannoma. Laryngoscope 2005;115: 1827–1832.
29 Lee DJ, Westra WH, Staecker H, Long D, Niparko JK: Clinical and histopathologic features of recurrent vestibular schwannomas (acoustic neuroma) after stereotactic radiosurgery. Otol Neurotol 2003;24:650–660.
30 Loeffler JS, Niemierko A, Chapman PH: Second tumors after radiosurgery: tip of the iceberg or a bump in the road? Neurosurgery 2003;52: 1436–1442.

Bruce E. Pollock, MD
Department of Neurological Surgery, Mayo Clinic
Rochester, MN 55905 (USA)
Tel. +1 507 284 5317, Fax +1 507 294 5206, E-Mail pollock.bruce@mayo.edu

Régis J, Roche P-H (eds): Modern Management of Acoustic Neuroma.
Prog Neurol Surg. Basel, Karger, 2008, vol 21, pp 228–237

Linear Accelerator Radiosurgery for Vestibular Schwannomas

William A. Friedman

Department of Neurological Surgery, University of Florida, Gainesville, Fla., USA

Abstract

Linear accelerator (LINAC) radiosurgery was developed in the 1980s. The treatment paradigm uses the rotating high-energy X-ray output of the LINAC to focus many hundreds of 'beam equivalents' on intracranial or spinal targets. At the University of Florida, 450 vestibular schwannomas have been treated. Tumor control has been achieved in 90% (5-year actuarial data). 99% of patients treated have required no further intervention. Since reducing the treatment dose to 1,250 cGy, in 1994, the incidence of facial and trigeminal nerve injury has been <1%. No instance of malignant tumor transformation has been observed. Other institutions using modern LINAC techniques report similar excellent results. We believe that radiosurgery is the treatment of choice for smaller vestibular schwannomas.

Stereotactic radiosurgery (SRS) is a minimally invasive treatment modality that delivers a large single dose of radiation to a specific intracranial target while sparing surrounding tissue. Unlike conventional fractionated radiotherapy, SRS does not maximally exploit the higher radiosensitivity of brain lesions relative to normal brain (therapeutic ratio). Its selective destruction is dependent mainly on sharply focused high-dose radiation and a steep dose gradient away from the defined target. The biological effect is irreparable cellular damage (probably via DNA strand breaks) and delayed vascular occlusion within the high-dose target volume. Because a therapeutic ratio is not required, traditionally radioresistant lesions can be treated. Since destructive doses are used, however, any normal structure included in the target volume is subject to damage.

The basis for SRS was conceived over 40 years ago by Lars Leksell [1]. He proposed the technique of focusing multiple beams of external radiation on a stereotactically defined intracranial target. The averaging of these intersecting beams results in very high doses of radiation to the target volume, but innocuously low doses to nontarget tissues along the path of any given beam. His team's implementation of this concept culminated in the development of the Gamma Knife. The modern Gamma Knife employs 201 fixed cobalt radiation sources in a fixed hemispherical array, such that all 201 photon beams are focused on a single point. The patient is stereotactically positioned in the Gamma Knife so that the intracranial target coincides with the isocenter of radiation. Using variable collimation, beam blocking, and multiple isocenters, the radiation target volume is shaped to conform to the intracranial target.

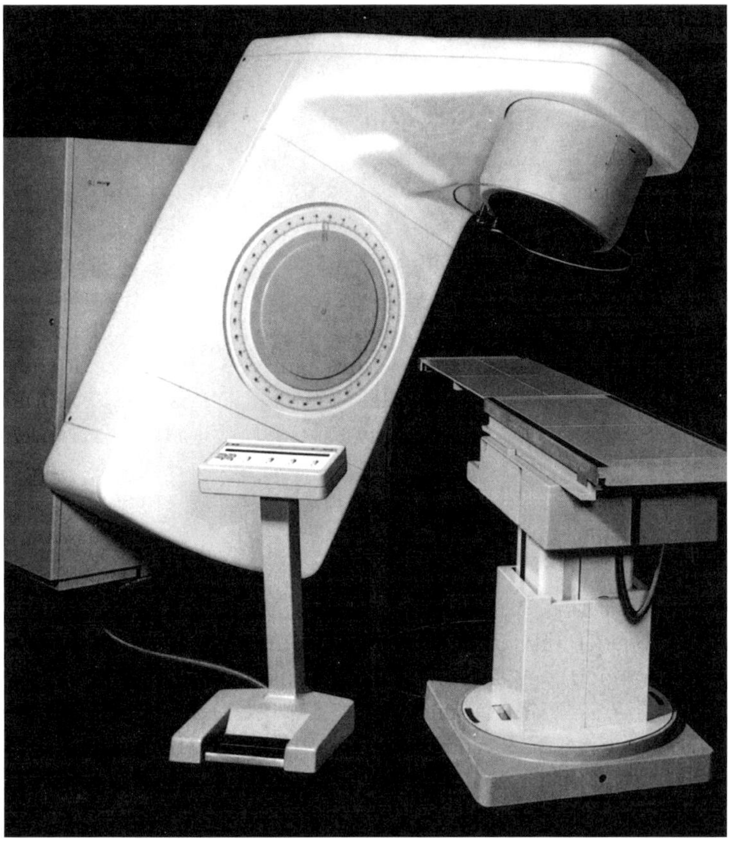

Fig. 1. LINACs are the preferred device, worldwide, for conventional radiotherapy. They accelerate electrons to near light speed, then collide them with a heavy metal (like tungsten) in the head of the machine. The collision mainly produces heat but a small percentage of the energy is converted into highly energetic photons. These photons, because they are electronically produced, are called 'X-rays'. The X-radiation is collimated and focused on the target.

An alternate radiosurgical solution using a linear accelerator (LINAC) was first described in 1984 by Betti and Derechinsky [2]. Colombo et al. [3] described such a system in 1985, and LINACs have subsequently been modified in various ways to achieve the precision and accuracy required for radiosurgical applications [4–7]. In 1986, a team composed of neurosurgeons, radiation physicists and computer programmers began development of the University of Florida LINAC-based radiosurgery system [8]. This system has been used to treat over 2,000 patients at the University of Florida since May 1988, and is in use at multiple sites worldwide. Many other commercial versions of radiosurgical systems are currently available, including the Brain Lab system, the Radionics (X-knife system), the Accuray (Cyberknife system), and others.

Most LINAC radiosurgical systems rely on the same basic paradigm: a collimated X-ray beam is focused on a stereotactically identified intracranial target. The gantry of the LINAC rotates around the patient, producing an arc of radiation focused on the target (fig. 1, 2). The patient couch is then rotated in the horizontal plane and another arc performed. In this manner, multiple noncoplanar arcs of radiation intersect at the target volume and produce a high target dose, with minimal radiation to surrounding brain. This dose concentration method is exactly analogous to the multiple intersecting beams of cobalt radiation in the Gamma Knife.

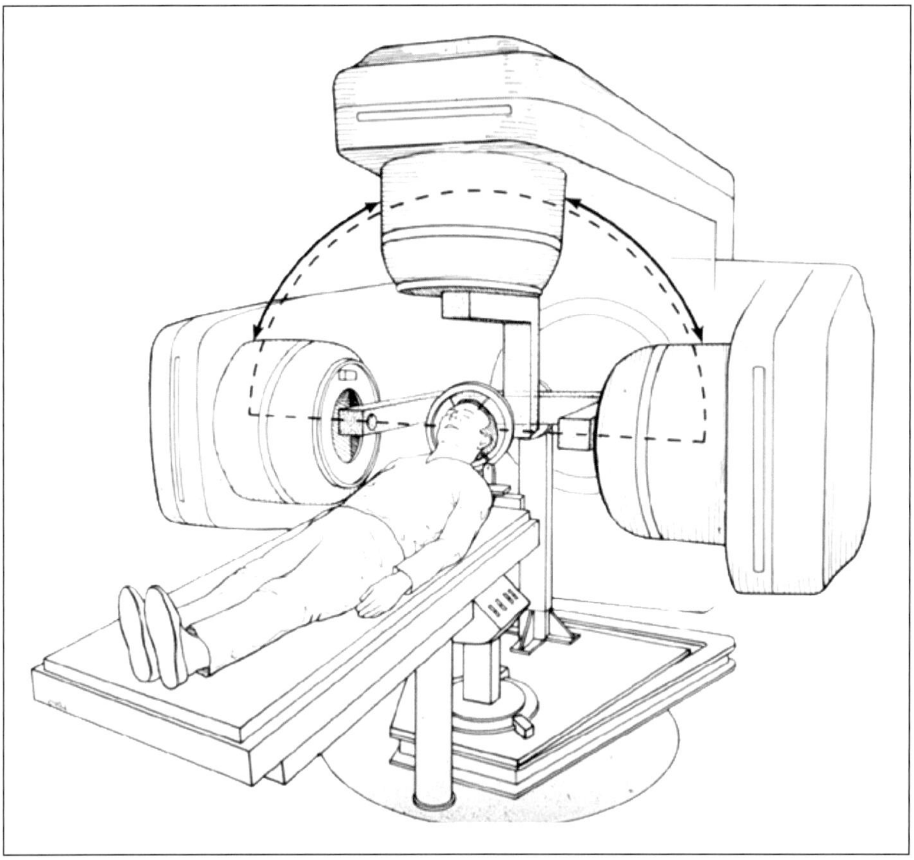

Fig. 2. This diagram shows an add-on device, designed to improve the accuracy of the LINAC, in place. The LINAC arcs around the patient, with its beam always focused on the stereotactically positioned target. The patient is then moved to a new horizontal (table) position, and another arc performed. The result is multiple, noncoplanar arcs of radiation, all converging on the target point.

The target dose distribution can be tailored by varying collimator sizes, eliminating undesirable arcs, manipulating arc angles, using multiple isocenters, and differentially weighting the isocenters [9]. In our center, multiple isocenters are used to achieve highly conformal dose distributions, exactly analogous to the Gamma Knife technique. Some LINAC systems use an alternative approach which relies upon a computer-driven multileaf collimator to generate nonspherical beam shapes which are conformal to the beam's eye view of the tumor. The multileaf collimator can be adjusted statically or dynamically as the LINAC rotates. Intensity modulation can be used to achieve dose distributions which are close to those seen with multiple isocenters and treatment time can be reduced.

Achievable dose distributions are similar for LINAC-based and Gamma Knife systems. With both systems, it is possible to achieve dose distributions that conform closely to the shape of the intracranial target, thus sparing the maximum amount of normal brain. Recent advances in stereotactic imaging and computer technology for dose planning, as well as refinements in radiation delivery systems have led to improved efficacy, fewer complications and a remarkable amount of interest in the various applications of SRS. Perhaps of equal importance is the fact that increasing amounts of scientific evidence have persuaded the majority of the international neurosurgical community that radiosurgery is a viable treatment option for selected patients suffering from a variety of challenging neurosurgical disorders.

This chapter will present a brief description of LINAC radiosurgical technique, followed by a detailed review of the experience with vestibular schwannoma treatment.

LINAC Radiosurgery Technique

Although the details of radiosurgical treatment techniques differ somewhat from system to system, the basic paradigm is quite similar everywhere. Below, is a detailed description of a typical radiosurgical treatment at the University of Florida.

Almost all radiosurgical procedures in adults are performed on an outpatient basis. The patient reports to the neurosurgical clinic the day before treatment for a detailed history and physical, as well as an in-depth review of the treatment options. If radiosurgery is deemed appropriate, the patient is sent to the Radiology Department for a volumetric magnetic resonance imaging (MRI) scan. A radiosurgical plan can be generated, in advance, using this MRI study. The next morning, the patient arrives at 7.00 a.m. A stereotactic head ring is applied under local anesthesia. No skin shaving or preparation is required. Subsequently, stereotactic CT scanning is performed. One-millimeter slices are obtained throughout the entire head. The patient is then transported to an outpatient holding area where he and his family have breakfast and relax until the treatment planning process is complete.

The stereotactic CT scan and the nonstereotactic volumetric MRI scan are transferred via Ethernet to the treatment-planning computer. The CT images are quickly processed so that each pixel has an anteroposterior, lateral, and vertical stereotactic coordinate, all related to the head ring previously applied to the patient's head. Using image fusion software, the nonstereotactic MRI is fused, pixel for pixel, with the stereotactic CT. The 'pre-plan' performed the day before is, likewise, fused to the stereotactic CT. Final dosimetry then begins and continues until the neurosurgeon, radiation therapist, and radiation physicist are satisfied that an optimal dose plan has been developed. A variety of options are available for optimizing the dosimetry. The fundamental goal is to deliver a radiation field that is precisely conformal to the lesion shape (fig. 3), while delivering a minimal dose of radiation to all surrounding neural structures.

When dose planning is complete, the radiosurgical device is attached to the LINAC. The patient then is attached to the device and treated. The head ring is removed and, after a short observation period, the patient is discharged. The radiosurgical device is disconnected from the LINAC, which is then ready for conventional usage. Close clinical and radiologic follow-up is arranged at appropriate intervals depending on the pathology treated and the condition of the patient.

Radiosurgery for Vestibular Schwannomas

Among benign intracranial tumors, vestibular schwannoma (acoustic neuroma) has been one of the most frequent targets for SRS. This common tumor (representing approximately 15% of all primary brain tumors) is a benign proliferation of Schwann cells arising from the myelin sheath of the vestibular branches of the VIIIth cranial nerve. These tumors are slightly more common in women, present at an average age of 50 years, and occur bilaterally in patients with neurofibromatosis type 2.

Leksell first used SRS to treat a vestibular schwannoma in 1969 [10]. SRS is a logical

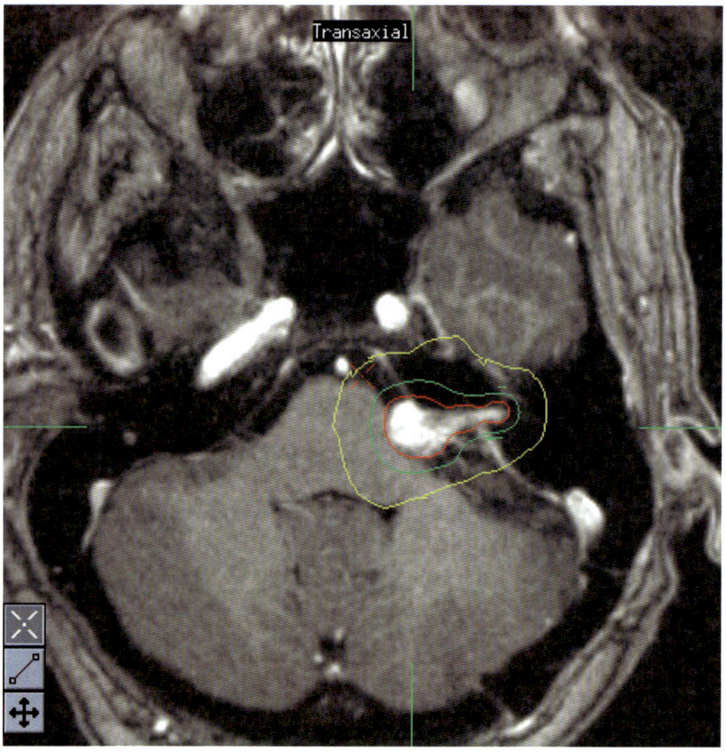

Fig. 3. In general, multiple isocenters are used to produce highly conformal dosimetry. Here, the red line is the prescription isodose, the green line is half of prescription, and the yellow line is 20% of prescription.

alternative treatment modality for this tumor for several reasons. A vestibular schwannoma is typically well demarcated from surrounding tissues on neuroimaging studies. The sharp borders of this noninvasive tumor make it a convenient match for the characteristically steep dose gradient produced at the boundary of a radiosurgical target. This allows the radiosurgeon to minimize radiation of normal tissue. Excellent spatial resolution on gadolinium-enhanced MRI facilitates radiosurgical dose planning. These tumors typically occur in an older population that may be less fit for microsurgical resection under general anesthesia. Finally, the location of these tumors at the skull base in close proximity to multiple critical neurologic structures (i.e. cranial nerves, brainstem) leads to appreciable surgical morbidity and rare mortality even in expert hands. This makes the concept of an effective, less invasive, less morbid alternative treatment that can be performed in a single day under local anesthesia quite attractive. Whether or not radiosurgery fits this description has been extensively debated.

Certainly, the role of radiosurgery is limited by its inability to expeditiously relieve mass effect in patients for whom this is necessary. The radiobiology of SRS also requires lower, potentially less effective doses for higher target volumes in order to avoid complications. This limits the use of SRS to the treatment of smaller tumors. Despite these limitations, there is a growing body of literature that substantiates the claim that radiosurgery is a safe and effective alternative therapy for vestibular schwannomas.

The published experience using LINAC-based radiosurgery for the treatment of vestibular schwannomas is relatively limited compared to the Gamma Knife literature. Foote et al. [11] performed an analysis of risk factors associated with radiosurgery for vestibular schwannoma at the

University of Florida. The aim of this study was to identify factors associated with delayed cranial neuropathy following radiosurgery for vestibular schwannoma and to determine how such factors may be manipulated to minimize the incidence of radiosurgical complications while maintaining high rates of tumor control. From July 1988 to June 1998, 149 cases of vestibular schwannoma were treated using LINAC radiosurgery at the University of Florida. In each of these cases, the patient's tumor and brainstem were contoured in 1-mm slices on the original radiosurgical targeting images. Resulting tumor and brainstem volumes were coupled with the original radiosurgery plans to generate dose-volume histograms. Various tumor dimensions were also measured to estimate the length of cranial nerve that would be irradiated. Patient follow-up data, including evidence of cranial neuropathy and radiographic tumor control, were obtained from a prospectively maintained, computerized database. The authors performed statistical analyses to compare the incidence of posttreatment cranial neuropathies or tumor growth between patient strata defined by risk factors of interest. One hundred and thirty-nine of the 149 patients were included in the analysis of complications. The median duration of clinical follow up for this group was 36 months (range 18–94 months). The tumor control analysis included 133 patients. The median duration of radiological follow up in this group was 34 months (range 6–94 months). The overall 2-year actuarial incidences of facial and trigeminal neuropathies were 11.8 and 9.5%, respectively. In 41 patients treated before 1994, the incidences of facial and trigeminal neuropathies were both 29%, but in the 108 patients treated since January 1994, these rates declined to 5 and 2%, respectively. An evaluation of multiple risk factor models showed that maximum radiation dose to the brainstem, treatment era (pre-1994 compared with 1994 or later), and prior surgical resection were all simultaneously informative predictors of cranial neuropathy risk. The radiation dose prescribed to the tumor margin could be substituted for the maximum dose to the brainstem with a small loss in predictive strength (fig. 3). The overall radiological tumor control rate (fig. 4) was 93% (59% tumors regressed, 34% remained stable, and 7.5% enlarged), and the 5-year actuarial tumor control rate was 87% (95% confidence interval 76–98%). Based on this study, the authors currently recommend a peripheral dose of 12.5 Gy for almost all acoustics, as that dose is most likely to yield long-term tumor control without causing cranial neuropathy.

Spiegelmann et al. [12, 13] have reported their experience. They reviewed the methods and results of linear accelerator radiosurgery in 44 patients with acoustic neuromas who were treated between 1993 and 1997. Computerized tomography scanning was selected as the stereotactic imaging modality for target definition. A single, conformally shaped isocenter was used in the treatment of 40 patients; two or three isocenters were used in 4 patients who harbored very irregular tumors. The radiation dose directed to the tumor border was the only parameter that changed during the study period: in the first 24 patients who were treated the dose was 15–20 Gy, whereas in the last 20 patients the dose was reduced to 11–14 Gy. After a mean follow-up period of 32 months (range 12–60 months), 98% of the tumors were controlled. The actuarial hearing preservation rate was 71%. New transient facial neuropathy developed in 24% of the patients and persisted to a mild degree in 8%. Radiation dose correlated significantly with the incidence of cranial neuropathy, particularly in large tumors (≥ 4 cm^3).

Several reports on smaller series of patients treated with LINAC-based radiosurgery for vestibular schwannomas have been published in recent years. Martens et al. [14] reported on 14 patients with at least 1-year of follow-up after radiosurgery on the LINAC unit in the University Hospital in Ghent, Belgium. A mean marginal dose of 19.4 Gy (range 16–20) was delivered to the 70% isodose

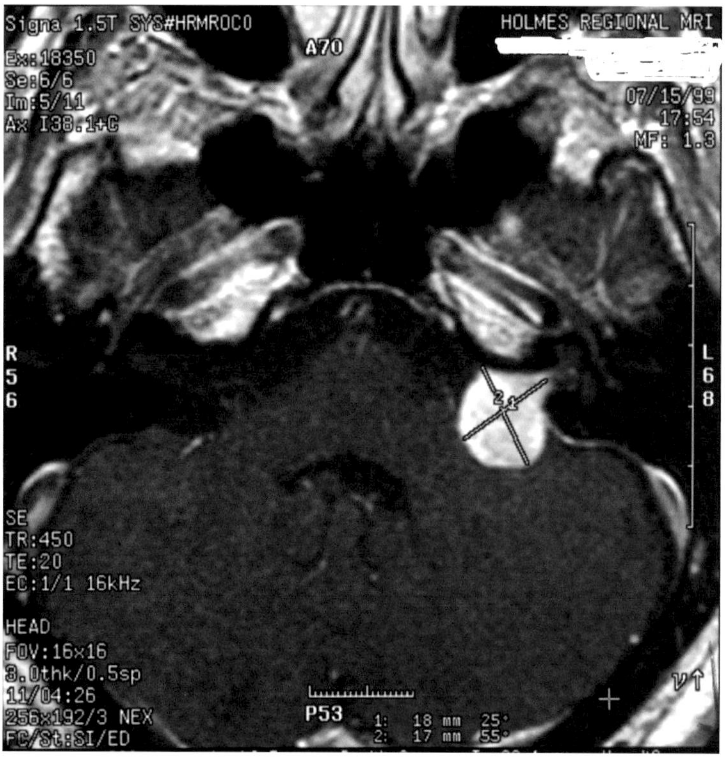

Fig. 4. Pretreatment MRI scan shows left-sided vestibular schwannoma.

line with a single isocenter. Mean follow-up duration was 19 months (range 12–24 months). During this relatively short follow-up interval, 100% radiographic tumor control has been achieved (29% regressed, 71% stable, zero enlarged). Rates of delayed facial and trigeminal neuropathy were 21 and 14%, respectively, and two of three facial nerve deficits resolved. Preoperative hearing was preserved 50% of the time.

Valentino and Raimondi [15] reported on 23 patients treated with LINAC radiosurgery in Rome, Italy. Five of these had neurofibromatosis and 7 (30%) had undergone previous surgery. Total radiation dose to the tumor margin ranged from 12 to 45 Gy (median 30 Gy) and was delivered in 1–5 sessions. One or two isocenters were used and mean duration of follow-up was 40 months (range 24–46 months). Results using this less conventional method of multisession radiosurgery were comparable to other radiosurgical techniques. Tumor control was achieved in 96% of patients (38% regressed, 58% remained stable, 4% enlarged), facial and trigeminal neuropathies each occurred at a rate of 4%, and 'hearing was preserved at almost the same level as that prior to radiosurgery in all patients'.

The use of LINAC radiosurgery for acoustics is briefly discussed in reports by Delaney et al. [16] and Barcia et al. [17]. In addition, fractionated stereotactic radiation therapy (SRT) has been used as an alternative management for vestibular schwannomas [1, 5]. This method is proposed as a way of exploiting the precision of stereotactic radiation delivery to minimize dose to normal brain, while employing lower fractionated doses in an effort to minimize complications. Thus far, most radiosurgeons feel that optimal results can be achieved with highly conformal single fraction radiosurgery, while sparing the patient the inconvenience of a prolonged treatment course.

'Fractionated' Radiosurgery for Vestibular Schwannoma

Although some would argue with the term 'fractionated radiosurgery', a number of groups have used multiple session treatments in an attempt to reduce complications, especially hearing loss. Varlotto et al. [18] treated 12 patients with vestibular schwannoma between June 1992 and October 1994. Follow-up ranged from 16 to 44 months. Patient age ranged from 27 to 70 (median: 45) years. Eight patients were treated with primary SRT and 4 patients were treated after primary surgical intervention for recurrent [3] or persistent [1] disease. Tumor volumes were 1.2–18.4 (median: 10.1) cm^3. Tumors received 1.8 Gy/day normalized to the 95% isodose line. Patients received a minimum prescribed dose of 54 Gy in 27–30 fractions over a 6-week period. After a median follow-up of 26.5 months, local control was obtained in 12 out of 12 lesions. Tumor regression was noted in 3 patients, and tumor stabilization was found in the remaining 9 patients. No patient developed a new cranial nerve deficit. One patient developed worsening of preexisting trigeminal neuropathy and another experienced a decrease in hearing. However, all 9 patients with useful hearing prior to SRT maintained useful hearing at last follow-up.

Fuss et al. [19] treated 51 patients with vestibular schwannoma with conventional fractionation. Mean total dose was 57.6 ± 2.5 Gy. Forty-two patients have been followed for at least 12 months and were subject of an outcome analysis. Mean follow-up was 42 months. Actuarial 2- and 5-year tumor control rates were 100 and 97.7%, respectively. Actuarial useful hearing preservation rate was 85% at 2 and 5 years. New hearing loss was diagnosed in 4 NF2 patients. Pretreatment normal facial nerve function was preserved in all cases. Two cases of new or impaired trigeminal nerve dysesthesia required medication. No other cranial nerve deficit was observed.

Williams [20] treated 80 consecutive patients (45 male, 35 female; age 56.8 ± 1.7 years). A prospective schedule permitted increased fractionation versus size. Seventy patients having AN <3.0 cm in diameter had 5 daily fractions of 5 Gy (25 Gy total) and 10 patients having AN ≥3 cm had 10 daily fractions of 3 Gy (30 Gy total). All treatments were prescribed to the 80% isodose and given via the dedicated 10 MeV accelerator. For both the larger and smaller AN, the percentage decrease in volume was similar. No tumor increased in size, no patient developed facial weakness and hearing was preserved.

Andrews et al. [21] compared the results of patients treated with radiosurgery on the Gamma Knife or fractionated radiotherapy from October 1994 through August 2000. Gamma Knife technique involved a fixed-frame multiple shot/high conformality single treatment, whereas LINAC technique involved daily conventional fraction treatments involving a relocatable frame, fewer isocenters, and high conformality established by noncoplanar arc beam shaping and differential beam weighting. Sixty-nine patients were treated on the Gamma Knife, and 56 patients were treated with radiation therapy. Three patients were lost to follow-up, and in the remaining 122 patients, mean follow-up was 119 ± 67 weeks for SRS patients and 115 ± 96 weeks for SRT patients. Tumor control rates were high (≥97%) for sporadic tumors in both groups. Cranial nerve morbidities were comparably low in both groups, with the exception of functional hearing preservation, which was 2.5-fold higher in patients who received conventional fractionation.

Most recently, Chang et al. [22] reported on 61 patients treated with the Cyberknife and followed for at least 36 months. They received either 18 or 21 Gy, in three fractions. Only one treated tumor progressed. Seventy-four percent of patients with serviceable hearing maintained it. No new trigeminal or facial complications developed.

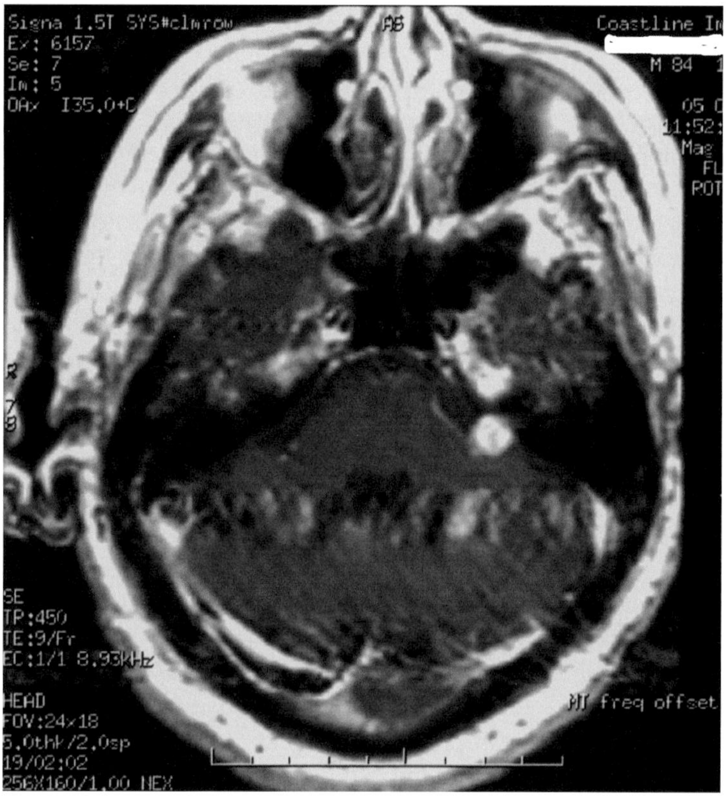

Fig. 5. Four years after treatment, the MRI scan shows the schwannoma to be much smaller.

The University of Florida Experience

As of September, 2005, the University of Florida experience with vestibular schwannomas comprised 392 patients. The indications for radiosurgery were: age >60 – 182, failed surgery – 81, preference – 123, medical infirmity – 6. The median treatment volume was 2 cm^3. Forty-two patients have been lost to follow-up. With a median follow-up of 32 months for the entire group, 111 tumors are unchanged, 169 are smaller (fig. 4, 5), and 13 tumors (4%) are larger. Only 4 patients have required surgery because of tumor growth after radiosurgery (1%). In other words, 99% of patients treated have not required subsequent surgery. Since 1994, when we reduced our treatment dose to 12.5 Gy, only 2% of patients have experienced facial or trigeminal neuropathy after treatment.

References

1 Leksell L: The stereotaxic method and radiosurgery of the brain. Acta Chir Scand 1951;102:316–319.

2 Betti OO, Derechinsky VE: Hyperselective encephalic irradiation with a linear accelerator. Acta Neurochir Suppl 1984;33:385–390.

3 Colombo F, Benedetti A, Pozza F, et al: External stereotactic irradiation by linear accelerator. Neurosurgery 1985;16:154–160.

4 Hartmann GH, Schlegel W, Sturm V, et al: Cerebral radiation surgery using moving field irradiation at a linear accelerator facility. Int J Radiation Oncology Biol Phys 1985;11: 1185–1192.

5 McGinley PH, Butker EK, Crocker IR, Landry JC: A patient rotator for stereotactic radiosurgery. Phys Med Biol 1990;35:649–657.
6 Podgorsak EB, Olivier A, Pla M, Lefebvre PY, Hazel J: Dynamic stereotactic radiosurgery. Int J Radiation Oncology Biol Phys 1988;14:115–126.
7 Winston KR, Lutz W: Linear accelerator as a neurosurgical tool for stereotactic radiosurgery. Neurosurgery 1988;22:454–464.
8 Friedman WA, Bova FJ: The University of Florida radiosurgery system. Surg Neurol 1989;32:334–342.
9 Friedman WA, Buatti JM, Bova FJ, Mendenhall WM: LINAC Radiosurgery – A Practical Guide. Berlin, Springer-Verlag, 1998.
10 Leksell L: A note on the treatment of acoustic tumors. Acta Chir Scand 1971;137:763–765.
11 Foote KD, Friedman WA, Buatti JM, Meeks SL, Bova FJ, Kubilis PS: Analysis of risk factors associated with radiosurgery for vestibular schwannoma. J Neurosurg 2001;95:440–449.
12 Spiegelmann R, Gofman J, Alezra D, Pfeffer R: Radiosurgery for acoustic neurinomas (vestibular schwannomas). Isr Med Assoc J 1999;1:8–13.
13 Spiegelmann R, Lidar Z, Gofman J, Alezra D, Hadani M, Pfeffer R: Linear accelerator radiosurgery for vestibular schwannoma. J Neurosurg 2001;94:7–13.
14 Martens F, Verbeke L, Piessens M, Van Vyve M: Stereotactic radiosurgery of vestibular schwannomas with a linear accelerator. Acta Neurochir 1994;62(Suppl):88–92.
15 Valentino V, Raimondi AJ: Tumour response and morphological changes of acoustic neurinomas after radiosurgery. Acta Neurochir 1995;133:157–163.
16 Delaney G, Matheson J, Smee R: Stereotactic radiosurgery: an alternative approach to the management of acoustic neuromas. Med J Austral 1992;156:440.
17 Barcia Salorio JL, Hernandez G, Ciudad J, Bordes V, Broseta J: Stereotactic radiosurgery in acoustic neurinoma. Acta NeurochirSuppl 1984;33: 373–376.
18 Varlotto JM, Shrieve DC, Alexander E, Kooy HM, Black PM, Loeffler JS: Fractionated stereotctic radiotherapy for the treatment of acoustic neuromas: preliminary results. Int J Radiat Biol 1996;36:141–145.
19 Fuss M, Debus J, Lohr F, et al: Conventionally fractionated stereotactic radiotherapy (FSRT) for acoustic neuromas. Int J Radiat Oncol Biol Phys 2000;48:1381–1387.
20 Williams JA: Fractionated stereotactic radiotherapy for acoustic neuromas: preservation of function versus size. J Clin Neurosci 2003;10:48–52.
21 Andrews DW, Suarez O, Goldman HW, et al: Stereotactic radiosurgery and fractionated stereotactic radiotherapy for the treatment of acoustic schwannomas: comparative observations of 125 patients treated at one institution. Int J Radiat Oncol Biol Phys 2001;50:1265–1278.
22 Chang SD, Gibbs IC, Sakamoto GT, Lee E, Oyelese A, Adler JR Jr: Staged stereotactic irradiation for acoustic neuroma. Neurosurgery 2005;56: 1254–1261; discussion 61–63.

William A. Friedman, MD
Department of Neurosurgery, University of Florida
PO Box 100265, MBI
Gainesville, FL 32610 (USA)
Tel. +1 352 392 4331, Fax +1 352 392 8413, E-Mail friedman@neurosurgery.ufl.edu

Régis J, Roche P-H (eds): Modern Management of Acoustic Neuroma.
Prog Neurol Surg. Basel, Karger, 2008, vol 21, pp 238–246

Radiotherapy of Cranial Nerve Schwannomas

John C. Flickinger · Steven Burton

Department of Radiation Oncology, University of Pittsburgh School of Medicine, Pittsburgh, Pa., USA

Abstract

Fractionated stereotactic radiotherapy is an attractive, low-morbidity alternative to surgical resection for managing cranial nerve schwannomas. So far, the outcomes reported from fractionated stereotactic radiotherapy seem roughly equivalent to contemporary radiosurgery series. However, a randomized, controlled clinical trial is needed to adequately compare these techniques.

Cranial nerve schwannomas are almost exclusively benign, slow-growing tumors that most commonly arise in the vestibular nerve. Whether they arise from the VIIIth cranial nerve (the most common site), or from less frequently affected cranial nerves, V, VII, or IX–XII, their behavior and response to radiation appear similar [1–5]. Since it is easier to draw conclusions from larger, more uniform series, this paper will focus on vestibular schwannomas.

Management options for newly diagnosed cranial nerve schwannomas include initial observation, operative resection, and radiation treatment, with single-fraction radiosurgery (RS) or fractionated radiotherapy. Because schwannomas can sometimes remain stable in size, for years, many physicians advocate initial observation of small acoustic schwannomas. Since hearing loss or other nerve injuries are usually irreversible and since complication risks from surgery or radiation increase with increasing tumor size, an argument can be made that most schwannoma patients are better served by early intervention, as long as the morbidity of active treatment is low. Compared to microsurgery, RS and radiotherapy of schwannomas have lower morbidity rates; while available information suggests similar long-term rates of tumor control for radiation and surgery, the very long-term (more than 10 year) results of both treatments are still very poorly known [6–27].

Evolution of Treatment Techniques

Radiation treatment and treatment planning techniques have evolved considerably over the last 20 years. This is particularly true for RS and radiotherapy of intracranial schwannomas. These changes include improved stereotactic imaging, treatment planning, and lower dose prescriptions. The early Swedish RS experience at Karolinska began with hand dose calculations. Tumor imaging started with pneumoencephalography and angiography, before moving to computed tomography (CT) and finally magnetic resonance imaging. By 1992, high-resolution stereotactic magnetic resonance imaging was being used for stereotactic targeting by Gamma Knife centers and image fusion techniques were being developed for use with stereotactic CT scans.

During the late 1980s and early 1990s, most RS centers limited the number of isocenters treated to the minimum possible. Treatment plans were not as conformal as today's plans, now that multiple isocenters are used freely. Faster treatment-planning programs that were fully integrated with imaging, made it easier to create elaborate, highly conformal, multi-isocenter treatment plans. Intensity-modulated radiotherapy (IMRT) also began to be introduced into radiotherapy practice around this time. Contrary to conventional 3-D treatment planning, where every beam treats the entire target volume, IMRT employs multiple fields, each of which may treat only a portion of the tumor at a time. In reality, multiple isocenter RS meets the definition of IMRT. Other developments have included noninvasive stereotactic techniques such as using noninvasive stereotactic frames and imaging, integrated radiotherapy with either robotic fluoroscopic-based guidance (example: Cyberknife) or CT (tomotherapy or CT scanners combined with linear accelerators).

Prescription doses for schwannoma RS have dropped over the last 20 years, without any apparent drop in tumor control documented so far. Much of the early experience at Karolinska used minimum% tumor doses of 20 Gy. Initially minimum tumor doses of 16–20 Gy were prescribed at Pittsburgh in the 1980s depending on the tumor volume. The most commonly used prescription doses (marginal doses) for RS today are in the range of 12–13 Gy [6]. How much RS or fractionated radiotherapy doses for acoustic neuroma doses can be lowered without compromising tumor control is unclear. Foote et al. [7] observed a trend ($p = 0.207$) toward poorer tumor control with RS doses less than 10 Gy in the University of Florida series. No large series defines tumor control for acoustic scwhannoma RS in the dose range of 5–9 Gy, where one would expect tumor control rates to fall off. Fractionated stereotactic radiotherapy (FSRT) has been used with doses as low as 18 Gy in 3 fractions and 20 Gy in five fractions [20, 22], while doses as low as 15 Gy in 5 fractions are being tested at Brown University.

It is presently almost impossible to perform any reliable dose-response analysis for either RS or fractionated radiotherapy of acoustic tumors. Unlike conventional large-field fractionated radiotherapy, where homogenous treatment volumes with margins of 10–20 mm are commonly added to the gross tumor or target volume (GTV) to form the planning treatment volume (PTV), it is unclear how best to define the minimum tumor dose for RS where the PTV = GTV. The prescription dose, also referred to as the marginal tumor dose or perhaps incorrectly as the minimum tumor dose, does not consistently correspond to the true absolute minimum tumor dose. One time the marginal dose may be prescribed to a treatment isodose covering 95% of the tumor, another time to 100%, and yet another time to 89% of the tumor, all at the same institution. In the past, most Gamma Knife plans were generated with only visual matching of the contour to the imaging without outlining the tumor target or analyzing the tumor dose-volume histogram. Contours of the GTV vary with imaging techniques used and vary between different physicians. This leads to uncertainties in assessing the minimum tumor doses within different RS and FSRT plans. This complicates assessing minimum tumor doses necessary for tumor control and determining what dose parameter (prescription/marginal dose, absolute minimum tumor dose, dose covering 99% of the tumor, mean tumor dose, etc.) best correlates with tumor control.

Radiobiological Rationale for Fractionation

Before RS was introduced, essentially all clinical radiotherapy to intracranial targets was highly fractionated. Lacking any data on the response of benign tumors to radiation, most radiation oncologists have assumed that increasing the number of fractions for a radiotherapy course to a benign tumor from one to 5–30 would decrease complications while maintaining tumor control. While this is found in analyzing dose-responses for cell culture of most malignant tumors, where α/βratios are higher than for surrounding normal brain or cranial nerves, it is not necessarily true for benign tumors, where there are no reliable radiobiological studies. Using an in vivo malignant tumor animal model, Garcia-Barros et al. [28] demonstrated that the single-fraction radiation response is determined primarily by the normal endothelial cells within the tumor vasculature (which appear to have a low α/βratio). Thus, the α/βratio of the tumor cells may be relatively unimportant in the radiation response, and may not be any different from that for normal tissue, which eliminates much of the classical radiobiological rationale for fractionating radiotherapy.

Comparison of Outcome with Single versus Multiple Fractions

Fortunately, acoustic schwannoma patients have two very good alternatives to surgical resection for controlling their tumors: RS and stereotactic fractionated radiotherapy. To compare acoustic schwannoma RS with stereotactic fractionated radiotherapy, long-term data for both tumor control and complications must be evaluated over a range of different doses. Proving the significance of any possible small differences in tumor control would take long follow-up and hundreds, if not thousands of patients, because of the low failure rates and relatively flat slope of the dose-response for control of acoustic schwannoma tumor control seen so far. If one unfairly compares the results of FSRT for acoustic schwannoma to the initial results of RS performed in the 1980s then fractionation would appear, at first glance, to lower complications. If one takes a closer look at outcome from RS using techniques since the early 1990s with lower dose prescriptions of 12–13 Gy, while paying attention to the variability in results of both FSRT and RS, along with the length and type of follow-up (example: audiogram versus phone call evaluation for hearing changes), the differences become unclear.

Recent Radiosurgery Series

Representative series of acoustic schwannoma patients managed with modern RS techniques are listed in table 1. Regis et al. [13] carefully documented a comparison of 110 surgery and 97 RS (prescription doses of 12–14 Gy) acoustic schwannoma patients with close follow-up (4 years minimum). With RS, facial nerve preservation was 100% (vs. 63% with microsurgery) and functional hearing preservation was 70%. A larger study from the same institution of 211 unilateral acoustic schwannoma patients reported a hearing preservation rate of 73%. They correlated improved hearing preservation with preoperative class 1 Gardner-Robertson hearing, multiple isocenter planning, and marginal tumor doses of less than 13 Gy. Stage 1 intracanalicular tumors with Gardner-Robertson class 1 hearing treated with doses less than 13 Gy had more than a 95% chance of functional hearing conservation at 2 years after RS.

The University of Pittsburgh reported on 313 patients with previously untreated unilateral acoustic schannomas who underwent Gamma Knife RS doses of 12–13 Gy (median = 13 Gy) between February 1991 and February 2001 [6]. Treatment volumes varied between 0.04–21.4 cm^3 (median = 1.1 cm^3). The median follow-up was 24 months, maximum follow-up was 115 months, and 36 patients had >60-month follow-up. The actuarial clinical tumor control rate (defined as no surgical intervention required) was 98.6 + 1.1% at 7 years. Two patients underwent tumor resection; one had solid tumor growth completely resected and the other required a partial resection because of an enlarging adjacent subarachnoid cyst, despite control of the irradiated tumor. The actuarial rates for unchanged facial strength, unchanged facial sensation, unchanged hearing-level, and useful hearing preservation were 100%, 95.6 + 1.8%, 70.3 + 5.8%, and 78.6 + 5.1%, respectively, at 7 years. Eight patients developed new trigeminal neuropathy (5–48 months after RS), 6 of whom developed numbness (actuarial rate: 2.5 + 1.5% at 7 years), while the other 2 developed new typical trigeminal neuralgia (actuarial rate: 1.9 + 1.5% at 7 years). The risk of developing post-RS trigeminal neuropathy of any type correlated with increasing tumor volume ($p = 0.038$).

Iwai et al. [9] reported the results of low-dose Gamma Knife RS (8–12 Gy, median = 12 Gy) in 51 consecutive acoustic schwannoma patients treated from 1992 to 1996 in Osaka. Follow-up varied from 19 to 96 months with a median of 60 months. The clinical tumor control rate (freedom from requirement for surgical resection) was 96%. The rates of patients being free from any new facial weakness or new facial numbness after RS were 100% for both endpoints, although 4% of patients with pre-existing trigeminal neuropathy developed increased facial numbness after RS. They found class 1–2 (serviceable) hearing preservation in 56% of patients following RS.

Other centers report results that are either better or worse despite seemingly similar RS techniques. Paek et al. [12] from Seoul, South Korea, reported a lower 52% rate of preserving useful/serviceable hearing (Gardner-Robertson grade 1–2) after Gamma Knife RS to a mean prescribed dose of 12.0 + 0.7 Gy (range: 11–14 Gy) in 25 acoustic schwannoma patients (mean follow-up: 45 months, range: 22–75 months). They correlated hearing loss with maximum dose to the cochlear nucleus within the brainstem. The mean value for the maximum cochlear nucleus dose was 11.1 + 3.9 Gy for patients losing hearing compared to 6.9 +4.5 Gy for those with preserved hearing. Their radiological tumor control was 92%, but the resection-free clinical tumor control was 100%. In contrast, Muacevic et al. [10] from Munich reported only a better 90% rate of hearing preservation following RS in 219 acoustic schwannoma patients (median follow-up: 6 years). It was unclear in their report whether this figure was based on audiometry at 6 months or at last follow-up. They also reported that transient facial weakness developed in 0.5% and transient facial numbness in 5.0% of patients. Rowe et al. [14] reported the Sheffield experience with Gamma Knife RS using a clearly higher median marginal dose of 15 Gy (range: 13–15 Gy) in 234 unilateral acoustic schwannomas with a mean follow up of 35 + 16 months. Despite the higher dose, Gardner-Robertson hearing levels were preserved in 75% of patients. Transient vestibular-cochlear symptoms developed in 13% of patients. Although facial weakness developed in 4.5%, it persisted in <1%. PreRS trigeminal symptoms improved in 3%, while new trigeminal neuropathy developed in 5% of patients and persisted in 1.5%. The actuarial rate of resection-free clinical tumor control rate was 96%.

Recent Fractionated Radiotherapy Series

Table 2 outlines the results for a number of representative series of FSRT for acoustic schwannoma. Williams reported the Johns Hopkins experience with FSRT in 125 acoustic schwannoma patients with >1-year follow-up [27]. They treated tumors smaller than 3.0 cm in diameter to 25 Gy given in 5 consecutive 5-Gy fractions (111 patients), while tumors >3.0 cm in diameter received 30 Gy in 10 fractions (14 patients). At the time of that report (with a median follow-up of 21 months, range: 12–68 months), tumor control and facial nerve preservation were both 100%. Hearing was preserved in approximately 70% of patients. Transient decreases in facial sensation developed after FSRT in 2 patients (2%).

Combs et al. [21] from Heidelberg reported on 106 acoustic schwannoma patients managed with FSRT to a median dose of 57.6 with 1.8 Gy fractions prescribed to a 90% isodose treatment volume encompassing the PTV. The median follow-up in their series was 48 months, with a range of 3–172 months. After 5 years, the actuarial tumor control was 93%. They reported a surprisingly high rate of 94% useful hearing preservation, but based that number on follow-up telephone questioning rather than audiograms. They reported a 98% rate of actuarial hearing preservation for non-NF2 patients compared to 68% for NF2 patients. Their rates for developing postradiation trigeminal and facial neuropathies were 3.4 and 2.3%, respectively.

The UCLA group reported their FSRT experience in 50 unilateral acoustic schwannoma patients irradiated to 54 Gy in 30 fractions to a 90% isodose treatment volume (PTV) that included a 1- to 3-mm margin around gross tumor [25]. All tumors were controlled with a median follow-up of 36 months (range: 6–74 months). They reported an unusually high rate of useful hearing preservation of 93%, but defined it as the ability to talk on the telephone with the affected ear. Audiograms were not routinely performed before or after RS. New facial numbness developed in one patient (2%) and facial weakness also in one patient (2%) after radiotherapy.

Sakamoto et al. [24] and Shirato et al. [26] from Hokkaido University in Sapporo, Japan, reported their experience with stereotactic fractionated radiotherapy to 44–50 Gy in 22–25 fractions in 65 acoustic schwannoma patients. The mean follow-up was 37 months with a range of 6–97 months. The 5-year actuarial tumor control rate for 44 patients with >2-year follow-up was 92%. Transient facial and trigeminal nerve problems developed after FSRT in 4.6and 9.2% of those 44 patients, respectively. They found that transient trigeminal nerve sequelae developed significantly more frequently in cystic solid tumors than solid tumors (25 vs. 2%).

Chang et al. [20] recently reported the Stanford Cyberknife experience. They evaluated 61 acoustic schwannoma patients treated to 18- or 21-Gy marginal doses in three fractions who had a minimum of 36 months follow-up (mean = 48 months). They controlled tumor growth in 60/61 (98%) and preserved serviceable hearing in 74% of patients at the latest follow-up. No patients developed facial weakness or numbness after FSRT, although transient facial twitching developed in 2 patients. Figures 1 and 2 show a typical Cyberknife plan for an acoustic schwannoma.

Bush et al. [19] evaluated the Loma Linda experience with fractionated proton beam radiotherapy in 29 acoustic schwannoma patients after 34 months median follow-up (range: 7–98 months). Patients with useful hearing (Gardner-Robertson grade 1–2) received 54 cobalt Gy equivalent (CGE) in 30 fractions. Tumors in patients with poorer hearing received 60 CGE in 30 fractions. No tumors progressed and required resection. Useful hearing was preserved in only 4/13 (31%) patients. No facial or trigeminal neuropathy developed after treatment. Other FSRT series are also listed in table 1 along with the FSRT arms of two series comparing RS with FSRT.

Single Institution Comparisons of Radiosurgery and Fractionated Radiotherapy

Jefferson University in Philadelphia and VU University Medical Center in Amsterdam both published single-institution comparisons of RS versus stereotactic fractionated radiotherapy for acoustic schwannomas [17, 18]. The Jefferson group compared 69 RS patients with 50 patients who underwent FSRT to 50 Gy/25 fractions [18]. Their first 25 acoustic schwannoma patients were treated using a linear accelerator. Fourteen patients without hearing underwent RS, while 11 with pre-treatment hearing underwent fractionated radiotherapy with 9 4-Gy fractions. The authors stated that the patients treated with 9 4-Gy fractions will be the subject of a separate report, but it is not clear how many LINAC RS patients

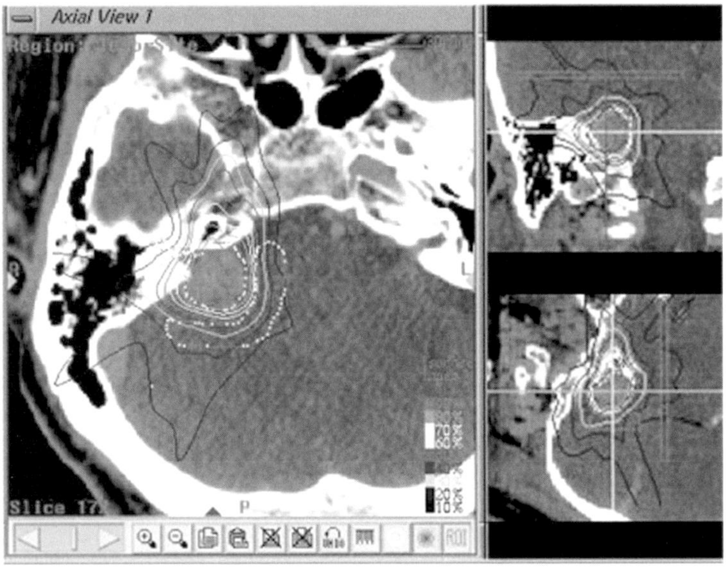

Fig. 1. Typical isodose plot of a Cyberknife RS treatment plan for a right-sided acoustic schwannoma.

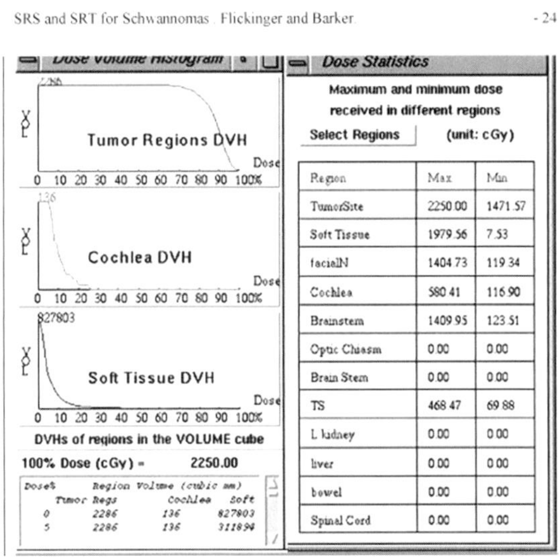

Fig. 2. Dose-volume histograms and dose statistics for the Cyberknife RS treatment plan shown in figure 1. The prescription dose was 18 Gy to the 80% isodose treatment volume in three fractions.

were included in the total of 69 RS patients. They state that they performed Gamma Knife RS '*almost* invariably' with a marginal dose of 12 Gy to the 50% isodose volume. Although some of the RS patients received higher prescription doses than 12 Gy, there are no details provided in the paper. The authors found facial and trigeminal neuropathy rates that were similar for the RS and fractionated radiotherapy groups (tables 1 and 2), but the rate of hearing loss was significantly higher in the RS group. Because follow-up was limited and because there were only a small number of patients with serviceable (useful) hearing in each group prior to radiation treatment (12 in the RS and 21 in the FSRT groups), it was by no means clear that the long-term hearing preservation will be significantly different between the groups. This study also does not rule out the possibility that hearing loss could develop more slowly after radiotherapy than RS, but with eventually the same rate of long-term hearing preservation.

Meijer et al. [17], from Amsterdam, also reported a single-institution comparison of linear accelerator RS with FSRT for acoustic schwannoma patients. They selected 49 edentulous patients (mean age = 63 years) for RS who were unable to reliably use the bite block for their relocatable/noninvasive FSRT frame. RS doses were either 10- or 12.5-Gy marginal dose prescribed

Table 1. Tumor control (freedom from resection or other intervention) and cranial nerve preservation rates in modern representative series for single-fraction RS of acoustic schwannomas

RS institution	Median marginal dose in Gy (range)	Patients	Median follow-up, months (range)	Tumor control %	Post-RS complications for cranial nerves, %		
					V	VII	VIII
Pittsburgh [16]	13 (12–13)	313	24 (1–115)	98.6	4	0	30
Sheffield [14]	15 (13–15)	234	35 + 16	96	5	4.5	25
Munich [10]	13 (10–15)	219	72 (24–120)	97	5	0.5	10[1]
Marseille [13]	12–14	97	? (36–108?)	97	4	0	30
Jefferson [18]	12	69	27 +15 (SE)	98	5	2	67
Osaka [9]	12 (8–12)	51	60 (8–96)	92	2	0	44
Amsterdam [17]	10 or 12.5	49	33 (12–107)	100	8	7	25
South Korea [12]	12 (11–14)	25	45 (22–75)	100	5	4	52

[1]The audiometric assessment time was unclear (6 months versus latest follow-up?).

Table 2. Tumor control and cranial nerve preservation rates for recent representative series for FSRT of acoustic schwannomas

Stereotactic fractionated radiotherapy institution	Median marginal tumor dose, Gy/fractions	Patients	Median follow-up (range) months	Tumor control	Complications in cranial nerves[1], %		
					V	VII	VIII
Heidelberg [21]	57.6 + 2.5/32	106	48 (3–172)	93	3.4	2.3	6[2]
UCLA [25]	54/30	50	36 (6–74)	100	2	2	7[2]
Stanford [20]	18–21/3	61	48 (36–?)	98	0	0	26
Staten Island [22]	20/4–5	38	24 (24–32)	100	0	3	23
Jefferson [18]	50/25	56	27 + 22 (SE)	92[2]	7	2	30[2]
Amsterdam [17]	20/4–5	80	33 (12–107)	94	2	3	39
Sapporo [24, 26]	36–50/20–23	65	37 (6–97)	92	12	5	53?
Johns Hopkins [27]	25/5, 30/10	125	21 (12–68)	100	0/2	0	30
Loma Linda (proton) [19]	54 or 60 CGE/30	29	34 (7–98)	100	0	0	69

[1]Temporary/permanent rates.
[2]Hearing assessed by follow-up questions rather than audiometry.

to the 80% isodose. Eighty patients (mean age = 43 years) with intact dentition (able to use the bite block for the relocatable stereotactic frame), underwent stereotactic fractionated radiotherapy to 20 Gy in 4–5 fractions prescribed to the 80% isodose volume. They found a higher rate of trigeminal neuropathy following RS than after stereotactic radiotherapy (8% RS vs. 2% FSRT at 5 years, $p = 0.048$). Five-year actuarial tumor control rates were similar (100% RS vs. 94% FSRT), as were rates of developing new facial neuropathy (7% RS vs. 3% FSRT), and hearing loss (25% RS vs. 39% FSRT). The rates of facial and trigeminal neuropathy for their RS group were higher than those in published low-dose RS results with Gamma Knife. It is possible that the RS treatment plans were not fully conformal.

Conclusion

FSRT appears to be an excellent alternative to microsurgical resection for management of small- to medium-sized acoustic schwannomas. Reviews of radiobiological data and published clinical series of acoustic schwannoma FSRT and RS results with current techniques cannot answer whether FSRT will live up to the hope of equal or better long-term tumor control with lower complications than RS. So far, the results of acoustic schwannoma RS and FSRT seem roughly equivalent. Ideally, a randomized, controlled clinical trial should be performed to adequately compare these techniques.

References

1 Mabanta SR, Buatti JM, Friedman WA, Meeks SL, Mendenhall WM, Bova FJ: Linear accelerator radiosurgery for nonacoustic schwannomas. Int J Radiat Oncol Biol Phys 1999;43:545–548.

2 Pan L, Wang EM, Zhang N, Zhou LF, Wang BJ, Dong YF, Dai JZ, Cai PW: Long-term results of Leksell gamma knife surgery for trigeminal schwannomas. J Neurosurg 2005; 102(suppl):220–224.

3 Pollock BE, Foote RL, Stafford SL: Stereotactic radiosurgery: the preferred management for patients with nonvestibular schwannomas? Int J Radiat Oncol Biol Phys 2002;15;52:1002–1007.

4 Pollock BE, Kondziolka D, Flickinger JC, Maitz A, Lunsford LD: Preservation of cranial nerve function after radiosurgery for nonacoustic schwannomas. Neurosurgery 1993;33: 597–601.

5 Zabel A, Debus J, Thilmann C, Schlegel W, Wannenmacher M: Management of benign cranial nonacoustic schwannomas by fractionated stereotactic radiotherapy. Int J Cancer 2001;96:356–362.

6 Flickinger JC, Kondziolka D, Niranjan A, Maitz A, Voynov G, Lunsford LD: Acoustic neuroma radiosurgery with marginal tumor doses of 12 to 13 Gy. Int J Radiat Oncol Biol Phys 2004;60:225–230.

7 Foote KD, Friedman WA, Buatti JM, et al: Analysis of risk factors associated with radiosurgery for vestibular schwannoma. Journal of Neurosurgery. 2001;95:440–449, S.

8 Inoue HK: Low-dose radiosurgery for large vestibular schwannomas: long-term results of functional preservation. J Neurosurg 2005;102(suppl):111–113.

9 Iwai Y, Yamanaka K, Shiotani M, Uyama T: Radiosurgery for acoustic neuromas: results of low-dose treatment. Neurosurgery 2003;53:282–287; discussion 287–288.

10 Muacevic A, Jess-Hempen A, Tonn JC, Wowra B: Results of outpatient gamma knife radiosurgery for primary therapy of acoustic neuromas. Acta Neurochir Suppl 2004;91:75–78.

11 Flickinger JC, Kondziolka D, Lunsford L: Fractionation of radiation treatment in acoustics. Rationale and evidence in comparison to radiosurgery. Neurochirurgie 2004;50:421–426.

12 Paek SH, Chung HT, Jeong SS, Park CK, Kim CY, Kim JE, Kim DG, Jung HW: Hearing preservation after gamma knife stereotactic radiosurgery of vestibular schwannoma. Cancer 2005;104:580–590.

13 Regis J, Pellet W, Delsanti C, Dufour H, Roche PH, Thomassin JM, Zanaret M, Peragut JC: Functional outcome after gamma knife surgery or microsurgery for vestibular schwannomas. J Neurosurg 2002;97:1091–1100.

14 Rowe JG, Radatz MW, Walton L, Hampshire A, Seaman S, Kemeny AA: Gamma knife stereotactic radiosurgery for unilateral acoustic neuromas. J Neurol Neurosurg Psychiatry 2003;74:1536–1542.

15 Weber DC, Chan AW, Bussiere MR, Harsh GR 4th, Ancukiewicz M, Barker FG 2nd, Thornton AT, Martuza RL, Nadol JB Jr, Chapman PH, Loeffler JS: Proton beam radiosurgery for vestibular schwannoma: tumor control and cranial nerve toxicity. Neurosurgery 2003;53:577–586.

16 Wowra B, Muacevic A, Jess-Hempen A, Hempel JM, Muller-Schunk S, Tonn JC: Outpatient gamma knife surgery for vestibular schwannoma: definition of the therapeutic profile based on a 10-year experience. J Neurosurg 2005;102(suppl):114–118.
17 Meijer OW, Vandertop WP, Baayen JC, Slotman BJ: Single-fraction vs. fractionated linac-based stereotactic radiosurgery for vestibular schwannoma: a single-institution study. Int J Radiat Oncol Biol Phys 2003;56:1390–1396.
18 Andrews DW, Suarez O, Goldman HW, Downes MB, Bednarz G, Corn BW, Werner-Wasik M, Rosenstock J, Curran WJ Jr: Stereotactic radiosurgery and fractionated stereotactic radiotherapy for the treatment of acoustic schwannomas: comparative observations of 125 patients treated at one institution. Int J Radiat Oncol Biol Phys 2001;50:1265–1278.
19 Bush DA, McAllister CJ, Loredo LN, Johnson WD, Slater JM, Slater JD: Fractionated proton beam radiotherapy for acoustic neuroma. Neurosurgery 2002;50:270–273; discussion 273–275.
20 Chang SD, Gibbs IC, Sakamoto GT, Lee E, Oyelese A, Adler JR Jr: Staged stereotactic irradiation for acoustic neuroma. Neurosurgery 2005;56:1254–1261; discussion 1261–1263.
21 Combs SE, Volk S, Schulz-Ertner D, Huber PE, Thilmann C, Debus J: Management of acoustic neuromas with fractionated stereotactic radiotherapy (FSRT): long-term results in 106 patients treated in a single institution. Int J Radiat Oncol Biol Phys 2005;63:75–81.
22 Lederman G, Lowry J, Wertheim S, Fine M, Lombardi E, Wronski M, Arbit E: Acoustic neuroma: potential benefits of fractionated stereotactic radiosurgery. Stereotactic & Functional Neurosurgery 1997;69:175–182.
23 Lin VY, Stewart C, Grebenyuk J, Tsao M, Rowed D, Chen J, Nedzelski J: Unilateral acoustic neuromas: long-term hearing results in patients managed with fractionated stereotactic radiotherapy, hearing preservation surgery, and expectantly. Laryngoscope 2005;115:292–296.
24 Sakamoto T, Shirato H, Takeichi N, Aoyama H, Fukuda S, Miyasaka K: Annual rate of hearing loss falls after fractionated stereotactic irradiation for vestibular schwannoma. Radiother Oncol 2001;60:45–48.
25 Selch MT, Pedroso A, Lee SP, Solberg TD, Agazaryan N, Cabatan-Awang C, DeSalles AA: Stereotactic radiotherapy for the treatment of acoustic neuromas. J Neurosurg 2004; 101(suppl 3):362–372.
26 Shirato H, Sakamoto T, Sawamura Y, Kagei K, et al: Comparison between observation policy and fractionated stereotactic radiotherapy (SRT) as an initial management for vestibular schwannoma. Int J Radiat Oncol Biol Phys 1999;44:545–550.
27 Williams JA: Fractionated stereotactic radiotherapy for acoustic neuromas. Int J Radiat Oncol Biol Phys 2002;54:500–504.
28 Garcia-Barros M, Paris F, Cordon-Cardo C, Lyden D, Rafii S, Haimovitz-Friedman A, Fuks Z, Kolesnick R: Tumor response to radiotherapy regulated by endothelial cell apoptosis. Science 2003;300:1155–1159.

John C. Flickinger, MD
Joint Radiation Oncology Center
200 Lothrop Street
Pittsburgh, PA 15213 (USA)
Tel. +1 412 647 3600, Fax +1 412 647 6029, E-Mail flickingerjc@upmc.edu

Régis J, Roche P-H (eds): Modern Management of Acoustic Neuroma.
Prog Neurol Surg. Basel, Karger, 2008, vol 21, pp 247–254

Future Perspectives in Acoustic Neuroma Management

Douglas Kondziolka · L. Dade Lunsford

Departments of Neurological Surgery and Radiation Oncology, Center for Image-Guided Neurosurgery, University of Pittsburgh, Pittsburgh, Pa., USA

Abstract

Management options for patients with vestibular schwannomas (acoustic neuromas) include observation, resection, stereotactic radiosurgery, or fractionated radiotherapy. In this report, we review our experience with radiosurgery over a 20-year interval, and discuss indications and expectations with the different approaches. There has been an evolution in available technologies, and an evolution in both patient and physician approaches to the management of this tumor. Patient decisions must be based on quality information from the peer-reviewed literature. Future concepts for radiosurgery are discussed.

For decades, the successful care of a patient with a vestibular schwannoma (acoustic neuroma), has been gratifying to the neurosurgeon. Decades ago, Kenneth McKenzie, Canada's first neurosurgeon, chose to have himself painted, with arm outstretched, pointing to an acoustic neuroma specimen within a glass jar, successfully removed. Such an accomplishment was considered one of the true achievements in neurosurgery.

Over the next decades, technical advances led to improved clinical outcomes. By the 1970s, use of the operating microscope significantly assisted safe tumor resection. Neurophysiological monitoring, improved anesthetic care, and new instrumentation, improved outcomes further. The goal of saving the life of the patient was changed to the avoidance of hemiplegia, and later the avoidance of facial weakness. In the 1990s, a new era of hearing preservation began.

Over that time, others were working to develop radical new concepts for tumor management. In 1971, Lars Leksell described the indications and technique of acoustic tumor radiosurgery, first performed in a patient 2 years before [1]. Since the initial radiosurgical concept (1951), many basic studies were performed to determine the effects of different radiosurgery doses in normal brain, particularly as they applied to functional radiosurgery. The management of selected patients with pituitary tumors and pineal region tumors, lesions that could be identified using plain X-rays or studies such as cisternography or ventriculography, ushered in a new era. Leksell was challenged by disorders that were associated with high rates of management morbidity, and surgery for an acoustic neuroma certainly met that criteria. Despite improvements in resection, hearing loss was the norm, facial weakness was common and hemiparesis, significant ataxia and death still occurred. In a large resection series reported by Olivecrona in 1967, the overall mortality was 22%, but in the smaller tumors, only 9%. Facial nerve function was preserved in only 21% of patients [2]. In 1957, Pool stated that acoustic neuroma resection was, 'not only one of the most exacting and laborious, but also one of the most dangerous and unpredictable operations in the entire neurosurgical repertoire'. In a 1969 series reported by House, 200 patients underwent surgery; there were 56 partial removals and a mortality rate of 7%. Leksell believed that stereotactic radiosurgery offered a new approach to this problem. Using his first generation gamma unit with 179 cobalt-60 radiation beams, the tumor was targeted with air or contrast encephalography. He stated that doses of 5–7 krad were administered to the center of the tumors in the first 3 patients.

Later, Norén et al. [3] reported a comprehensive evaluation of the initial Swedish patient series. He and his colleagues described 14 patients who were managed over a 6-month period in 1975, who had at least 4 years of follow-up. Two of these patients had prior partial resections. Radiosurgical planning was aided by preoperative CT scanning, metrizamide cisternography and in some cases, pneumoencephalography. These patients received a radiosurgical dose at the tumor margin that varied between 7 and 45 Gy. Such high doses may have followed work from an early laboratory study that evaluated human vestibular schwannoma cells in culture irradiated with 30–150 Gy [4]. On imaging after radiosurgery, 8 tumors decreased in size, 2 were unchanged and 3 had increased. Later, questions were raised regarding the accuracy of early radiosurgery targeting with such crude imaging and calculations performed without computer assistance.

The modern era of acoustic tumor radiosurgery was ushered in at the University of Pittsburgh under Dr. L. Dade Lunsford. As the fifth center in the world to use the Gamma Knife, and the first in the United States to install a 201-source unit, radiosurgery was performed using higher resolution imaging techniques. Lunsford began a commitment to rigid outcomes evaluations, publication and presentation of results, and education. An early evaluation of results [5, 6] was reported. Lunsford was also the first to report the economic benefits of radiosurgery, noting an average 65% reduction in hospital charges compared to the cost of microsurgical removal. Within 2 years, both Linskey et al. [7] (n = 26 patients) and Kondziolka et al. [8] (n = 85 patients) reported the expanding Pittsburgh experience. In the latter paper, Kondziolka noted a 3% development of new trigeminal deficits and a 20% onset of facial weakness, although these usually were mild and transient [8]. In that report, 11 patients had excellent preradiosurgery hearing and at follow-up 6 were unchanged. This report was the first to emphasize the role of radiosurgery as primary management to achieve preservation of cranial nerve function. Prior to that time, radiosurgery had been seen as a therapeutic tool to reduce overall treatment risks particularly for elderly patients, those with concomitant medical problems, or those that had already failed surgery. The concept that radiosurgery could be used in younger patients in order to provide effective treatment with lower risks than those associated with resection was novel. Reports on acoustic neuroma radiosurgery then spread outside the neurosurgical or otolaryngology literature. Flickinger et al. [9] published a comprehensive review of the Pittsburgh experience in *Cancer*. Noren continued his detailed review of the Stockholm experience with a report on 254 patients managed from 1969 through 1991 with a minimum follow-up of 12 months [10].

Evolution of Radiosurgery Techniques

Prior reports in this monograph have focused on the evolution of radiosurgical techniques. These changes included improvements in stereotactic imaging, dose planning, and refinements in dose prescription. Tumor imaging (beginning with pneumoencephalography and angiography, and even early-generation CT), was inadequate for fully defining the tumor by today's standards. The intracanalicular portion of the tumor was usually not covered in the plan. The early radiosurgery dose plans were not created with the assistance of computers, and the calculation of the integral dose with multiple isocenters was likely an estimate.

By 1992, high-resolution stereotactic MR imaging was used for targeting by many Gamma Knife centers [11–13]. Because treatment planning programs were faster and fully integrated with imaging, elaborate, highly conformal, multi-isocenter treatment plans could be developed in minutes. Surgeons began using 6–13 isocenters in more than half the patients to achieve high conformality [14]. The stereotactic use of multiple isocenters to achieve conformality represents the most precise and ultimate form of intensity-modulated irradiation. By 1994, some linac centers were adopting multiple isocenter techniques, switching to multiple static conformal fields to improve conformality, or switching to fractionated techniques with lower radiation doses [15]. Later years saw the introduction of inverse treatment planning wherein the computer itself was programmed to indentify a treatment volume based on three-dimensional tracing of the tumor volume. Such a method may not be intuitive for the physician, and has not been shown to improve results.

Prescription doses for radiosurgery declined until the early 1990s. Initially minimum tumor doses of 16–20 Gy were prescribed at Pittsburgh according to tumor volume. Prescription doses were lowered slowly, because of the fear of compromising long-term tumor control for lower morbidity. So far that has not occurred. Since 1992, the most commonly used prescription doses (marginal doses) today are in the range of 12–13 Gy, with no known compromise in tumor control seen so far in prospective analysis [16–20]. How much further radiosurgery doses for vestibular schwannoma may be safely lowered is unclear [21, 22]. Fractionated stereotactic radiotherapy has been used with doses as low as 20 Gy in five fractions. The single-session equivalent for a dose of 20 Gy in five fractions predicted by the linear quadratic formula with alpha/beta ratios of 0, 2.5, or 5 would be 8.9, 9.2, or 11.1 Gy, respectively. Arguing against using doses this low, is the observation by Foote of a trend ($p = 0.207$) for poorer tumor control with radiosurgery doses less than 10 Gy in the University of Florida series [23]. Results for modern Gamma Knife radiosurgery techniques are found in recently published series from Pittsburgh, Baltimore, Marseille, and Osaka [18, 21, 22, 24–26].

Current Management Options

Patients with acoustic neuromas have several management options including observation, surgical resection, stereotactic radiosurgery, and fractionated radiation therapy [27]. Many patients choose between radiosurgery and resection based on their own specific goals and their understanding of possible results. The expected results after modern microsurgical resection are well reported [28–34]. The decision can be difficult for some patients and easier for others, depending on the sources of information given to the patient [35]. These include discussions with surgeons and other physicians, written material from peer-reviewed medical journals, handouts from support groups, internet-based reports (of variable reliability), and discussions between patients. A decision analysis study concluded that radiosurgery would be a more desirable choice for most patients [36]. We believe that information provided from the peer-reviewed medical literature is the most reliable for patient education. Nevertheless, some patients become confused by what they perceive as conflicting opinions amongst physicians.

We do not favor observation for younger patients with acoustic neuromas. Yamamoto et al.

[37] followed 12 patients who chose observation. A significant increase in tumor volume was found in 7 patients during a mean observation period of 19 months. Most schwannomas will show demonstrative tumor growth within 5 years of follow-up, although the growth rate during this period may be variable. On the other hand, we commonly see patients who have been followed with serial imaging, in an attempt to delay the use of a specific procedure for as long as possible. Unfortunately, many demonstrate a significant decline in hearing function during this time, and therefore lose the opportunity for hearing preservation.

Resection is indicated for patients with larger tumors which have caused major neurological deficits from brain compression. In the future, as is the case now, the surgeon together with the patient will discuss the options of attempted complete tumor removal or planned subtotal removal followed by radiosurgery. The patient may specifically request that tumor be left along the facial or cochlear nerves, rather than attempting a dissection in that area. Since it is clear that the consistency and vascularity of tumors in different patients can vary widely, intraoperative decision making is important to obtain the best functional outcome. For tumors that seem more adherent to cranial nerves or more vascular, a decision to perform a partial removal may be wise.

Surgeons perform stereotactic radiosurgery for small or medium-sized tumors with the goals of preserved neurological function and prevention of tumor growth. The long-term outcomes of radiosurgery, particularly with Gamma Knife technique, have proven its role in the primary or adjuvant management of this tumor. Fractionated radiation therapy has been suggested by some as an alternative for selected patients with larger tumors for whom microsurgery may not be feasible, or for some patients in an attempt to preserve cranial nerve function. At present, the available published data do not support the conclusion that fractionated radiation therapy provides any advantage [38]. In some reports, the results have been poorer, but this may reflect selection of patients with larger tumors. The results will vary depending on tumor size, radiation dose, conformality, and the unknown factors of nerve-related ischemia or individual tumor differences. Patients who receive low biologic doses of irradiation may have low rates of early side effects, but should be expected to have higher rates of later tumor growth, and concomitant neuropathy. Some centers also offer radiosurgery, but most do not.

Patients with neurofibromatosis type 2 pose specific challenges, particularly in regard to preservation of hearing and other cranial nerve function [39]. The primary clinical issues for all patients include avoiding tumor-related or treatment-related mortality, prevention of further tumor-related neurologic disability, minimizing treatment risks such as spinal fluid leakage, infections, or cardiopulmonary complications, maintaining regional cranial nerve function (facial, trigeminal, cochlear, and glossopharyngeal/vagal), avoiding hydrocephalus, maintaining quality of life and employment, and reducing cost. All choices should strive to meet all of these goals. Several reports and surveys evaluated patient outcomes, particularly in regard to quality of life [40–42]. Our single-center analysis of outcomes following radiosurgery or resection showed either equal or better results with Gamma Knife radiosurgery [43].

Issues in Decision Making

When we evaluate patients with acoustic tumors, many ask the following two questions. First, is the tumor more difficult to resect if radiosurgery fails? The answer to this is not clear [44, 45]. Few patients have required resection, and the opinions of the surgeons we have asked indicated that some tumors were less difficult, some about the same, and some more difficult. A tumor may be less difficult if it has lost much of its blood supply. In a report on this issue that included 13 patients who had resection after radiosurgery, 8 were thought to be more difficult. However, 5 of these 8 patients had failed resection *before* they had radiosurgery [45]. Second, patients inquire about the risk of delayed malignant transformation. Malignant schwannomas are rare, but have been reported de novo, after prior resection [46, 47], and after irradiation. We answer that this is always a risk after irradiation, but that the risk should be very low [48]. We have not seen this yet in any of our 7,500 patients during our first 18 years experience with radiosurgery, but quote the patient an estimated risk of 1:1,000, significantly less than the risks for developing cancer on their own or for the risk of death after resective surgery. One report from Japan found a malignant tumor 4 years after resection, and 6 months following radiosurgery. The time interval after irradiation was too short to be causative [46]. A second report noted the development of a temporal lobe glioblastoma 7.5 years after radiosurgery for a nearby acoustic neuroma. The temporal lobe had received a low radiation dose [47]. In contrast, we have a patient who had initial resection and irradiation of a frontal lobe astrocytoma, and years later this patient developed an acoustic neuroma. Is there a relationship? Were these tumors related in some oncogenetic way, or were they radiation related?

Is there a specific role for fractionated radiation? Optimally, appropriate doses of radiation should be delivered precisely to the tumor and the regional brain structures should be spared of radiation. This is not usually the case with fractionated techniques where larger volumes of regional tissue are irradiated [49–56]. We believe that any advantage in fractionation in limiting toxicity only makes sense if the target volume contains normal brain or nerve. Sophisticated stereotactic radiosurgical instruments allow regional brain or nerve to be spared through frame-based, single-session, image guidance. Some centers have used a more extensive fractionation regimen over weeks [38], whereas others have used limited fraction numbers over a few days [57]. At present, the available data do not show that fractionation provides any useful advantage over radiosurgical techniques that have been in use for the last 14 years. In order to confirm a significant difference, a prospective trial likely would require hundreds of patients in each arm to detect a difference.

Future Concepts

It is clear that more and more patients are choosing radiosurgery for their acoustic neuroma [58]. The technology is becoming increasingly available and patients in many countries are demanding it. It is reasonable to believe that as more outcomes studies are published, fewer patients will choose to undergo surgical resection. There are now four matched cohort studies (nonrandomized) that compare Gamma Knife radiosurgery to resection [24, 25, 43]. Consistent across all four studies is that clinical outcomes are better or equal after radiosurgery.

In the future, clinical results following radiosurgery could be improved in several ways. First, studies that define the lower dose limit may enable us to better meet the goal of tumor growth arrest with functional preservation. Although there is now much data for the tumor margin dose of 12 Gy, future studies might evaluate the 10- to 11-Gy range. Second, pharmacological radioprotection during irradiation has been evaluated in normal brain and experimental tumor models, but has not reached the clinical setting. Agents such as the 21-aminosteroid family of drugs work through membrane stabilization and free radical scavenging effects, particularly in endothelial cells [59, 60]. The drug tirilizad has been tested in subarachnoid hemorrhage and spinal cord injury and is free of significant side effects. It should be tested in tumor radiosurgery.

Third, can we halt an adverse radiation effect once it occurs? We should test new anti-inflammatory agents such as the cyclooxygenase-2 inhibitors to see if they are as effective in the brain as they are with joint inflammation. Animal models may be useful to test effects [61]. Fourth, we should work to develop new management strategies for patients with large tumors that include planned tumor resection followed by radiosurgery for the residual mass. This would hopefully lead to improved neurologic outcomes in patients with the most difficult tumors. Fifth, we should perform studies that evaluate the effects of radiation on adjacent anatomic structures such as the cochlea [62].

As the number of patients who choose radiosurgery or radiotherapy increases, there will be occasional patients with tumors that continue to grow despite irradiation. In some the enlargement may be minimal and transient, likely related to radiation effects on the tumor and the replacement of tumor with granulation tissue. In a recent report by Pollock et al, such transient enlargements were quantified and recommendations made for continued observation in most patients [63]. Some patients will exhibit a small expansion of the tumor volume, and then no further change. These patients do not require additional procedures, but do require continued observation. In others with continued tumor growth, the possibility of a second radiosurgery may be raised. Although there are little available data after a second radiosurgery, we have used this approach in a few patients with good early results (up to 4 years at present). Stereotactic radiosurgery has transformed the management of patients with acoustic neuromas with proven and consistent longer-term results [64, 65]. New biological approaches for schwannomas that target molecular or genetic tumor substrates will represent the next revolution.

References

1 Leksell L: A note on the treatment of acoustic tumors. Acta Chir Scand 1971;137:763–765.

2 Olivecrona H: The surgical treatment of intracranial tumors. Handbuch der Neurochirurgie, Springer, Heidelberg, 1967, volume 4.

3 Norén G, Arndt J, Hindmarsh T: Stereotactic radiosurgery in cases of acoustic neurinoma: Further experiences. Neurosurgery 1983;13:12–22.

4 Anniko M, Arndt J, Noren G: The human acoustic neurinoma in organ culture II. Tissue changes after gamma irradiation. Acta Otolaryngol 1981;91:223–235.

5 Kamerer D, Lunsford LD, Moller M: Gamma knife: An alternative treatment for acoustic neurinomas. Annals Otol Rhinol Laryngol 1988;97:631–635.

6 Lunsford LD, Goodman M: Stereotactic radiosurgery for acoustic neurinomas. Surg Forum 1988;39:505–507.

7 Linskey M, Lunsford LD, Flickinger JC: Radiosurgery for acoustic neurinomas. Early experience. Neurosurgery 1990;26:736–745.

8 Kondziolka D, Lunsford LD, Coffey R, Flickinger JC: Cranial nerve preservation after stereotactic radiosurgery of acoustic neurinomas. Surg Forum 1990;41:508–510.

9 Flickinger JC, Lunsford LD, Coffey RJ, Linskey ME, Bissonette DJ, Maitz AH, Kondziolka D: Radiosurgery of acoustic neurinomas. Cancer 1991;67:345–353.

10 Hirsch A, Noren G: Audiological findings after stereotactic radiosurgery in acoustic neurinomas. Acta Otolaryngol 1988;106:244–251.

11 Forster D, Kemeny A, Pathak A, Walton L: Radiosurgery: a minimally interventional alternative to microsurgery in the management of acoustic neuroma. Br J Neurosurg 1996;10:169–174.

12 Kondziolka D, Dempsey PK, Lunsford LD, et al: A comparison between magnetic resonance imaging and computed tomography for stereotactic coordinate determination. Neurosurgery 1992;30:402–407.

13 Linskey ME, Lunsford LD, Flickinger JC: Neuroimaging of acoustic nerve sheath tumors after stereotaxic radiosurgery. AJNR 1991;12:1165–1175.

14 Flickinger JC, Kondziolka D, Lunsford LD, et al: Evolution in technique for vestibular schwannoma radiosurgery and effect on outcome. Int J Radiat Oncol Biol Phys 1996;36:275–280.

15 Varlotto JM, Shrieve DC, Alexander E 3rd, et al: Fractionated stereotactic radiotherapy for the treatment of acoustic neuromas: preliminary results. Int J Radiat Oncol Biol Phys 1996;36:141–145.

16 Flickinger JC, Kondziolka D, Lunsford LD: Dose and diameter relationships for facial, trigeminal, and acoustic neuropathies following acoustic neuroma radiosurgery. Radiother Oncol 1996;41:215–219.
17 Flickinger JC, Kondziolka D, Niranjan A, Lunsford LD: Results of acoustic neuroma radiosurgery: An analysis of 5 years experience using current methods. J Neurosurg 2001;94:1–6.
18 Flickinger JC, Kondziolka D, Niranjan A, et al: Acoustic neuroma radiosurgery with marginal tumor doses of 12 to 13 Gy. Int J Radiat Oncol Biol Phys, 2004, in press.
19 Ogunrinde OK, Lunsford LD, Flickinger JC, Kondziolka D: Cranial nerve preservation after stereotactic radiosurgery of small acoustic tumors. Arch Neurol 1995;52:73–79.
20 Ogunrinde OK, Lunsford LD, Flickinger JC, et al: Stereotactic radiosurgery for acoustic tumors in patients with useful preoperative hearing: Results at two years. J Neurosurg 1994;80:1011–1017.
21 Iwai Y, Yamanaka K, Shiotani M, Uyama T: Radiosurgery for acoustic neuromas: results of low-dose treatment. Neurosurgery 2003;53:282–287.
22 Petit JH, Hudes RS, Chen T, et al: Reduced dose radiosurgery for vestibular schwannomas. Neurosurgery 2001;49:1299–1307.
23 Foote KD, Friedman WA, Buatti JM, et al: Analysis of risk factors associated with radiosurgery for vestibular schwannoma. J Neurosurg 2001;95:440–449.
24 Regis J, Pellet W, Delsanti C, Dufour H, Roche PH, Thomassin JM, Zanaret M, Peragut JC: Functional outcome after gamma knife surgery or microsurgery for vestibular schwannomas. J Neurosurg 2002;97:1091–1100.
25 Myrseth E, Moller P, Pederson PH, Vassbotn F, Lund-Johansen M: Vestibular schwannomas: Clinical results and quality of life after microsurgery or gamma knife radiosurgery. Neurosurgery 2005;56:927–935.
26 Hasegawa T, Kida Y, Kobayashi T, Yoshimoto M, Mori Y, Yoshida J: Long-term outcomes in patients with vestibular schwannomas treated using gamma knife surgery: 10 year follow up. J Neurosurg 2005;102:10–16.
27 Bederson JB, von Ammon K, Wichmann W, et al: Conservative treatment of patients with acoustic tumors. Neurosurgery 1991;28:646–651.
28 Brennan JW, Rowed D, Nedzelski J, Chen J: Cerebrospinal fluid leak after acoustic neuroma surgery: influence of tumor size and surgical approach on incidence and response to treatment. J Neurosurg 2001;94:217–233.
29 Cerullo LJ, Grutsch JF, Heiferman K, et al: The preservation of hearing and facial nerve function in a consecutive series of unilateral vestibular nerve schwannoma surgical patients. Surg Neurol 1993;39:485–493.
30 Gardner G, Robertson JH: Hearing preservation in unilateral acoustic neuroma surgery. Ann Otol Rhinol Laryngol 1988;97:55–66.
31 Gormley WB, Sekhar LN, Wright D, et al: Acoustic neuromas: results of current surgical management. Neurosurgery 1997;41:50–60.
32 Mazzoni A, Calabrese V, Moschini L: Residual and recurrent acoustic neuroma in hearing preservation procedures: Neuroradiologic and surgical findings. Skull Base Surg 1996;6:105–112.
33 Post KD, Eisenberg MB, Catalano PJ: Hearing preservation in vestibular schwannoma surgery: what factors influence outcome? J Neurosurg 1995;83:191–196.
34 Samii M, Matthies C: Management of 1000 vestibular schwannomas (acoustic neuromas): Surgical management and results with an emphasis on complications and how to avoid them. Neurosurgery 1997;40:11–23.
35 Ross IB, Tator CH: Stereotactic radiosurgery for acoustic neuroma: A Canadian perspective. Can J Neurol Sci 1998;25:310–314.
36 Hudgins WR: Patients attitude about outcomes and the role of gamma knife radiosurgery in the treatment of vestibular schwannomas. Neurosurgery 1994;34:459–465.
37 Yamamoto M, Hagiwara S, Ide M, et al: Conservative management of acoustic neurinomas: Prospective study of long-term changes in tumor volume and auditory function. Min Invasiv Neurosurg 1998;41:86–92.
38 Chan AW, Black PM, Ojemann R, Barker FG, Kooy H, Lopes VV, McKenna MJ, Shrieve DC, Martuza RL, Loeffler JS: Stereotactic radiotherapy for vestibular schwannomas: Favorable outcome with minimal toxicity. Neurosurgery 2005;57:60–70.
39 Subach B, Kondziolka D, Lunsford LD, Bissonette D, Flickinger JC, Maitz A: Stereotactic radiosurgery in the management of acoustic neuromas associated with neurofibromatosis – type II. J Neurosurg 1999;90:815–822.
40 Martin HC, Sethi J, Lang D, et al: Patient-assessed outcomes after excision of acoustic neuroma: postoperative symptoms and quality of life. J Neurosurg 2001;94:211–216.
41 Wiegand DA, Fickel V: Acoustic neuroma – the patients perspective: subjective assessment of symptoms, diagnosis, therapy, and outcome in 541 patients. Laryngoscope 1989;99:179–187.
42 Wiegand DA, Ojemann R, Fickel V: Surgical treatment of acoustic neuroma (vestibular schwannoma) in the United States: report from the Acoustic Neuroma Registry. Laryngoscope 1996;106:58–66.
43 Pollock BE, Lunsford LD, Kondziolka D, et al: Outcome analysis of acoustic neuroma management: A comparison of microsurgery and stereotactic radiosurgery. Neurosurgery 1995;36:215–229.
44 Pollock B, Lunsford LD, Flickinger J, Clyde B, Kondziolka D: Vestibular schwannoma management. Part I. Failed microsurgery and the role of delayed stereotactic radiosurgery. J Neurosurg 1998;89:944–948.
45 Pollock B, Lunsford LD, Kondziolka D, Sekula R, Subach B, Foote RL, Flickinger J: Vestibular schwannoma management. Part II. Failed radiosurgery and the role of delayed microsurgery. J Neurosurg 1998;89:949–955.
46 Hanabusa K, Morikawa A, Murata T, Taki W: Acoustic neuroma with malignant transformation. Case report. J Neurosurg 2001;95:518–521.
47 Shamisa A, Bance M, Nag S, et al: Glioblastoma multiforme occurring in a patient treated with gamma knife surgery. Case report. J Neurosurg 2001;94:816–821.

48 Comey C, McLaughlin M, Jho H, et al: Death from a malignant cerebellopontine angle triton tumor despite stereotactic radiosurgery. J Neurosurg 1998;89:653–658.
49 Andrews DW, Suarez O, Goldman HW, et al: Stereotactic radiosurgery and fractionated radiotherapy for the treatment of acoustic schwannomas: comparative observations of 125 patients treated at one institution. Int J Radiat Oncol Biol Phys 2001;50:1265–1278.
50 Bush DA, McAllister CJ, Loredo LN, Johnson WD, Slater JM, Slater JD: Fractionated proton beam radiotherapy for acoustic neuroma. Neurosurgery 2002;50:270–273.
51 Fuss M, Debus J, Lohr F, Huber P, Rhein B, Engenhart-Cabillic R, Wannenmacher M: Conventionally fractionated stereotactic radiotherapy (FSRT) for acoustic neuromas. Int J Radiat Oncol Biol Phys 2000;48:1381–1387.
52 Maire JP, Floquet A, Darrouzet V, Guerin J, Bebear JP, Caudry M: Fractionated radiation therapy in the treatment of stage 3 and 4 cerebellopontine angle neurinomas: Preliminary results in 20 cases. Int J Radiat Oncol Biol Phys 1992;23:147–152.
53 Meijer OW, Vandertop WP, Baayen JC, Slotman BJ: Single-fraction vs. fractionated linac-based stereotactic radiosurgery for vestibular schwannoma: a single-institution study. Int J Radiat Oncol Biol Phys 2003;56: 1390–1396.
54 Sawamura Y, Shirato H, Sakamoto T, et al: Management of vestibular schwannoma by fractionated stereotactic radiotherapy and associated cerebrospinal fluid malabsorption. J Neurosurg 2003;99:685–692.
55 Wallner KE, Sheline GE, Pitts LH, Wara WM, Davis RL, Boldrey EB: Efficacy of irradiation for incompletely excised acoustic neurilemomas. J Neurosurg 1987;67:858–863.
56 Williams JA: Fractionated stereotactic radiotherapy for acoustic neuromas. Stereotact Funct Neurosurg 2002;78:17–28.
57 Chang SD, Gibbs I, Sakamoto G, Lee E, Oyelese A, Adler J: Staged stereotactic irradiation for acoustic neuroma. Neurosurgery 2005;56: 1254–1263.
58 Pollock BE, Lunsford LD, Noren G: Vestibular schwannoma management in the next century: A radiosurgical perspective. Neurosurgery 1998;43: 475–483.
59 Kondziolka D, Somaza S, Martinez AJ, Jacobsohn J, Lunsford LD, Maitz AH, Flickinger JC: Radioprotective effects of the 21-aminosteroid U74389G for stereotactic radiosurgery. Neurosurgery 1997;41:203–208.
60 Kondziolka D, Mori Y, Martinez AJ, McLaughlin M, Flickinger JC, Lunsford LD: Beneficial effects of the radioprotectant 21-aminosteroid U-74389G in a radiosurgery rat malignant glioma model. Int J Radiat Oncol Biol Phys 1999;44:179–184.
61 Linskey ME, Martinez AS, Kondziolka D, et al: The radiobiology of human acoustic schwannoma xenografts after stereotactic radiosurgery evaluated in the subrenal capsule of athymic mice. J Neurosurg 1993;78:645–653.
62 Linskey ME, Johnstone P, O'Leary M, Goetsch S: Radiation exposure of normal temporal bone structures during stereotactically guided gamma knife surgery for vestibular schwannomas. J Neurosurg 2003;98:800–806.
63 Pollock BE: Management of vestibular schwannomas that enlarge after stereotactic radiosurgery: Treatment recommendations based on a 15 year experience. Neurosurgery 2006;58: 241–248.
64 Kondziolka D, Lunsford LD, McLaughlin M, et al: Long-term outcomes after acoustic tumor radiosurgery. The physicians and patients perspective. New Engl J Med 1998;339:1426–1433.
65 Kondziolka D, Nathoo N, Flickinger JC, Niranjan A, Maitz AH, Lunsford LD: Long-term results after radiosurgery for benign intracranial tumors. Neurosurgery 2003;53:815–822.

Douglas Kondziolka, MD
Suite B-400, UPMC Presbyterian, Department of Neurological Surgery
200 Lothrop St.
Pittsburgh, PA 15213 (USA)
Tel. +1 412 647 6782, Fax +1 412 647 0989, E-Mail kondziolkads@upmc.edu

Author Index

Subject Index